Clinical Advances in Dentistry

Clinical Advances in Dentistry

Editor: Edgar Weston

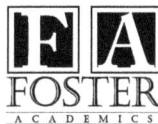

FA FOSTER
ACADEMICS

www.fosteracademics.com

www.fosteracademics.com

FA FOSTER
ACADEMICS

Cataloging-in-Publication Data

Clinical advances in dentistry / edited by Edgar Weston.
    p. cm.
Includes bibliographical references and index.
ISBN 978-1-63242-519-5
1. Dentistry. 2. Clinical medicine. I. Weston, Edgar.
RK51 .C55 2018
617.6--dc23

Foster Academics,
118-35 Queens Blvd., Suite 400,
Forest Hills, NY 11375, USA

ISBN 978-1-63242-519-5 (Hardback)

Contents

Preface..IX

Chapter 1   **A Conservative Esthetic Approach using Enamel Recontouring and Composite Resin Restorations**..1
Paula Mathias, Emily Vivianne Freitas da Silva, Thaiane Rodrigues Aguiar, Aline Silva Andrade and Juliana Azevedo

Chapter 2   **Reestablishing the Function and Esthetics in Traumatized Permanent Teeth with Large Apical Lesion**..6
Alexandra Rubin Cocco, Ângelo Niemczewski Bobrowski, Rudimar Antônio Baldissera, Luiz Fernando Machado Silveira and Josué Martos

Chapter 3   **Treatment of a Developmental Groove and Supernumerary Root using Guided Tissue Regeneration Technique**..11
Zahra Alizadeh Tabari, Hamed Homayouni, Tahere Pourseyediyan, Armita Arvin, Derrick Eiland and Nima Moradi Majd

Chapter 4   **Peripheral Calcifying Epithelial Odontogenic Tumour Mimicking a Gingival Inflammation: A Diagnostic Dilemma**...16
Danielle Lima Corrêa de Carvalho, Alan Motta do Canto, Fernanda de Paula Eduardo, Letícia Mello Bezinelli, André Luiz Ferreira Costa and Paulo Henrique Braz-Silva

Chapter 5   **Solitary Plasmacytoma in the Mandible Resembling an Odontogenic Cyst/Tumor**.............................20
Fatemeh Rezaei, Hesamedin Nazari and Babak Izadi

Chapter 6   **Prosthetic Management of a Child with Hypohidrotic Ectodermal Dysplasia: 6-Year Follow-Up**..25
Antonione Santos Bezerra Pinto, Moara e Silva Conceição Pinto, Cinthya Melo do Val, Leonam Costa Oliveira, Cristhyane Costa de Aquino and Daniel Fernando Pereira Vasconcelos

Chapter 7   **Successful Fitting of a Complete Maxillary Denture in a Patient with Severe Alzheimer's Disease Complicated by Oral Dyskinesia**..31
Hiromitsu Morita, Akie Hashimoto, Ryosuke Inoue, Shohei Yoshimoto, Masahiro Yoneda and Takao Hirofuji

Chapter 8   **Oral Rehabilitation and Management for Secondary Sjögren's Syndrome in a Child**............................36
Tatiana Kelly da Silva Fidalgo, Carla Nogueira, Marcia Rejane Thomas Canabarro Andrade, Andrea Graciene Lopez Ramos Valente and Patricia Nivoloni Tannure

Chapter 9   **A Rare Malignant Peripheral Nerve Sheath Tumor of the Maxilla Mimicking a Periapical Lesion**..41
José Alcides Arruda, Pamella Álvares, Luciano Silva, Alexandrino Pereira dos Santos Neto, Cleomar Donizeth Rodrigues, Antônio Caubi, Marcia Silveira, Sandra Sayão and Ana Paula Sobral

Chapter 10   **Esthetic Rehabilitation of Anterior Teeth with Copy-Milled Restorations: A Report of Two Cases**..46
Sapna Rani, Jyoti Devi, Chandan Jain, Parul Mutneja and Mahesh Verma

Chapter 11   **Minimally Invasive Laminate Veneers: Clinical Aspects in Treatment Planning and Cementation Procedures**..51
R. K. Morita, M. F. Hayashida, Y. M. Pupo, G. Berger, R. D. Reggiani and E. A. G. Betiol

Chapter 12   **Sclerotherapy of Intraoral Superficial Hemangioma**..64
Resmije Ademi Abdyli, Yll Abdyli, Feriall Perjuci, Ali Gashi, Zana Agani and Jehona Ahmedi

Chapter 13   **Mandibular Canal Widening and Bell's Palsy: Sequelae of Perineural Invasion in Oral Cancer**..69
Gopinath Thilak Parepady Sundar, Vishwanath Sherigar, Sameep S. Shetty, Shree Satya and Sourabh M. Gohil

Chapter 14   **An Endocrine Jaw Lesion: Dentist Perspective in Diagnosis**....................................73
Lavanya Kalapala, Surapaneni Keerthi sai, Suresh Babburi, Aparna Venigalla, Soujanya Pinisetti, Ajay Benarji Kotti and Kiranmai Ganipineni

Chapter 15   **Geminated Maxillary Lateral Incisor with Two Root Canals**....................................78
Nayara Romano, Luis Eduardo Souza-Flamini, Isabela Lima Mendonça, Ricardo Gariba Silva and Antonio Miranda Cruz-Filho

Chapter 16   **Apical Revascularization after Delayed Tooth Replantation: An Unusual Case**...................83
Marília Pacífico Lucisano, Paulo Nelson-Filho, Lea Assed Bezerra Silva, Raquel Assed Bezerra Silva, Fabricio Kitazono de Carvalho and Alexandra Mussolino de Queiroz

Chapter 17   **Regional Odontodysplasia with Generalised Enamel Defect**....................................88
A. M. Al-Mullahi and K. J. Toumba

Chapter 18   **A Conservative Approach to a Peripheral Ameloblastoma**...93
Rocco Borrello, Elia Bettio, Christian Bacci, Marialuisa Valente, Stefano Sivolella, Sergio Mazzoleni and Mario Berengo

Chapter 19   **Effectiveness of Long Term Supervised and Assisted Physiotherapy in Postsurgery Oral Submucous Fibrosis Patients**...98
S. Kale, N. Srivastava, V. Bagga and A. Shetty

Chapter 20   **Tardive Dyskinesia, Oral Parafunction and Implant-Supported Rehabilitation**...................103
S. Lumetti, G. Ghiacci, G. M. Macaluso, M. Amore, C. Galli, E. Calciolari and E. Manfredi

Chapter 21   **A Case of Primary Combined Squamous Cell Carcinoma with Neuroendocrine (Atypical Carcinoid) Tumor in the Floor of the Mouth**...110
Kenji Yamagata, Kazuhiro Terada, Fumihiko Uchida, Naomi Kanno, Shogo Hasegawa, Toru Yanagawa and Hiroki Bukawa

Chapter 22   **Nondestructive Microcomputed Tomography Evaluation of Mineral Density in Exfoliated Teeth with Hypophosphatasia**...116
Sachiko Hayashi-Sakai, Takafumi Hayashi, Makoto Sakamoto, Jun Sakai, Junko Shimomura-Kuroki, Hideyoshi Nishiyama, Kouji Katsura, Makiko Ike, Yutaka Nikkuni, Miwa Nakayama, Marie Soga and Taichi Kobayashi

Chapter 23   **World's First Clinical Case of Gene-Activated Bone Substitute Application**..122
I. Y. Bozo, R. V. Deev, A. Y. Drobyshev, A. A. Isaev and I. I. Eremin

Chapter 24   **Soft Tissue Schwannomas of the Hard Palate and the Mandibular Mentum**......................................128
Cennet Neslihan Eroglu, Serap Keskin Tunc and Omer Gunhan

Chapter 25   **Autogenous Tooth Fragment Adhesive Reattachment for a Complicated Crown Root Fracture: Two Interdisciplinary Case Reports**......................................132
Antonello Francesco Pavone, Marjan Ghassemian, Manuele Mancini, Roberta Condò, Loredana Cerroni, Claudio Arcuri and Guido Pasquantonio

Chapter 26   **Cholesterol Granuloma in Odontogenic Cyst: An Enigmatic Lesion**..139
Mala Kamboj, Anju Devi and Shruti Gupta

Chapter 27   **Treatment of Class III Malocclusion: Atypical Extraction Protocol**..144
Fernando Pedrin Carvalho Ferreira, Maiara da Silva Goulart, Renata Rodrigues de Almeida-Pedrin, Ana Claudia de Castro Ferreira Conti and Maurício de Almeida Cardoso

Chapter 28   **A Novel Procedure for the Immediate Reconstruction of Severely Resorbed Alveolar Sockets for Advanced Periodontal Disease**......................................153
Mario Aimetti, Valeria Manavella, Luca Cricenti and Federica Romano

Chapter 29   **Coverage Root after Removing Peripheral Ossifying Fibroma: 5-Year Follow-Up Case Report**......................................158
Paulo S. G. Henriques, Luciana S. Okajima, Marcelo P. Nunes and Victor A. M. Montalli

Chapter 30   **Oral Health Characteristics and Dental Rehabilitation of Children with Global Developmental Delay**......................................164
Saurabh Kumar, Deepika Pai and Runki Saran

Chapter 31   **Cone Beam CT in Diagnosis and Surgical Planning of Dentigerous Cyst**..168
Naira Figueiredo Deana and Nilton Alves

Chapter 32   **Free Gingival Graft to Increase Keratinized Mucosa after Placing of Mandibular Fixed Implant-Supported Prosthesis**......................................174
Danny Omar Mendoza Marin, Andressa Rosa Perin Leite, Lélis Gustavo Nícoli, Claudio Marcantonio, Marco Antonio Compagnoni and Elcio Marcantonio Jr.

Chapter 33   **Necrotizing Sialometaplasia of the Hard Palate in a Patient Treated with Topical Nonsteroidal Anti-Inflammatory Drug**......................................179
Alessandro Gatti, Emanuele Broccardo, Giuseppe Poglio and Arnaldo Benech

Chapter 34   **Differential Diagnosis of Parotid Lipoma in a Breast Ca Patient**..183
Melda Misirlioglu, Yagmur Yilmaz Akyil, Mehmet Zahit Adisen and Alime Okkesim

Chapter 35   **A Giant-Cell Lesion with Cellular Cannibalism in the Mandible: Case Report and Review of Brown Tumors in Hyperparathyroidism**......................................187
Lorenzo Azzi, Laura Cimetti, Matteo Annoni, Diego Anselmi, Lucia Tettamanti and Angelo Tagliabue

Chapter 36   **Laser Photobiomodulation for a Complex Patient with Severe Hydroxyurea-Induced Oral Ulcerations**... 195
Marco Cabras, Adriana Cafaro, Alessio Gambino, Roberto Broccoletti,
Ercole Romagnoli, Davide Marina and Paolo G. Arduino

Permissions

List of Contributors

Index

Preface

Dentistry is that branch of medicine which deals with the treatment and prevention of various diseases and disorders occurring in the oral cavity and oral mucosa. It is divided into different specialties namely, endodontics, oral implantology, orthodontics, geriodontics, pedodontics, veterinary dentistry, etc. The aim of this text is to provide the reader with a detailed overview of this complex field. The subject deals with topics like root canal, oral and maxillofacial surgery, dental implants, etc. Some of the diverse topics covered in the text address the varied branches that fall under this category. The extensive content of the book provides the readers with a thorough understanding of the subject of dentistry. For all those who are interested in the subject, this book can prove to be an essential guide.

Various studies have approached the subject by analyzing it with a single perspective, but the present book provides diverse methodologies and techniques to address this field. This book contains theories and applications needed for understanding the subject from different perspectives. The aim is to keep the readers informed about the progresses in the field; therefore, the contributions were carefully examined to compile novel researches by specialists from across the globe.

Indeed, the job of the editor is the most crucial and challenging in compiling all chapters into a single book. In the end, I would extend my sincere thanks to the chapter authors for their profound work. I am also thankful for the support provided by my family and colleagues during the compilation of this book.

Editor

A Conservative Esthetic Approach Using Enamel Recontouring and Composite Resin Restorations

Paula Mathias,[1] **Emily Vivianne Freitas da Silva,**[2] **Thaiane Rodrigues Aguiar,**[1] **Aline Silva Andrade,**[3] **and Juliana Azevedo**[4]

[1]Department of Clinical Dentistry, School of Dentistry, Federal University of Bahia, Salvador, BA, Brazil

[2]Department of Dental Materials and Prosthodontics, Aracatuba Dental School, Universidade Estadual Paulista, UNESP, Aracatuba, SP, Brazil

[3]Department of Restorative Dentistry, Araraquara Dental School, Universidade Estadual Paulista, UNESP, Araraquara, SP, Brazil

[4]Department of Clinical Dentistry, School of Dentistry, Bahiana School of Medicine and Public Health, Salvador, BA, Brazil

Correspondence should be addressed to Paula Mathias; pmathias@yahoo.com

Academic Editor: Zühre Akarslan

Conservative clinical solutions, predictable esthetic, and immediate outcomes are important concepts of restorative dentistry. The aim of this case study was to recognize the selective enamel removal as an interesting conservative alternative to achieve optimal esthetic results and discuss the clinical protocol. This clinical report described an alternative esthetic and conservative treatment to transform the long and sharp aspect of the maxillary canines with a slightly aggressive aspect into features of slightly curved teeth with delicate lines. An accurate diagnostic and esthetic analysis of the smile was initially performed. The selective enamel removal was performed, and direct composite restoration was strategically placed. Clinical assessment showed good esthetic outcomes, enabling a smile harmony with an immediate, simple, and lower-cost technique. Practitioners should be exposed to conservative approaches to create esthetic smiles based on the selective enamel removal technique combined with composite resin.

1. Introduction

The esthetic demand for a Perfect Smile has been growing fast year-after-year, as an important way to improve the patient acceptance with tooth appearance especially related to color changes and alignment [1–3]. Overall, patients are more confident after dental treatment, which positively affect their personal lives and professional relationships [4–6]. On the other hand, esthetic treatment is always accompanied by unique expectations with regard to the final outcomes.

Facial esthetics are guided by the harmony of soft tissue, gingival esthetics, microesthetics, and macroesthetics [7–9]. To improve the dental esthetic appearance, restorative approach can be combined with interdisciplinary treatment, such as periodontal and orthodontic treatment [3, 10]. However, these techniques require time due to the healing process and changes of the alveolar bone.

Although interdisciplinary evaluation and treatment are crucial in achieving optimum smile composition, under-standing the patient's wishes is essential to the success of therapy [3, 10]. Therefore, to cater to the patient requirement for improved dental esthetic results in the shortest possible time, selective enamel recontouring and direct restorations seem to be a good alternative [2, 11–15].

Minimally invasive treatment can be performed using selective enamel recontouring since the removal of a slight amount of enamel is only superficial, without dentin exposure and hence no postoperative sensitivity [2, 16]. In addition, the main advantage of this treatment is restoring a more natural teeth appearance using a relatively simple, immediate, and low-cost manner [2]. Thus, the aim of this article was to describe a successful conservative technique when changes in the shape of teeth are required for optimal esthetic results.

2. Clinical Report

A 26-year-old female patient complained about the elongated and protruded aspect of her maxillary canine (Figure 1).

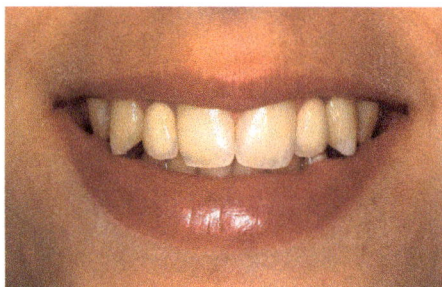

FIGURE 1: Initial clinical aspect showing the relationship between sharp maxillary canines and lips. Incisal thirds of the canines are projected in the vestibular direction, compromising tooth alignments and the harmony of smile.

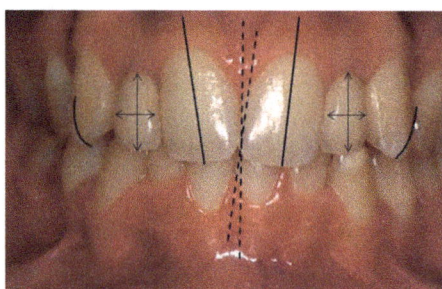

FIGURE 2: Frontal view showing the mid sagittal line alteration between the midline of the maxillary and mandibular arches (dotted lines); changes in the long axis of the maxillary central incisors (unbroken lines); disharmony in the height-width ratio of the lateral incisor crowns (crossed arrows); more prominent incisal thirds of the maxillary canines projected in the labial direction with sharp appearance (schematic drawing with curved lines pointing out the sharp aspect of canines).

The patient agreed to treatment and signed an informed consent. An interview of her medical history was performed and no concern was revealed. After clinical examination and esthetic analysis, some alterations were noted: midline variation between the maxillary and mandibular dental arches; changes in the axial inclination of maxillary central incisors; disharmony between the height-width ratio of dental crowns on the lateral incisors; more pronounced proclined maxillary canines with a sharp aspect, giving her smile a more aggressive appearance and masculine characteristic (Figure 2).

Concerning the gingival esthetics, a cervical gingival gap in the region of the lateral incisors was observed in an intraoral photograph; however, it was not revealed in the smile photography. Therefore, since the patient did not complain about this aspect, no periodontal intervention for esthetic purpose was performed. In spite of recognizing the benefits of an orthodontic treatment, the patient reported satisfaction with the other aspects related to her smile and the color of her teeth. In addition, she was looking for immediate esthetic results and a minimally invasive manner. She also pointed out that she sought dental treatment at that time only to solve the esthetics of her smile as described before. It is emphasized out that the patient has dental implants and their

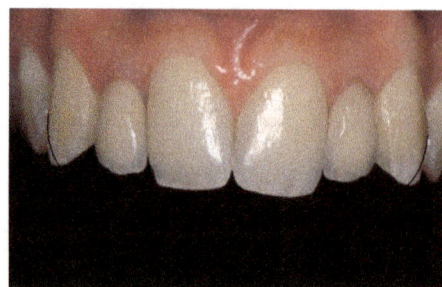

FIGURE 3: Frontal view of selective enamel recontouring of canine maxillary using a guide in order to reduce the buccal inclination, especially in the incisal third, and obtain an incisal angle more rounded.

respective implant supported dentures in the region of tooth #1.2 and tooth #2.2 (maxillary lateral incisors).

Initially, occlusal contacts were verified with articulating paper. When the canine guidance was observed, the option taken in order to attend the patient's demand was not to perform any wear in the incisal and palatine surface. As a result, the selective enamel recontouring was planned without reduction of the length of the tooth. To control this procedure, the guide was done with graphite on each tooth (#1.3 and #2.3) (Figures 3 and 4). The enamel recontouring was performed with diamond tip (#9138, KG Sorensen, Cotia, SP, Brazil), at high speed under constant water irrigation. Afterwards, decreasing granulation of aluminum oxide discs (Sof-lex Pop-on, 3M ESPE, St. Paul, MN, USA) was used to refine and polish the enamel surface.

The reduction of the buccal inclination of the incisal third as well as the rounding of incisal edge towards the palatine surface was performed. As shown, the flat area of the buccal surface was reduced in the cervical-incisal direction, giving the teeth a less elongated appearance. In addition, the enamel recontouring promoted better alignment between the incisal third of maxillary canines and incisors. Moreover, the enhanced space in the buccal corridor makes the smile more attractive.

To give the canines a more rounded aspect, which characterizes a more feminine smile, composite resin restorations in the cervical to middle third of the buccal surface of the maxillary canines were planned [8]. Moreover, an additional small direct restoration was indicated at the distal incisal angle fractured of the permanent central incisor (#1.1). The composite resin selection was performed positioning small increments of the selected composite over the teeth, followed by its polymerization [17]. Afterwards, a relative isolation was provided using labial retractor, gingival retraction cord, and cotton rolls. Then, etching enamel with phosphoric acid 37% was performed followed by the application of the adhesive systems (Adper Scotchbond Multipurpose Primer/Adhesive, 3M ESPE). The resin composite (Supreme XT Shade A3-E, 3M ESPE) was applied in the cervical to middle third of the canines in order to reproduce the buccal enamel. For fractured incisor, the resin composite shades A2B and A2E (Supreme XT, 3M ESPE) were used to restore the edge and the external enamel, respectively. All materials were used in

(a)

(b)

(c)

(d)

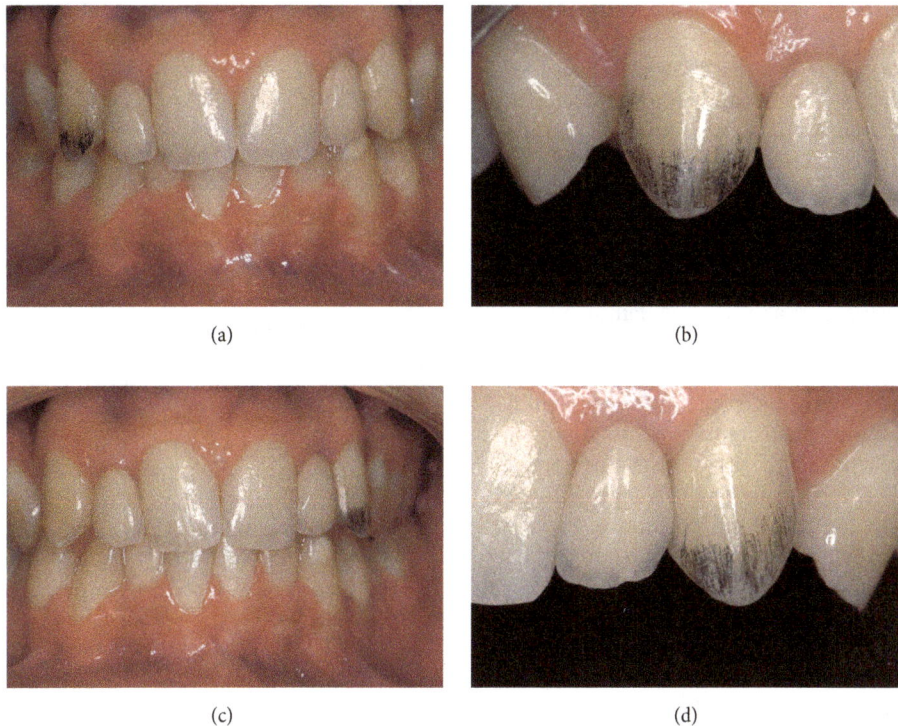

FIGURE 4: Different view of the guide of selective enamel recontouring of canine maxillary. (a) Marking on the most prominent third of the buccal face of tooth #13. (b) An approximate view of the teeth after enamel recontouring. (c) Marking on the most prominent third of the buccal face of tooth #23. (d) An approximate view of the teeth after enamel recontouring. Note on the proximal saliencies, greater wear was performed in the cervical direction in order to prevent them from remaining more projected and therefore outstanding in the smile.

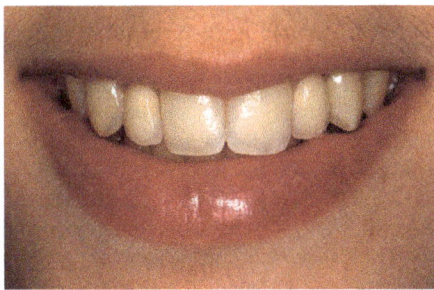

FIGURE 5: Final aspect after performing the finishing and polishing procedures, in which more harmonious and rounded contours, more in keeping with the patient's face and gender, may be observed.

accordance with the manufacturer's instructions and light-activated using a light emitted diode unit (Bluephase, Ivoclar-Vivadent, Schaan, Liechtenstein).

Afterwards, the restorations were polished with decreasing grits of aluminum oxide discs. In the smile photograph, the obtainment of more harmonious shapes and sizes of maxillary canines can be observed (Figure 5).

3. Discussion

The improvement in self-esteem, quality of life, and social acceptance are important factors that induce the patient seeking esthetic dental treatment [4–6]. Optimizing smiles guided by preservation of tooth structure, immediate results, and eventual future replacements are a changeling in restorative dentistry field [18]. Although new techniques and restorative materials are constantly being developed, a conservative and reversible approach to improve the smile design can be obtained by implementing a relative simple technique based on selective enamel removal and composite resin restoration.

In this case presentation, we reported a predictable plan treatment to transform the sharp and aggressive aspect of maxillary canines into more rounded and harmonious design according to the patient's face and gender. Regarding the dental esthetic principles, tooth size, shape, and proportion between height and width of crowns are the most easy perceptible factors in the smile [7]. Moreover, dental morphology should be harmonious with the gender characteristics to make a more natural smile [8, 19]. The feminine tooth shows characteristics such as slightly curved, smooth, delicate lines and absence of sharp angles. In contrast, masculine teeth are more angular and have straight lines, giving them an aspect of force and greater aggressiveness [8].

Reshaping performed with restorative techniques such as selective enamel recontouring or additional composite resin has shown advantages. For instance, allow greater preservation of healthy tooth structure, few clinical sessions, and reduced cost when compared to indirect restorations [3, 11, 12, 15, 20, 21]. It is emphasized that, in spite of being a simple technique, it depends on adequate treatment planning including knowledge of tooth morphology and dental/dentofacial esthetic common sense principles [22, 23].

After treatment, canine crowns showed a more adequate volume and depth. These morphology characteristics improve the smile attractiveness [8]. Other studies have shown that enamel recontouring is a safe and widely used procedure for the realignment of teeth, especially in canine teeth with rounded salience and large quantities of enamel in the buccal surface [2, 11, 12]. With regard to enamel removal, this aspect is significantly relevant, since wear can lead to tooth sensitivity, which occurs as a result of dentin exposure.

Selective enamel removal procedures have limitations, especially when compared with orthodontic treatment, since their indications are concerned. Orthodontic treatment can achieve the functional and esthetic requirements, minimizing and avoiding the wear of tooth [24]. On the other hand, if the patient is not inclined to receive this type of therapy and minor changes in the shape and position of the tooth are present, one of the alternative solutions to enhance the esthetic appearance of the smile is the enamel removal combined or not with direct restoration.

The patient's choice of treatment options is fundamental for the success of any procedure and it must be respected since it involves their psychological, physical, and financial aspects [25]. The patient in the present clinical case did not agree to have previous orthodontic therapy for tooth realignment. Therefore, tooth recontouring became a more feasible treatment option, taking into consideration the biological and functional concepts of dental structure preservation and esthetic demand. At the end of the procedure, the patient's satisfaction with the harmony obtained in her smile was achieved and undoubtedly functioned as an important instrument in the final evaluation of the result obtained.

In conclusion, the tooth recontouring techniques based on selective enamel removal and composite resin restorations provide a minimally invasive protocol with excellent esthetic result. This is an interesting restorative alternative based on a relatively simple treatment and lower-cost technique compared to traditional all ceramic restorations.

Competing Interests

The authors declare that they have no competing interests.

References

[1] W. Okuda, "Developing a road map for success in esthetics," *General Dentistry*, vol. 61, no. 6, pp. 10–12, 2013.

[2] D. Dietschi, "Optimizing smile composition and esthetics with resin composites and other conservative esthetic procedures," *European Journal of Esthetic Dentistry*, vol. 3, no. 1, pp. 14–29, 2008.

[3] L. Claman, M. A. Alfaro, and A. Mercado, "An interdisciplinary approach for improved esthetic results in the anterior maxilla," *Journal of Prosthetic Dentistry*, vol. 89, no. 1, pp. 1–5, 2003.

[4] K. A. Kolawole, O. O. Ayeni, and V. I. Osiatuma, "Psychosocial impact of dental aesthetics among university undergraduates," *International Orthodontics*, vol. 10, no. 1, pp. 96–109, 2012.

[5] J. A. Olsen and M. R. Inglehart, "Malocclusions and perceptions of attractiveness, intelligence, and personality, and behavioral intentions," *American Journal of Orthodontics and Dentofacial Orthopedics*, vol. 140, no. 5, pp. 669–679, 2011.

[6] M. M. Tin-Oo, N. Saddki, and N. Hassan, "Factors influencing patient satisfaction with dental appearance and treatments they desire to improve aesthetics," *BMC Oral Health*, vol. 11, article 6, 2011.

[7] N. C. Davis, "Smile design," *Dental Clinics of North America*, vol. 51, no. 2, pp. 299–318, 2007.

[8] M. Bhuvaneswaran, "Principles of smile design," *Journal of Conservative Dentistry*, vol. 13, no. 4, pp. 225–232, 2010.

[9] S. Shetty, V. Pitti, C. Satish Babu, G. Surendra Kumar, and K. Jnanadev, "To evaluate the validity of recurring esthetic dental proportion in natural dentition," *Journal of Conservative Dentistry*, vol. 14, no. 3, pp. 314–317, 2011.

[10] J. R. Calamia, J. B. Levine, M. Lipp, G. Cisneros, and M. S. Wolff, "Smile design and treatment planning with the help of a comprehensive esthetic evaluation form," *Dental Clinics of North America*, vol. 55, no. 2, pp. 187–209, 2011.

[11] A. Thordarson, B. U. Zachrisson, and I. A. Mjör, "Remodeling of canines to the shape of lateral incisors by grinding: a long-term clinical and radiographic evaluation," *American Journal of Orthodontics and Dentofacial Orthopedics*, vol. 100, no. 2, pp. 123–132, 1991.

[12] B. U. Zachrisson and I. A. Mjör, "Remodeling of teeth by grinding," *American Journal of Orthodontics*, vol. 68, no. 5, pp. 545–553, 1975.

[13] Y. Wang, Y. Sa, S. Liang, and T. Jiang, "Minimally invasive treatment for esthetic management of severe dental fluorosis: a case report," *Operative Dentistry*, vol. 38, no. 4, pp. 358–362, 2013.

[14] N. Malhotra, K. Mala, and S. Acharya, "Resin-based composite as a direct esthetic restorative material," *Compendium of Continuing Education in Dentistry*, vol. 32, no. 5, pp. 14–23, 2011.

[15] S. Ardu, N. Benbachir, M. Stavridakis, D. Dietschi, I. Krejci, and A. Feilzer, "A combined chemo-mechanical approach for aesthetic management of superficial enamel defects," *British Dental Journal*, vol. 206, no. 4, pp. 205–208, 2009.

[16] D. Edelhoff and J. A. Sorensen, "Tooth structure removal associated with various preparation designs for anterior teeth," *Journal of Prosthetic Dentistry*, vol. 87, no. 5, pp. 503–509, 2002.

[17] F. P. S. Nahsan, R. F. L. Mondelli, E. B. Franco et al., "Clinical strategies for esthetic excellence in anterior tooth restorations: understanding color and composite resin selection," *Journal of Applied Oral Science*, vol. 20, no. 2, pp. 151–156, 2012.

[18] Z. Akarslan, B. Sadik, H. Erten, and E. Karabulut, "Dental esthetic satisfaction, received and desired dental treatments for improvement of esthetics," *Indian Journal of Dental Research*, vol. 20, no. 2, pp. 195–200, 2009.

[19] L. R. Paranhos, C. S. Lima, R. H. da Silva, E. Daruge Júnior, and F. C. Torres, "Correlation between maxillary central incisor crown morphology and mandibular dental arch form in normal occlusion subjects," *Brazilian Dental Journal*, vol. 23, pp. 149–153, 2012.

[20] D. Wolff, T. Kraus, C. Schach et al., "Recontouring teeth and closing diastemas with direct composite buildups: a clinical evaluation of survival and quality parameters," *Journal of Dentistry*, vol. 38, no. 12, pp. 1001–1009, 2010.

[21] M. Gresnigt and M. Ozcan, "Esthetic rehabilitation of anterior teeth with porcelain laminates and sectional veneers," *Journal of the Canadian Dental Association*, vol. 77, article b143, 2011.

[22] J. R. Greenberg and M. C. Bogert, "A dental esthetic checklist for treatment planning in esthetic dentistry," *Compendium of Continuing Education in Dentistry*, vol. 31, no. 8, pp. 630–638, 2010.

[23] S. Siéssere, M. Vitti, L. G. de Sousa, M. Semprini, and S. C. H. Regalo, "Educational material of dental anatomy applied to study the morphology of permanent teeth," *Brazilian Dental Journal*, vol. 15, no. 3, pp. 238–242, 2004.

[24] D. R. Bloom and J. N. Padayachy, "Smile lifts—a functional and aesthetic perspective," *British Dental Journal*, vol. 200, no. 4, pp. 199–203, 2006.

[25] C. H. Chu, C. F. Zhang, and L. J. Jin, "Treating a maxillary midline diastema in adult patients—a general dentist's perspective," *Journal of the American Dental Association*, vol. 142, no. 11, pp. 1258–1264, 2011.

Reestablishing the Function and Esthetics in Traumatized Permanent Teeth with Large Apical Lesion

Alexandra Rubin Cocco,[1] **Ângelo Niemczewski Bobrowski,**[2] **Rudimar Antônio Baldissera,**[1] **Luiz Fernando Machado Silveira,**[3] **and Josué Martos**[3]

[1]*Department of Operative Dentistry, School of Dentistry, Federal University of Pelotas, Pelotas, RS, Brazil*
[2]*Department of Oral and Maxillofacial Surgery, School of Dentistry, Federal University of Pelotas, Pelotas, RS, Brazil*
[3]*Department of Semiology and Clinics, Faculty of Dentistry, University Federal of Pelotas, Pelotas, RS, Brazil*

Correspondence should be addressed to Josué Martos; josue.sul@terra.com.br

Academic Editor: Daniel Torrés-Lagares

Dental trauma is a challenge for dental integrity and can lead to pulp necrosis. The clinical case reports the diagnosis of a maxillary right central incisor traumatized and its multidisciplinary treatment. Calcium hydroxide material was used to perform the processing apexification. An apical surgery was carried out to remove the apical periodontitis and to return the aesthetics to the patient; internal and external tooth whitening in maxillary right central incisor was performed. We conclude that surgery associated with the root filling in the central incisor led to a successful completion. Moreover, it is of utmost importance to demonstrate the interaction between the various areas of dentistry.

1. Introduction

The eruption of permanent teeth occurs between 6 and 16 years [1], and any factor that interferes in this physiological process can interfere with root development [2]. A classic example of this interference is the occurrence of dental trauma. Most of these injuries happen before the complete formation of the dental root, predisposing as an immediate consequence a pulp inflammation or pulp necrosis [3]. In addition to the resulting inflammation the complete destruction of the Hertwig's epithelial root sheath may occur, causing an outage of root formation.

Moreover, consequences may be generated with incomplete root formation as such invasion of bacteria favors the formation of periapical lesions [4]. The presence of apical periodontitis will promote the formation of cysts in all cases and the conventional endodontic treatment alone will not be enough [5]. In these clinical situations, multidisciplinary interventions may be required.

In this context, the use of apexification technique has been recommended to induce a calcified root barrier to open apex or incomplete root apical development associate with pulp necrosis [6, 7]. Calcium hydroxide is the most common material used to induce the formation of apical hard tissue [8, 9], with success rates of 74–100% [1, 8, 10]. The mineral trioxide aggregate (MTA), due to showing favorable properties including biocompatibility [11–13], has also been used for the same purpose, showing similar results [10]. Other treatment recommended in cases of incomplete root formation is revascularization. A study performed revascularization/revitalization therapy in traumatized anterior teeth and it had a high clinical success rate in one-year follow-up [14].

The paper presents a case report of a patient with large periapical lesion that was treated by apical curettage followed by the apexification technique using calcium hydroxide medication and final root canal sealing with MTA.

2. Case Presentation

A 21-year-old female patient sought dental care due to bulging in the palate region, as well as dissatisfaction with the color of your maxillary right central incisor.

The patient reported having suffered a facial trauma in an anterior-superior direction arising caused by a stone impact. The trauma resulted in a fractured maxillary right central

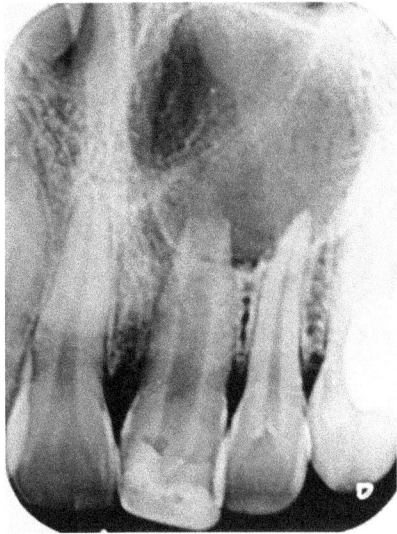

FIGURE 1: Initial radiograph of the maxillary right central incisor.

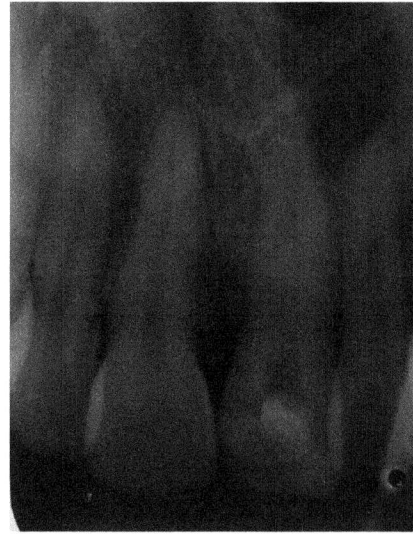

FIGURE 2: Intracanal medication of calcium hydroxide.

incisor, in addition to a mucous fistula appearance in the region after some time. She highlighted a new history of trauma in the same region in the past three years of the first event.

During clinical examination, a light mobility in teeth maxillary right central incisor (11) was verified, in addition to an expansion of about 2 cm^2 of the palatal cortical bone and presenting hard consistency. Palpation in the palate with light pressure had drainage of large amounts of purulent secretion. Diagnostic evaluation showed negative response to pulp sensitivity tests in the upper right central incisor, but the adjacent teeth showed pulp normality. By radiographic examination a circumscribed lesion in the apical region of the maxillary right central incisor with presumed periapical cyst and an incomplete apical root formation was observed (Figure 1).

The clinical planning highlighted the need for surgical intervention in the apical region of the central incisor associated with endodontic therapy and later following a second stage of the treatment comprising the cosmetic/restorative procedures.

Endodontic treatment started with complete rubber dam isolation without dental clamps of tooth maxillary right central incisor (11) and endodontic access following copious irrigation of the pulp chamber and cervical third. The root canal was cleaned with endodontic K-files (Dentsply-Maillefer, Ballaigues, Switzerland) until the working length was reached, and it was copiously irrigated with sodium hypochlorite (NaOCl) at 2.5% alternated with 17% EDTA, aspirated, and dried with absorbent cones. After root canal preparation the application of calcium hydroxide paste was performed. Intracanal medication of calcium hydroxide (Callen, SS White, Rio de Janeiro, RJ, Brazil) was applied prior to the surgical procedure and sealed with glass ionomer restorative material (Figure 2).

After performing antisepsis, local anesthesia, and incision the mucoperiosteum flap displacement was done and osteotomy was carried out to allow access to the affected

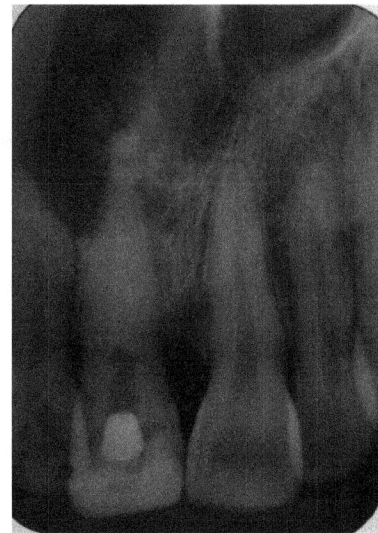

FIGURE 3: Postsurgical aspect.

area. It was possible to perform the excision of the periapical process and a careful curettage of the apical area. The biopsy of the specimen identified dense fibrous connective tissue, exhibiting intense inflammatory infiltrate and diffuse lymphocytic, confirming the diagnosis of periapical cyst. After a week of paraendodontic surgery, the patient had no asymmetry of the alveolar mucosa in the palate as well as exudation. Radiographically, the operated area and the need of new root application of calcium hydroxide paste were evident (Figure 3).

After six months, the operative procedures for permanent obturation of the root canal of the central incisor were started. After the removal of intracanal calcium hydroxide, the root canal final filling with cone rolled technique associated with a MTA-based endodontic cement was performed (MTA-Fillapex, Angelus, Londrina, PR, Brazil) (Figure 4).

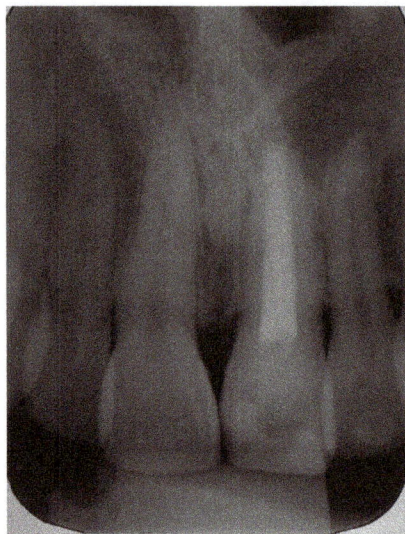

FIGURE 4: Root canal final filling with a MTA-based endodontic cement.

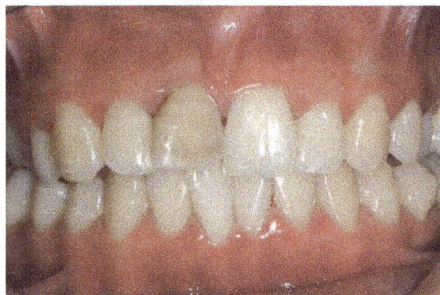

FIGURE 5: Crown darkening of maxillary right central incisor.

The crown darkening of tooth maxillary right central incisor (11) observed by the color scale (Vitapan 3D-Master, Vita Zahnfabrik GmbH, Germany) provided the use of dental office whitening technique (Figure 5). The clinical office whitening procedure began with the application of a light-cured gingival barrier at the cervical region of the tooth to be cleared to the protection of gingival tissue (Gingi Dam, Villevie, Dentalville, Joinville, Brazil). A twist-pen applicator with hydrogen peroxide at 35% was used (Mix One Supreme, Villevie, Dentalville, Joinville, Brazil) following the manufacturer's instructions. A layer of gel based on hydrogen peroxide (Mix One Supreme, Villevie, Dentalville, Joinville, SC, Brazil) was applied using external crown application only.

Three applications of whitening product were performed during forty-five minutes in one unique clinical session, and, at the end of the proposed treatment, a satisfactory change was observed in the chromatic aspect in the color of the central incisor (Figure 6). The clinical and radiographic follow-up shows a satisfactory outcome for the dental specialties involved in this treatment.

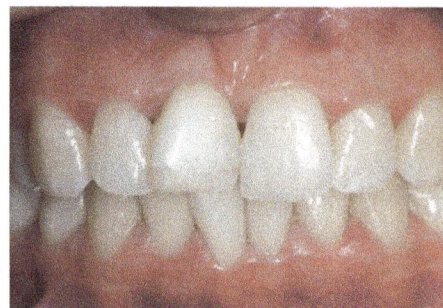

FIGURE 6: Final result after bleaching procedure.

3. Discussion

The multidisciplinary integration is very important for planning and executing a dental treatment. In this clinical report success with the approach can be seen through the interaction of distinct areas like surgical, endodontic, and operative dentistry.

After surgical removal of the lesion, the endodontic technique of apexification was performed. This technique consists in applying a biocompatible material into the root canal to establish an apical stop allowing the root filling in future to induce root formation and subsequent closing of the apical foramen. This is possible due to the deposit of mineralized hard tissue composed of osteocement, osteodentin, or bone or a combination of these three tissues at apical level [6, 7].

Currently, other technique has been widely used for immature teeth with nonvital pulp as the revascularized/revitalized teeth. This technique induces apexogenesis. It is new treatment modality that uses, instead of tissue replacement using artificial substitutes, tissue regeneration [1, 15]. However, this technique was not used in this study and due to the absence of well conducted long-term studies the technique raises several questions, among which is whether the technique serves as a permanent treatment or whether filling of the canal space is recommended. In our knowledge, there is only one study with one year follow-up [14]. It is necessary to have more studies in the long term.

However, apexification treatment has been a routine procedure to treat and preserve such teeth for many decades [15, 16]. The process of apexification forms an apical barrier, so that the subsequent condensation of the filling material canal can be adequately achieved [17]. Traditionally, the most common material used is calcium hydroxide, due to their biological stimulation capability, their osteogenic potential, and their antibacterial action [17–21]. These properties are related to the highly released and extremely reactive hydroxyl ions. These ions cause damage to the bacterial citoplasmatic membrane, denaturing their proteins and providing irreversible damage to their DNA [17–21].

Calcium hydroxide has been used successfully in the apical barrier formation in 74–100% of cases [8, 9]. Some studies show that 86% of treated teeth showed a survival rate between 5 and 13 years [22–24]. However, this material has been replaced by the MTA because it is necessary to do various changes, generating a time-consuming treatment, which can vary between 3 and 17 months [9].

For the root canal filling, sealer Fillapex MTA was used. This material has some satisfactory properties such as good seal and good apical barrier consistency forming hard tissue [11, 12]. In addition, it promotes the efficient apical seal in the dentin and cementum, facilitating biological repair and regeneration of the periodontal ligament.

Regarding the bleaching procedures, scientific evidence shows that free radicals of hydrogen peroxide not catalyzed for tooth whitening are those that can cause the phenomenon of external cervical root resorption due to the inflammatory process. The cementoenamel junction is the point of fragility of the tooth structure because it can expose the dentin. In an attempt to prevent the spread of bleaching products on the outer surface at the cementoenamel junction and prevent an inflammatory response in the surrounding periodontal tissues, a protection or a gingival barrier was used at the cervical level before applying the bleaching product [7].

In view of these considerations it is important to note that when the tooth has been traumatized and requires bleaching, the first choice should be to use external application [7]. As an added precaution, the bleaching treatment was not made using hydrogen peroxide associated with heat, and the hydrogen peroxide was only applied to the external enamel surface.

4. Conclusion

Through a multidisciplinary approach, it was possible to obtain a clinical success of the case presented by restoring the function and aesthetics of the patient.

Competing Interests

The authors declare that there is no conflict of interests regarding the publication of this paper.

References

[1] M. Rafter, "Apexification: a review," *Dental Traumatology*, vol. 21, no. 1, pp. 1–8, 2005.

[2] G. T.-J. Huang, "A paradigm shift in endodontic management of immature teeth: conservation of stem cells for regeneration," *Journal of Dentistry*, vol. 36, no. 6, pp. 379–386, 2008.

[3] J. O. Andreasen and T. R. Pitt Ford, "A radiographic study of the effect of various retrograde fillings on periapical healing after replantation," *Endodontics & Dental Traumatology*, vol. 10, no. 6, pp. 276–281, 1994.

[4] G. Sundqvist, "Taxonomy, ecology, and pathogenicity of the root canal flora," *Oral Surgery, Oral Medicine, Oral Pathology*, vol. 78, no. 4, pp. 522–530, 1994.

[5] P. N. R. Nair, U. Sjögren, G. Krey, K.-E. Kahnberg, and G. Sundqvist, "Intraradicular bacteria and fungi in root-filled, asymptomatic human teeth with therapy-resistant periapical lesions: a long-term light and electron microscopic follow-up study," *Journal of Endodontics*, vol. 16, no. 12, pp. 580–588, 1990.

[6] G. De-Deus and T. Coutinho-Filho, "The use of white Portland cement as an apical plug in a tooth with a necrotic pulp and wide-open apex: a case report," *International Endodontic Journal*, vol. 40, no. 8, pp. 653–660, 2007.

[7] L. Mattge, C. B. Xavier, L. F. M. Silveira, M. F. Damian, and J. Martos, "Endodontic treatment in avulsed permanent teeth with immature apex," *Journal of Endodontics*, vol. 33, pp. 121–129, 2015.

[8] E. C. Sheehy and G. J. Roberts, "Use of calcium hydroxide for apical barrier formation and healing in non-vital immature permanent teeth: a review," *British Dental Journal*, vol. 183, no. 7, pp. 241–246, 1997.

[9] D. Finucane and M. J. Kinirons, "Non-vital immature permanent incisors: factors that may influence treatment outcome," *Endodontics and Dental Traumatology*, vol. 15, no. 6, pp. 273–277, 1999.

[10] S. Chala, R. Abouqal, and S. Rida, "Apexification of immature teeth with calcium hydroxide or mineral trioxide aggregate: systematic review and meta-analysis," *Oral Surgery, Oral Medicine, Oral Pathology, Oral Radiology, and Endodontology*, vol. 112, no. 4, pp. e36–e42, 2011.

[11] M. Torabinejad, C.-U. Hong, S.-J. Lee, M. Monsef, and T. R. Pitt Ford, "Investigation of mineral trioxide aggregate for root-end filling in dogs," *Journal of Endodontics*, vol. 21, no. 12, pp. 603–608, 1995.

[12] M. Torabinejad, T. F. Watson, and T. R. Pitt Ford, "Sealing ability of a mineral trioxide aggregate when used as a root end filling material," *Journal of Endodontics*, vol. 19, no. 12, pp. 591–595, 1993.

[13] G. De Deus, R. Ximenes, E. D. Gurgel-Filho, M. C. Plotkowski, and T. Coutinho-Filho, "Cytotoxicity of MTA and Portland cement on human ECV 304 endothelial cells," *International Endodontic Journal*, vol. 38, no. 9, pp. 604–609, 2005.

[14] T. M. A. Saoud, A. Zaazou, A. Nabil, S. Moussa, L. M. Lin, and J. L. Gibbs, "Clinical and radiographic outcomes of traumatized immature permanent necrotic teeth after revascularization/revitalization therapy," *Journal of Endodontics*, vol. 40, no. 12, pp. 1946–1952, 2014.

[15] A. L. Frank, "Therapy for the divergent pulpless tooth by continued apical formation," *The Journal of the American Dental Association*, vol. 72, no. 1, pp. 87–93, 1966.

[16] G. T.-J. Huang, "Apexification: the beginning of its end," *International Endodontic Journal*, vol. 42, no. 10, pp. 855–866, 2009.

[17] G. H. Yassen, J. Chin, A. G. Mohammedsharif, S. S. Alsoufy, S. S. Othman, and G. Eckert, "The effect of frequency of calcium hydroxide dressing change and various pre- and inter-operative factors on the endodontic treatment of traumatized immature permanent incisors," *Dental Traumatology*, vol. 28, no. 4, pp. 296–301, 2012.

[18] C. R. Barthel, L. G. Levin, H. M. Reisner, and M. Trope, "TNF-α release in monocytes after exposure to calcium hydroxide treated *Escherichia coli* LPS," *International Endodontic Journal*, vol. 30, no. 3, pp. 155–159, 1997.

[19] J. Jiang, J. Zuo, S.-H. Chen, and L. S. Holliday, "Calcium hydroxide reduces lipopolysaccharide-stimulated osteoclast formation," *Oral Surgery, Oral Medicine, Oral Pathology, Oral Radiology, and Endodontics*, vol. 95, no. 3, pp. 348–354, 2003.

[20] E. Kontakiotis, M. Nakou, and M. Georgopoulou, "In vitro study of the indirect action of calcium hydroxide on the anaerobic flora of the root canal," *International Endodontic Journal*, vol. 28, no. 6, pp. 285–289, 1995.

[21] K. E. Safavi and F. C. Nichols, "Alteration of biological properties of bacterial lipopolysaccharide by calcium hydroxide treatment," *Journal of Endodontics*, vol. 20, no. 3, pp. 127–129, 1994.

[22] M. Thäter and S. C. Maréchaux, "Induced root apexification following traumatic injuries of the pulp in children: follow-up

study," *ASDC Journal of Dentistry for Children*, vol. 55, no. 3, pp. 190–195, 1988.

[23] H. S. Chawla, "Apexification: follow-up after 6–12 years," *Journal of the Indian Society of Pedodontics and Preventive Dentistry*, vol. 8, no. 1, pp. 38–40, 1991.

[24] I. Ballesio, E. Marchetti, S. Mummolo, and G. Marzo, "Radiographic appearance of apical closure in apexification: follow-up after 7-13 years," *European journal of paediatric dentistry*, vol. 7, pp. 29–34, 2006.

Treatment of a Developmental Groove and Supernumerary Root Using Guided Tissue Regeneration Technique

Zahra Alizadeh Tabari,[1] **Hamed Homayouni,**[2] **Tahere Pourseyediyan,**[1] **Armita Arvin,**[3] **Derrick Eiland,**[4] **and Nima Moradi Majd**[5]

[1]*Department of Periodontics, Dental School, Qazvin University of Medical Sciences, Qazvin 34157-59811, Iran*
[2]*Department of Endodontics, Dental School, Qazvin University of Medical Sciences, Qazvin 34157-59811, Iran*
[3]*Department of Endodontics, Dental School, Yazd University of Medical Sciences, Yazd 8914881167, Iran*
[4]*Dental Emergency Department, Howard University College of Dentistry, Washington, DC 20001, USA*
[5]*Dental Research Laboratory, Howard University College of Dentistry, Washington, DC 20001, USA*

Correspondence should be addressed to Armita Arvin; arvinarmita85@gmail.com

Academic Editor: Ali I. Abdalla

Introduction. The radicular groove is a developmental groove which is usually found on the palatal or lateral aspects of the maxillary incisor teeth. The present case is a maxillary lateral incisor with a small second root and a deep radicular groove. The developmental groove caused a combined periodontal-endodontic lesion. *Methods.* Case was managed using a combined treatment procedure involving nonsurgical root canal therapy and surgical periodontal treatment. After completion of root canal treatment, guided tissue regeneration (GTR) was carried out using decalcified freeze dried bone allograft (DFDBA) and a bioabsorbable collagenous membrane. Tooth also was splinted for two months. *Results.* After 12 months the tooth was asymptomatic. The periapical radiolucency disappeared and probing depth did not exceed 3 mm. *Conclusion.* Combined treatment procedure involving nonsurgical root canal therapy and surgical periodontal regenerative treatment can be a predictable technique in treating combined endodontic-periodontal lesions caused by radicular groove.

1. Introduction

The radicular groove is a developmental groove which is usually found on the palatal or lateral aspects of the maxillary incisor teeth. It is a linear depression that sometimes reaches the apex [1]. The groove is a rare anomaly with prevalence rate of 2.8–8.5% and generally presents on the maxillary lateral incisors [2].

Radicular grooves have been classified into three groups based on their severity. Type I, the groove is limited to the coronal third of the root. Type II, the groove is extended beyond the coronal third of the root but it is shallow and pulp is not exposed. Type III, the groove is long and deep, it is extended beyond the coronal third of the root, and root canal system is involved [3].

It has been stated that the radicular groove is analogous to the pathogenesis of dens invaginatus because it happens due to a slight in-folding of the enamel organ and Hertwig's epithelial root sheath cells during odontogenesis [4].

Radicular groove can be an appropriate habitat for microorganisms and plaque accumulation. Therefore, a local inflammation and deep periodontal pocket are general findings. A deep pocket that reaches to the root apex can affect the pulp vitality and causes a combined periodontal-endodontic lesion [5].

In order to treat a radicular groove the following procedures have been suggested: curettage of the affected periodontal tissues [6], sealing the groove with a biocompatible material [7], saucerization of the groove [7], root canal therapy when an endodontic lesion is present [8], and

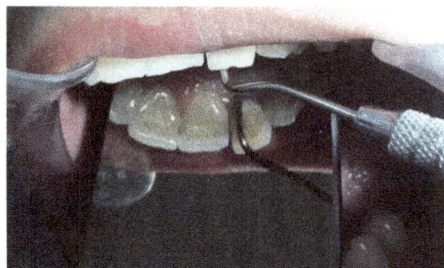

FIGURE 1: Preoperative photograph; a 7 mm localized pocket was detected on the palatal of tooth #10.

surgical techniques (i.e., guided tissue regeneration therapy and intentional replantation) [9, 10].

Although most anatomical studies have shown that maxillary incisors always have a single root, there are case reports suggesting lateral incisor with two [11, 12] and three root canals [13]. The term "supernumerary root" has been used to describe the development of increased number of roots on a tooth compared with the classical description in dental anatomy [14].

The aim of the present paper is to report a case involving a maxillary lateral incisor with a small second root and a Type III deep radicular groove which caused a combined periodontal-endodontic lesion. Therefore, a combined treatment procedure involving nonsurgical root canal therapy and surgical periodontal treatment was required.

2. Case Report

A 32-year-old female patient presented to endodontic department of Qazvin School of Dentistry with a chief complaint of mobility of maxillary left lateral incisor. Clinical examination was performed. A 7 mm localized pocket was detected on the palatal of tooth #10 (Figure 1). Probing depth of the mesial, distal, and buccal gingival sulcus was within normal limits. Tooth #10 did not respond to electric pulp test (Analytic Technology, Redmond, WA, USA), cold test (Roeko Endo-Frost; Roeko, Langenau, Germany), percussion, and palpation; it also had grade I mobility. Periapical radiograph and cone beam computed tomography (CBCT) were taken (Figure 2). CBCT revealed a radicular groove on tooth #10 and a large radiolucency in relation to left lateral incisor. A supernumerary root was also observed in the radiographs.

Considering patient's history, clinical and radiographic examination, the lesion was provisionally diagnosed as necrotic pulp and localized periodontitis secondary to the radicular groove.

Treatment options were presented to the patient including a combined procedure involving endodontic and periodontal regenerative treatments. She was informed that due to length and depth of the radicular groove, long-term prognosis of tooth #10 is questionable. A written informed consent was obtained and the patient was scheduled for endodontic treatment.

3. Endodontic Treatment

At the patient's return, local anesthesia was administered using local infiltration (supraperiosteal) technique with a cartridge of lidocaine (2% lidocaine with 1/80000 epinephrine; Darupakhsh, Tehran, Iran); after proper isolation, access cavity on tooth #10 was prepared. Canal preparation was performed using the ProTaper system (Dentsply Maillefer, Ballaigues, Switzerland) according to the manufacturer's instructions. An attempt was made to negotiate the second root canal, but no canal opening was found for the supernumerary root. Sodium hypochlorite 2.5% (Kimia Tehran Acid, Tehran, Iran) was used as irrigating solution. Canal was obturated using lateral compaction technique with gutta-percha (Gapadent Co., LTD, Korea) and AH26 sealer (DeTrey, Dentsply, Konstanz, Germany). The access cavity was sealed with Cavit (Coltosol, AriaDent, Tehran, Iran) (Figure 3).

4. Surgical Procedure

The surgical area was made aseptic and local anesthesia was administered (2% lidocaine with 1/80000 epinephrine; Darupakhsh, Tehran, Iran). Sulcular incisions were placed on the labial side from #9 to #11; to increase the access a releasing incision was also made on the distal of #11. A full thickness mucoperiosteal flap was raised on labial and palatal aspects to access the radicular groove (Figure 4). Granulation tissues were removed using curettage and root planning was carried out; then the supernumerary root was cut off and groove was saucerized. No canal opening was found on the area of removed root. The supernumerary root and surrounding tissue were sent to the lab for histologic examination. Then, guided tissue regeneration (GTR) was carried out using decalcified freeze dried bone allograft (DFDBA) with particle size of 500 to 1000 μm (Cenobone, Tissue Regeneration Corporation, Kish Island, Iran) and a 20 × 25 mm (0.4 to 0.6 mm thickness) bioabsorbable collagenous membrane (Cenomembrane, Tissue Regeneration Corporation, Kish Island, Iran) (Figure 5). The flap was repositioned and stabilized with sutures. The tooth was restored using composite resin and immobilized with a semirigid splint. The splint was initially placed on the buccal aspect of the tooth, but due to esthetic consideration, after four weeks, it was removed and placed lingually. The patient was prescribed a chlorhexidine gluconate mouth rinse and 4 × 400 mg Ibuprofen plus 3 × 500 mg amoxicillin daily for a week. Sutures were removed two weeks after the surgery, but the splint was remained for two months. No mobility was detected after splint removal.

The histologic examination results revealed that the structure of supernumerary root has no abnormality, no dysplastic cell is detected, and the surrounding tissue consists of connective tissue and inflammatory cells (Figure 6).

Twelve months' follow-up revealed absence of signs and symptoms, and probing depth did not exceed 3 mm and radiographic examination indicated disappearance of the radiolucency around the tooth #10 due to bone grafting and simultaneous bone regeneration (Figure 7).

5. Discussion

Combined endodontic-periodontal lesions are real clinical dilemmas due to difficulty of making a differential diagnosis

(a)

(b)

(c)

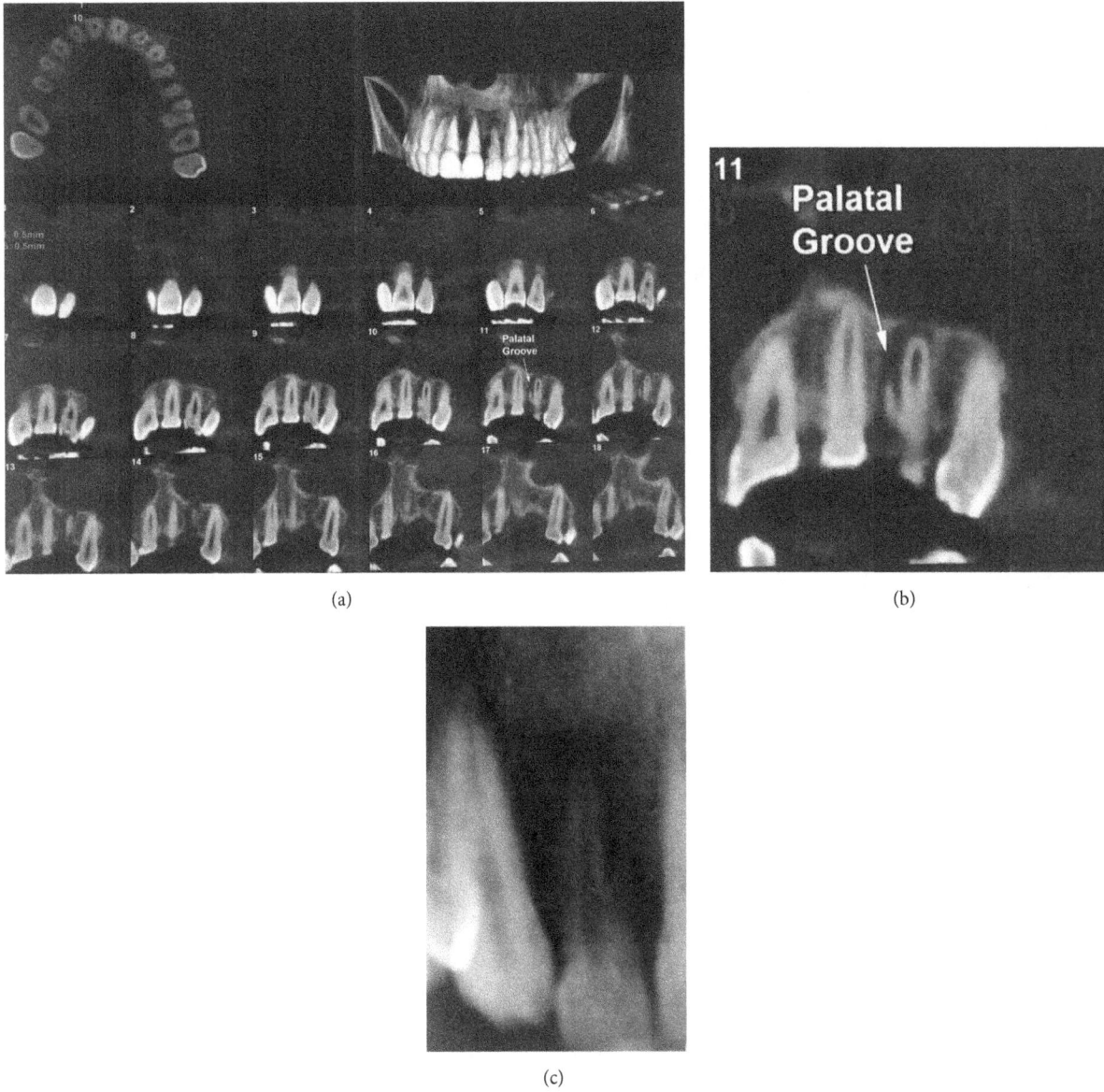

FIGURE 2: (a) Preoperative cone beam computed tomography (CBCT); (b) CBCT revealed a radicular groove on tooth #10; (c) preoperative periapical radiograph, there is a large radiolucency in relation to left lateral incisor.

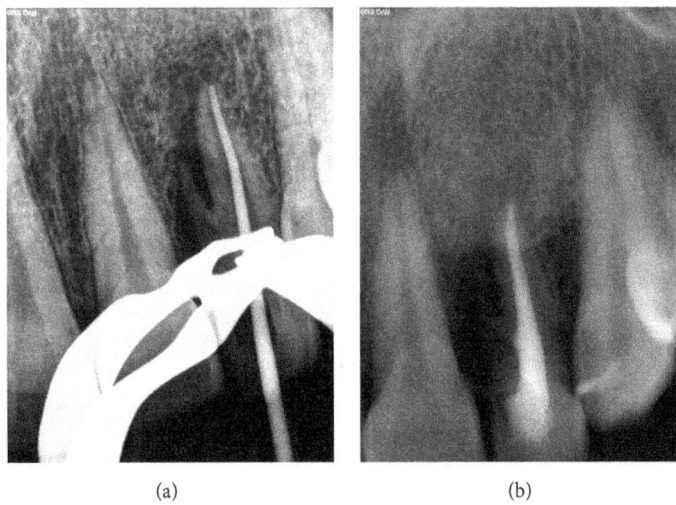

(a)

(b)

FIGURE 3: Toot #10 was endodontically treated.

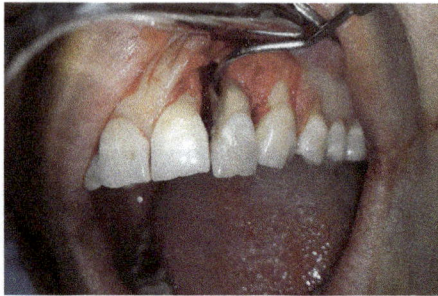

FIGURE 4: A full thickness mucoperiosteal flap was raised on labial and palatal aspects of tooth #10 to access the radicular groove.

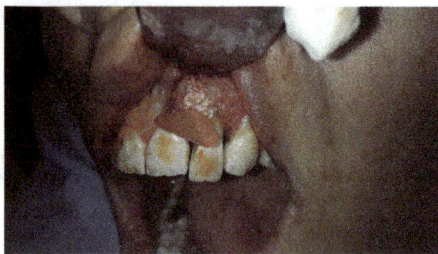

FIGURE 5: Guided tissue regeneration (GTR) was carried out using decalcified freeze dried bone allograft (DFDBA) and a bioabsorbable collagenous membrane.

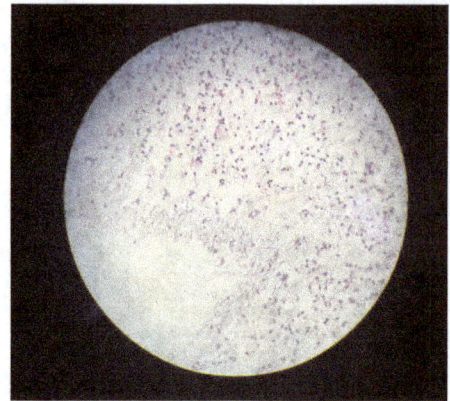

FIGURE 6: The histologic examination results revealed that the surrounding tissue consists of connective tissue and inflammatory cells and root structure is normal.

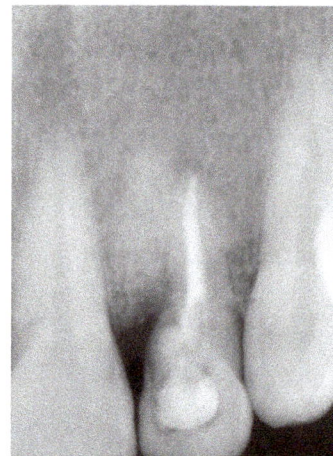

FIGURE 7: 12 months' follow-up radiograph indicated disappearance of the radiolucency around the tooth #10 due to bone grafting and simultaneous bone regeneration.

and deciding a prognosis. One of the serious factors that causes this kind of combined lesions is radicular groove. These developmental grooves act as "plaque trap" and initiating factor in localized gingivitis and periodontitis [15]. In cases with more complicated grooves (Type III), focal attachment loss may extend apically and result in a hopeless periodontal prognosis. It has been stated that long lasting deep periodontal pocket can secondarily lead to pulp necrosis and develop a combined endodontic-periodontal lesion [16].

The key factor to achieve success in management of this type of anomalies is accurate diagnosis [17]. Therefore, to obtain a three-dimensional image of the tooth and to determine its accurate prognosis, a CBCT image was taken.

Kerezoudis et al. [18] suggested the following treatment modalities to manage radicular grooves:

(1) Surgical removal of granulation tissue and irritants

(2) Gingivectomy and apically positioned flap

(3) Surgical exposure and flattening of the groove by grinding, with or without application of guided tissue regeneration techniques

(4) Placing amalgam restoration in the groove

(5) Orthodontic extrusion of the tooth

Although shallow grooves which are located entirely on the crown can be corrected by odontoplasty and curettage of granulation tissue, more complicated radicular grooves that are associated with severe periodontal breakdown and extensive periapical lesion need surgical intervention [19].

In our case, due to presence of deep periodontal pocket and severe attachment loss, surgical procedure was performed. After flattering and odontoplasty of the groove, the anatomy of the root was favorable. That is why no restorative material was used to restore the groove.

Regenerative periodontal therapy aims to predictably restore the periodontal tissue and leads to formation of a new cementum with inserting periodontal ligament fibers [20].

Therefore, to enhance the periodontal attachment of the tooth in the present case, DFDBA was used. It has been stated that DFDBA is a scaffold for bone formation and is able to be converted into bone [21]. Also, to provide epithelial exclusion and allow periodontal ligament, cementum, and bone to regenerate [22], a collagenous membrane was placed over the defect.

The applied treatment regimen was successful as it can be observed on the follow-up radiography. After 12 months the subjected tooth was asymptomatic, and a 3 mm healthy gingival sulcus was restored in relation to the radicular groove.

6. Conclusion

Combined treatment procedure involving nonsurgical root canal therapy and surgical periodontal regenerative treatment can be a predictable technique in treating combined endodontic-periodontal lesions caused by radicular groove.

Competing Interests

The authors declare that there are no competing interests regarding the publication of this article.

References

[1] M. F. D. C. Albaricci, B. E. C. de Toledo, E. P. Zuza, D. A. S. Gomes, and E. P. Rosetti, "Prevalence and features of palato-radicular grooves: an in-vitro study," *Journal of the International Academy of Periodontology*, vol. 10, no. 1, pp. 2–5, 2008.

[2] S. A. Schwartz, M. A. Koch, D. E. Deas, and C. A. Powell, "Combined endodontic-periodontic treatment of a palatal groove: a case report," *Journal of Endodontics*, vol. 32, no. 6, pp. 573–578, 2006.

[3] Y.-C. Gu, "A micro-computed tomographic analysis of maxillary lateral incisors with radicular grooves," *Journal of Endodontics*, vol. 37, no. 6, pp. 789–792, 2011.

[4] K. W. Lee, E. C. Lee, and K. Y. Poon, "Palato-gingival grooves in maxillary incisors. A possible predisposing factor to localised periodontal disease," *British Dental Journal*, vol. 124, no. 1, pp. 8–14, 1968.

[5] J. H. S. Simon, D. H. Glick, and A. L. Frank, "Predictable endodontic and periodontic failures as a result of radicular anomalies," *Oral Surgery, Oral Medicine, Oral Pathology*, vol. 31, no. 6, pp. 823–826, 1971.

[6] E. Schäfer, R. Cankay, and K. Ott, "Malformations in maxillary incisors: case report of radicular palatal groove," *Dental Traumatology*, vol. 16, no. 3, pp. 132–137, 2000.

[7] G. Zucchelli, M. Mele, and L. Checchi, "The papilla amplification flap for the treatment of a localized periodontal defect associated with a palatal groove," *Journal of Periodontology*, vol. 77, no. 10, pp. 1788–1796, 2006.

[8] T. G. Gound and G. I. Maze, "Treatment options for the radicular lingual groove: a review and discussion," *Practical Periodontics and Aesthetic Dentistry*, vol. 10, no. 3, pp. 369–375, 1998.

[9] M. P. Rethman, "Treatment of a palatal-gingival groove using enamel matrix derivative," *Compendium of Continuing Education in Dentistry*, vol. 22, no. 9, pp. 792–797, 2001.

[10] D. A. Johns, V. Y. Shivashankar, K. Shobha, and M. Johns, "An innovative approach in the management of palatogingival groove using Biodentine ™ and platelet-rich fibrin membrane," *Journal of Conservative Dentistry*, vol. 17, no. 1, pp. 75–79, 2014.

[11] J. D. Pecora and S. V. Santana, "Maxillary lateral incisor with two roots—case report," *Brazilian Dental Journal*, vol. 2, no. 2, pp. 151–153, 1992.

[12] A. J. Dexton, D. Arundas, M. Rameshkumar, and K. Shoba, "Retreatodontics in maxillary lateral incisor with supernumerary root," *Journal of Conservative Dentistry*, vol. 14, no. 3, pp. 322–324, 2011.

[13] S. V. Walvekar and J. M. Behbehani, "Three root canals and dens formation in a maxillary lateral incisor: a case report," *Journal of Endodontics*, vol. 23, no. 3, pp. 185–186, 1997.

[14] B. W. Neville, D. D. Damm, C. M. Allen, and J. E. Bouquot, *Oral and Maxillofacial Pathology*, W.B. Saunders, Philadelphia, Pa, USA, 2nd edition, 2002.

[15] S.-L. Oh, A. F. Fouad, and S.-H. Park, "Treatment strategy for guided tissue regeneration in combined endodontic-periodontal lesions: case report and review," *Journal of Endodontics*, vol. 35, no. 10, pp. 1331–1336, 2009.

[16] P. Castelo-Baz, I. Ramos-Barbosa, B. Martín-Biedma, A. B. Dablanca-Blanco, P. Varela-Patiño, and J. Blanco-Carrión, "Combined endodontic-periodontal treatment of a palatogingival groove," *Journal of Endodontics*, vol. 41, no. 11, pp. 1918–1922, 2015.

[17] A. Sooratgar, M. Tabrizizade, M. Nourelahi, Y. Asadi, and H. Sooratgar, "Management of an endodontic-periodontic lesion in a maxillary lateral incisor with palatal radicular groove: a case report," *Iranian Endodontic Journal*, vol. 11, no. 2, pp. 142–145, 2016.

[18] N. P. Kerezoudis, G. J. Siskos, and V. Tsatsas, "Bilateral buccal radicular groove in maxillary incisors: case report," *International Endodontic Journal*, vol. 36, no. 12, pp. 898–906, 2003.

[19] K. Attam, R. Tiwary, S. Talwar, and A. K. Lamba, "Palatogingival groove: endodontic-periodontal management—case report," *Journal of Endodontics*, vol. 36, no. 10, pp. 1717–1720, 2010.

[20] A. Sculean, D. Nikolidakis, and F. Schwarz, "Regeneration of periodontal tissues: combinations of barrier membranes and grafting materials—biological foundation and preclinical evidence: a systematic review," *Journal of Clinical Periodontology*, vol. 35, no. 8, supplement, pp. 106–116, 2008.

[21] J. A. Keestra, O. Barry, L. D. Jong, and G. Wahl, "Long-term effects of vertical bone augmentation: a systematic review," *Journal of Applied Oral Science*, vol. 24, no. 1, pp. 3–17, 2016.

[22] C. C. Villar and D. L. Cochran, "Regeneration of periodontal tissues: guided tissue regeneration," *Dental Clinics of North America*, vol. 54, no. 1, pp. 73–92, 2010.

Peripheral Calcifying Epithelial Odontogenic Tumour Mimicking a Gingival Inflammation: A Diagnostic Dilemma

Danielle Lima Corrêa de Carvalho,[1] Alan Motta do Canto,[1,2] Fernanda de Paula Eduardo,[1] Letícia Mello Bezinelli,[1] André Luiz Ferreira Costa,[3] and Paulo Henrique Braz-Silva[1]

[1]*Department of Stomatology, Division of General Pathology, School of Dentistry, University of São Paulo, São Paulo, SP, Brazil*
[2]*Unit of Oral and Maxillofacial Surgery, Santa Casa de São Paulo, School of Medical Sciences, São Paulo, SP, Brazil*
[3]*Department of Orthodontics and Radiology, University of São Paulo, São Paulo, SP, Brazil*

Correspondence should be addressed to Paulo Henrique Braz-Silva; pbraz@usp.br

Academic Editor: Adriano Loyola

The calcifying epithelial odontogenic tumour (CEOT) is an extremely rare benign neoplasia, accounting for approximately 1% of all odontogenic tumours. CEOT can have two clinical manifestations: central or intraosseous (94% of the cases) and peripheral or extraosseous (6% of the cases). Although the latter is less common, the peripheral variant has been described as an insidious lesion, since it is usually asymptomatic and may be erroneously mistaken with gingival hyperplasia, hamartomas, or even metastasis of malignant neoplasia. We report a case of a young male patient presenting with a peripheral CEOT in the mandibular posterior region, mimicking a located gingival inflammation.

1. Introduction

The calcifying epithelial odontogenic tumour (CEOT) is a rare odontogenic neoplasia characterised by the presence of amyloid material, which can present calcified [1]. This entity, earlier known as "Pindborg Tumour," has an epithelial origin and accounts for approximately 1 percent of all odontogenic tumours, affecting the mandibular bone in the majority of the cases [1].

Although the intraosseous variant is more common (94% of the cases), studies have shown evidence that this neoplasia affects exclusively soft tissues [1, 2]. Peripheral CEOT is extremely rare and accounts for approximately 13.3 percent of the cases of all peripheral tumours [3]. According to the studies, these tumours derive from epithelial remnants of the dental lamina or from the gingival surface [2].

Differently from the central variant, the peripheral CEOT is more prevalent in females, occurring between the third and fourth decades of life and involving the anterior maxillary region [4, 5]. These tumours are usually asymptomatic and tend to be less aggressive, causing only alterations in soft tissues. They respond to surgical treatment and do not relapse if properly treated [4].

The objective of this study is to describe a case of an uncommon peripheral CEOT in the posterior mandibular region as well as to perform a brief review of the literature.

2. Case Presentation

An 18-year-old male patient was referred for evaluation because of an asymptomatic increase in gingival volume, which was lasting for one month. On the clinical exam, the gingiva showed an exophytic lesion with erythematous and irregular surface located in the buccal region, between premolar and first lower molar, and measuring approximately 5×5 mm (Figure 1). The patient reported no pain in the region and oral hygiene was regularly performed, with the involved bone region showing no clinical or imagenological alterations. There was no history of local trauma. As medical history, the patient had acute lymphoblastic leukemia, which was successfully treated by means of chemotherapy 1 year earlier than the emergence of the lesion.

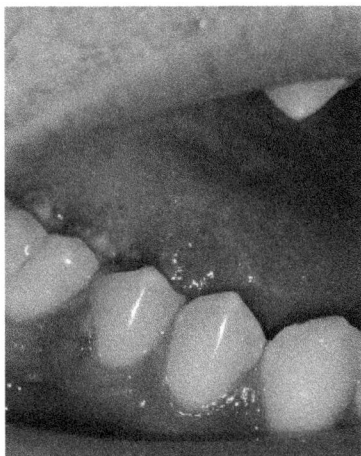

FIGURE 1: Clinical features of the lesion.

Considering the lesion's dimensions and aspects suggesting a benign behavior, an excisional biopsy of the region was performed under local anaesthesia. The haematoxylin-eosin stained histological sections showed proliferation of fusiform cells arranged either in bundles or randomly, including intense deposition of amorphous material among them. This substance had an eosinophilic appearance compatible with amyloid deposition associated with strings and islets of odontogenic epithelium dispersed through the neoplasia. The specimen was positive to Congo red under polarized light, showing the amyloid origin of the eosinophilic material. The mucosal lining epithelium showed areas of ulceration and neutrophilic infiltration (Figure 2).

Based on the clinical, radiological, and histopathological characteristics, the case was diagnosed as a peripheral CEOT. The patient was regularly followed up for one year and no sign of relapse was found.

3. Discussion

Calcifying epithelial odontogenic tumours are rare neoplasia accounting for a small percentage of all odontogenic tumours. Studies report that there are about 200 cases worldwide [6].

In addition to the rarity of these tumours, the peripheral variant is even more uncommon. Interestingly, 24 related cases were found in the PubMed database [1, 7].

In a recent literature review, Shetty et al. (2014) reported that peripheral CEOT is more common among females in the third and fourth decade of life (mean age of 37.33 years), usually affecting the anterior region of the maxilla [4]. Although the majority of the lesions are unilateral, studies have reported cases of bilateral lesions and tumours in maxilla and mandible simultaneously [2, 8]. However, as well as in our case report, some authors describe a higher rate of this variant among males, affecting areas of canines and premolars in the mandible [1, 2].

With regard to the origin of this neoplasia, it is believed that these tumours only stem from the dental lamina epithelium due to its association with teeth enclosed within the bone. Nevertheless, because of the presence of the gingival variant, other possible origins have been discussed and reported in other studies [4]. As soft tissues are exclusively affected, it has been strongly demonstrated that these tumours can also stem from basal cells of the oral epithelium, which persist in the region following disintegration of epithelial remnants (rests of Serres) [4].

With regard to the differential diagnosis, the peripheral CEOT can resemble clinically or histologically several other lesions such as peripheral odontogenic tumours, odontogenic carcinoma with dentinoid, clear cell odontogenic carcinoma with dentinoid, minor salivary gland tumours, tumour metastasis, reactive hyperplasia, and acute gingival inflammations [9]. According to Shetty et al. (2016), presence of amyloid material, calcifications, absence of mitoses, immunohistochemical positivity to cytokeratin 14, and absence of S-100 protein expression can help to perform a final diagnosis [1]. In addition to these characteristics, the positivity to Congo red under polarized light can be useful for diagnosing and differentiating other lesions [1, 8].

The histopathological aspect of peripheral CEOT is well characterised, consisting of epithelial cells with cytoplasmatic eosinophilic content and amorphous amyloid substance with spots of calcification organized in concentric lamellas [5]. These cells can occasionally have an empty and vacuolated cytoplasm (clear cell variant) and mimic clear cell carcinomas. These cells contain an abundant amount of glycogen and can also have Langerhans cells in some cases. According to the authors, due to higher aggressiveness of the clear cell tumours, CEOTs presenting this cell variation can exhibit greater tissue destruction and higher trend for relapse [10].

Although authors have described the potential reoccurrence of clear cell CEOT [9], studies showed evidence that soft tissue variants are less severe neoplasia as they usually have small sizes (i.e., 0.5 to 2 cm), preserve osseous tissue, and do not tend to relapse if properly removed [1]. Only one case described by Shetty et al. (2014) showed an atypical presentation of peripheral CEOT with great dimensions and calcifications and was treated through maxillectomy [4].

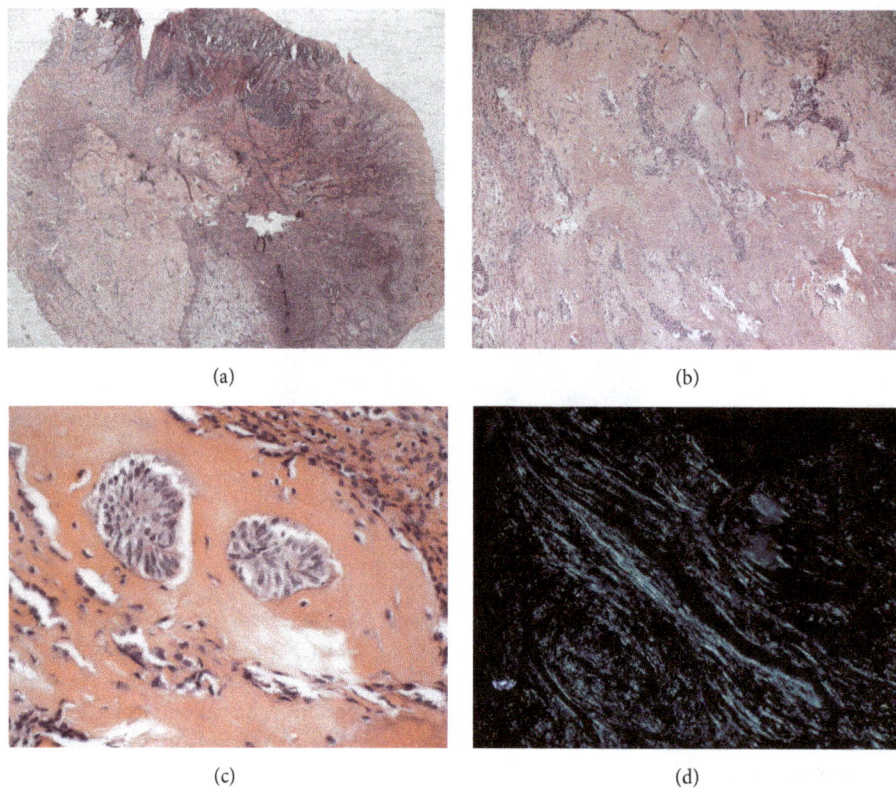

(a)

(b)

(c)

(d)

FIGURE 2: Histopathological features of the peripheral CEOT. (a) A general overview of the lesion, showing the mucosal lining epithelium with areas of ulceration and inflammatory cells infiltration. Proliferation of odontogenic epithelial cells organized in strands, cords, and nests and amyloid-like material (H & E, original magnification: ×25). ((b) and (c)) Strands, cords, and nests of odontogenic epithelial cells dispersed through the amyloid material (H & E, original magnification: ×40 (b), ×100 (c)). (d) Amyloid stained by Congo red showing apple-green birefringence in polarized light (original magnification: ×40).

Despite these characteristics in the present case as well as elsewhere, there are a few cases with evidence of relapse [1, 4, 8].

4. Conclusion

Due to the above-cited characteristics, the changes in gingival mucosa should be thoroughly examined because of the possibility of development of soft tissue peripheral neoplasia. Moreover, peripheral CEOTs have clinical similarities with several soft tissue lesions and thus their differentiation regarding other pathologies is of extreme importance for adequate treatment and follow-up.

Competing Interests

The authors declare that they have no competing interests.

References

[1] S. J. Shetty, T. Pereira, and R. S. Desai, "Peripheral clear cell variant of calcifying epithelial odontogenic tumor: case report and review of the literature," *Head and Neck Pathology*, 2016.

[2] M. G. de Oliveira, A. C. M. Chaves, F. Visioli et al., "Peripheral clear cell variant of calcifying epithelial odontogenic tumor affecting 2 sites: report of a case," *Oral Surgery, Oral Medicine, Oral Pathology, Oral Radiology, and Endodontology*, vol. 107, no. 3, pp. 407–411, 2009.

[3] A. Buchner, P. W. Merrell, and W. M. Carpenter, "Relative frequency of peripheral odontogenic tumors: a study of 45 new cases and comparison with studies from the literature," *Journal of Oral Pathology and Medicine*, vol. 35, no. 7, pp. 385–391, 2006.

[4] D. Shetty, B. V. Jayade, G. Jayade, and K. Gopalkrishnan, "Peripheral calcifying epithelial odontogenic tumor—case report," *Journal of Oral Biology and Craniofacial Research*, vol. 4, no. 2, pp. 147–150, 2014.

[5] G. D. Houston and C. B. Fowler, "Extraosseous calcifying epithelial odontogenic tumor: report of two cases and review of the literature," *Oral Surgery, Oral Medicine, Oral Pathology, Oral Radiology, and Endodontics*, vol. 83, no. 5, pp. 577–583, 1997.

[6] S. Caliaperoumal, S. Gowri, and J. Dinakar, "Pindborg tumor," *Contemporary Clinical Dentistry*, vol. 7, no. 1, pp. 95–97, 2016.

[7] M. L. Tejasvi, B. B. Balaji, K. Pramkusam, G. Donempudi, and H. Bhayya, "Gingival calcifying epithelial tumor—a rare case report," *Kathmandu University Medical Journal*, vol. 12, no. 47, pp. 215–218, 2014.

[8] A. C. Abrahão, D. R. Camisasca, B. R. M. V. Bonelli et al., "Recurrent bilateral gingival peripheral calcifying epithelial odontogenic tumor (Pindborg tumor): A Case Report," *Oral Surgery, Oral Medicine, Oral Pathology, Oral Radiology and Endodontology*, vol. 108, no. 3, pp. e66–e71, 2009.

[9] A. Afrogheh, J. Schneider, N. Mohamed, and J. Hille, "Calcifying epithelial odontogenic tumour with clear langerhans cells: a novel variant, report of a case and review of the literature," *Head and Neck Pathology*, vol. 8, no. 2, pp. 214–219, 2014.

[10] M. J. Hicks, C. M. Flaitz, M. E. K. Wong, R. K. McDaniel, and P. T. Cagle, "Clear cell variant of calcifying epithelial odontogenic tumor: case report and review of the literature," *Head and Neck*, vol. 16, no. 3, pp. 272–277, 1994.

5

Solitary Plasmacytoma in the Mandible Resembling an Odontogenic Cyst/Tumor

Fatemeh Rezaei,[1] Hesamedin Nazari,[2] and Babak Izadi[3]

[1]*Department of Oral Medicine, School of Dentistry, Kermanshah University of Medical Sciences, Kermanshah, Iran*
[2]*Department of Oral and Maxillofacial Surgery, School of Medicine, Kermanshah University of Medical Sciences, Kermanshah, Iran*
[3]*Department of Pathology, School of Medicine, Kermanshah University of Medical Sciences, Kermanshah, Iran*

Correspondence should be addressed to Hesamedin Nazari; hesamedin_nazari@yahoo.com

Academic Editor: Leandro N. de Souza

A 46-year-old male patient referred to Department of Oral Medicine, with the primary chief complaint of a painless swelling in the right side of mandibular. A panoramic radiograph revealed a well-defined, multilocular radiolucent bony lesion with thin and straight septa in the right side of mandible extending from distal of canine to mesial of third molar. Histological examination showed a solid proliferation of atypical plasmacytoid cells, which was indicative of plasmacytoma. A systemic workup for the final diagnosis was performed to rule out multiple myeloma.

1. Introduction

The plasmacytoma is a neoplastic and monoclonal proliferation of plasma cells that usually arises within bones [1, 2]. Most of the lesions present centrally within a single bone, and it occurs most frequently in the spine, vertebrae, femur, and pelvis [3, 4]. Infrequently, it is seen in soft tissue, in which case, the term extramedullary plasmacytoma is used. The upper respiratory tract, especially the nasal cavity, oropharynx, nasopharynx, and sinuses, is frequently involved. It has a longer survival rate [5, 6]. However, the extramedullary plasmacytoma can convert to plasmacytoma of bone and myeloma, both of which are associated with a poorer prognosis [7, 8].

The male to female ratio of solitary plasmacytoma is approximately 2 : 1, with an average age of 55 years [9, 10]. The localization of solitary plasmacytoma of bone in head and neck is very rare and usually occurs in the sinonasal tract [11]. Approximately 12% to 15% of solitary plasmacytomas of the bone occur in the jaw and they are commonly involved in the posterior body of the mandible that can extend to angle and ramus [10].

2. Case Presentation

A 46-year-old male patient presented to the Department of Oral Medicine, Kermanshah University of Medical Sciences in 2015 with the primary chief complaint of a painless swelling in the right side of mandibular bone that he had first noticed 2 months before (Figure 1). He had medical history of epilepsy and seizures so he has consumed phenytoin and lamotrigine for about 13 years. He did not use tobacco, alcohol, or other intravenous drugs. His general health was good without fatigue, fever, or weight loss. Neurologic examination of cranial nerves V and VII was normal without visible skin changes or drainage. He had no complaint of paresthesia or anesthesia. Maximum opening of the mouth was 4 cm, without deviation or clicking on the temporomandibular joint. Intraorally, the involved area had firm consistency without tenderness and was covered by normal mucosa (Figure 2).

He had generalized periodontitis and bone loss. Second molars premolars were mobile (grade II) and oral hygiene was poor. The third molar of the right mandible was nonvital but the other teeth on the same side were vital. There was no

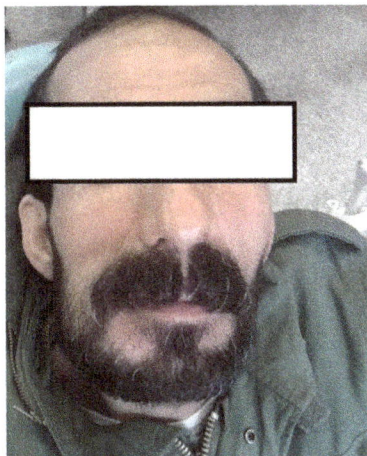

FIGURE 1: Swelling in the right side of mandibular bone.

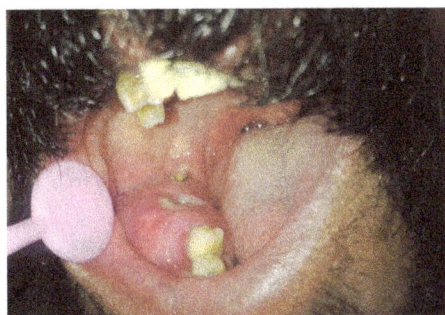

FIGURE 2: Clinical appearance of the expansion in the right side of mandible.

evidence of palpable submandibular, submental, or cervical lymphadenopathy.

A panoramic radiograph revealed a well-defined, multilocular radiolucent bony lesion with thin and straight septa in the right side of mandible extending from distal of canine to mesial of third molar. Resorption of the roots of the adjacent mandibular teeth did not occur (Figure 3).

Magnetic resonance imaging (MRI) was ordered to reveal the invasion and destruction of the lesion to the soft tissues. It revealed an expansile destructive lesion measuring about $4.4 * 6.3$ mm is noted in right side of mandibular bone with extension to right side hypoglossus and mylohyoid muscles as well as outer subcutaneous fat and skin and right buccinators and master spaces.

2.1. Differential Diagnosis. An expansile multilocular radiolucent lesion in a middle-aged adult brings to mind a number of lesions that should be included in a differential diagnosis. The most common lesions based on the clinical manifestation and radiographic feature included odontogenic myxoma, ameloblastoma, and odontogenic keratocyst.

Odontogenic myxoma is an uncommon benign mesenchymal odontogenic tumor arising from the dental papilla, follicle, or the periodontal ligament [12]. It commonly involves the mandibular premolar and molar regions. It is most frequently seen in patients in the second to the third decades

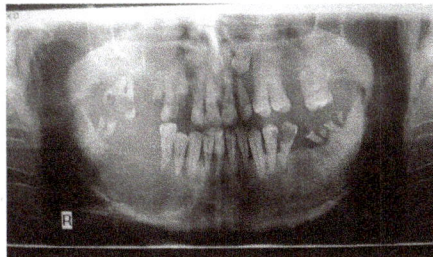

FIGURE 3: Panoramic radiograph demonstrating a large multilocular radiolucent lesion of the right mandible.

of life [13]. Odontogenic myxoma often grows without symptoms, most commonly presenting as a painless swelling [14]. Radiographically, its appearance ranges from unilocular to multilocular radiolucency with variable trabecular pattern giving rise to soap bubble, tennis racket, or honey comb appearance. Ideally, the septa that cause the multilocular feature are thin and straight, producing a tennis racket or stepladder pattern [15, 16]. Locating several straight septa in panoramic feature propelled us to this tumor as a first diagnosis.

Ameloblastoma is one of the most frequent odontogenic tumors [17]. It is most commonly seen in adults in the third to fourth decade but may be found in patients over a wide age range [18, 19]. Ameloblastoma most often presents as a hard painless intraoral swelling or as an incidental finding on routine dental imaging [20]. The radiographic features of conventional ameloblastoma are classified as unilocular or multilocular radiolucencies with well-defined borders [21].

The keratocystic odontogenic tumor (KOT) occurs in the 2nd and 3rd decade in the posterior body or in the ascending ramus of the mandible [22, 23]. The radiographic appearance of KOT may range from a small unilocular radiolucency to a large multilocular radiolucency. Multiple KOTs are associated with Nevoid basal cell carcinoma syndrome [24].

3. Diagnosis

Aspiration of lesion was nonproductive, so excluding the possibility of vascular and cystic lesions.

An incisional biopsy of the bony lesion was performed under local anesthesia without significant bleeding.

Histological examination on hematoxylin and eosin (H&E) staining showed a solid proliferation of atypical plasmacytoid cells with eccentric nuclei and basophilic cytoplasm, which was indicative of plasmacytoma (Figure 4).

In Complete Blood Count test (CBC and Diff test), white blood cell (WBC: 3600 cells/mL), red blood cell (RBC: $3.9 * 10^6$ cells/mL), hemoglobin (Hb: 12.9 g/dL), and hematocrit (HCT: 36.6%) were low but Mean Corpuscular Volume (MCV: 92.9 fL) and platelet (171000/mL) were in the normal range. In biochemistry test, urea (37 mg/dL) and creatinine (1 mg/dL) were normal and hypercalcaemia was not found so renal insufficiency was ruled out. Serum immunoelectrophoresis showed an increase in M-protein [immunoglobulin (IgG) κ type] and also a decrease in albumin of plasma and albumin/globulin ratio was lower than normal.

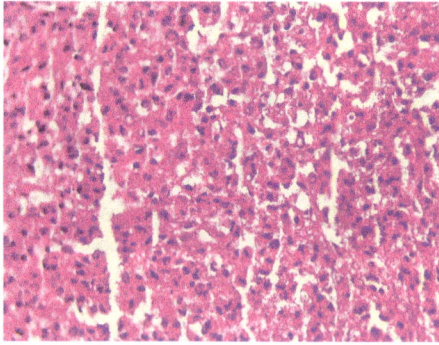

FIGURE 4: Diffuse infiltration of neoplastic large plasmablastic cells with pleomorphism and nuclei with one or several nucleoli (hematoxylin and eosin, original magnification ×40).

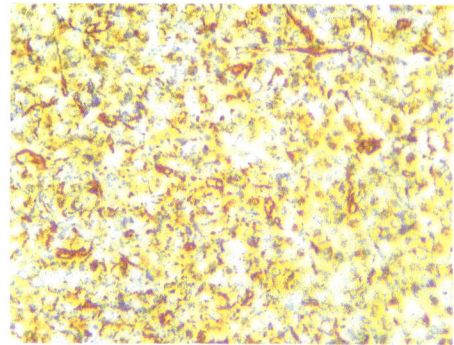

FIGURE 6: Immunohistochemical staining showing immunopositivity for vimentin (×40).

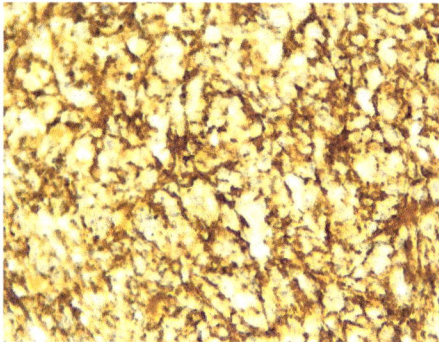

FIGURE 5: Immunohistochemical staining showing immunopositivity for CD138 (×40).

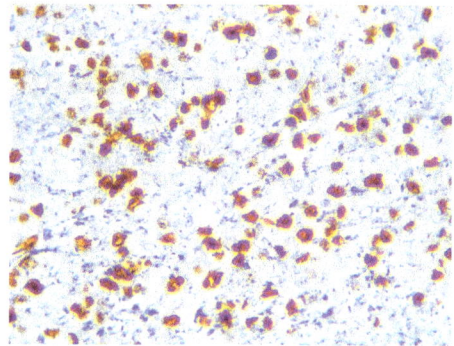

FIGURE 7: Immunohistochemical staining showing immunopositivity for Ki67 (×40).

A systemic workup for the final diagnosis was performed to rule out multiple myeloma. Radiographic survey including posteroanterior and lateral skull views was performed and showed no additional osteolytic lesion.

In immunohistochemical painting, CD138, vimentin, Ki67, and EMA were positive (Figures 5–8). But the immunohistochemical painting was negative for LCA, CK, CD3, CD20, CD1, NSE.

The patient was referred to haematooncologist. Bone marrow aspiration and trephine biopsy revealed hypercellular marrow with 6% plasma cell.

4. Discussion

Oral manifestations of solitary plasmacytoma of jaw include localized pain in the jaws and teeth, paresthesia, swelling, soft tissue masses, mobility and migration of teeth, hemorrhage, and pathological fracture. Fatigue and fever are the most common systemic symptoms [25, 26]. Our patient just had expansion in posterior mandible and mobility and migration of his teeth were probably due to aggressive periodontitis. He did not report history of pain or paresthesia in the jaws and teeth. Asymptomatic solitary bone plasmacytoma of the jaw is very rare but such a clinical form without pain has been described previously [27].

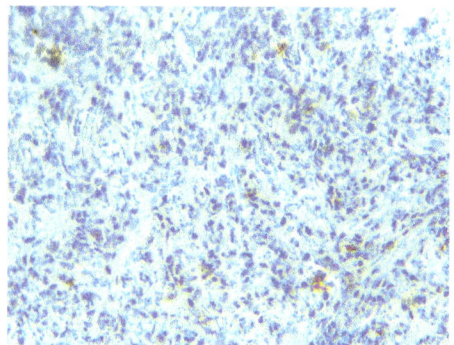

FIGURE 8: Immunohistochemical staining showing immunopositivity for EMA (×40).

Solitary plasmacytoma of the mandible also has various radiographic findings: from well-defined, unilocular radiolucency or "punched-out" appearance similar to multiple myeloma (MM) to ill-defined destructive radiolucencies with ragged borders but without periosteal reaction [28–30]. The radiographic feature of the present case was well-defined, multilocular radiolucency with several straight septa that resembled odontogenic myxoma.

Diagnosis is based on the presence of malignant proliferation of plasma cells in the biopsy.

Histological features of solitary plasmacytoma are identical to MM, Sheets, or clusters of atypical monoclonal plasma cells with various types of differentiation [28, 29].

Bone marrow biopsies are performed to ensure the disease is localized. In solitary and extramedullary plasmacytoma, there will not be an increase of monoclonal plasma cells in bone marrow [28, 30]. Bone marrow aspiration in our patient revealed 6% plasma cell.

A typical antibody is composed of two immunoglobulin (Ig) heavy chains and two Ig light chains. A monoclonal protein (M-protein) is an abnormal immunoglobulin (IgG) light chain that is produced in excess by an abnormal clonal proliferation of plasma cells [31, 32]. Diagnosis of this present case was confirmed as solitary plasmacytoma, because laboratory examination showed the presence of M-protein [immunoglobulin (IgG) κ type] on serum electrophoresis. 25% to 50% of patients show a monoclonal gammopathy on evaluation by serum protein immunoelectrophoresis, although the amount of abnormal protein is much less than seen with MM reflecting the lower tumor burden [31, 32].

In immunohistochemical painting, CD138, vimentin, and EMA were positive. Also Ki67 was positive in 70% of tumoral cells. The results of the present case are in accordance with some studies who reported that these atypical cells react positively for CD138 and k-light chain, whereas staining with CD20, CD1, and NSE is essentially negative which ruled out epithelial, muscle, neural, histiocytic, and salivary gland origin of the tumor cells [6, 31].

An early diagnosis of solitary plasmacytoma of bone is essential to patient survival rate. It may represent the first manifestation of MM and conversion to MM occurring in about 70% of cases at an average of 20.7 months after initial diagnosis [28, 29]. So a systemic workup should be obtained early after diagnosis of the lesion to rule out the existence of this systemic disease [32, 33].

The patient did not show typical complications of MM, such as bone pain, skeletal destruction with osteolytic lesions, pathological fractures, limited mobility, hypercalcaemia, renal failure, and end-organ/tissue damage [34, 35].

CBC and Diff test showed WBC, RBC, Hb, and HCT were lower than normal range; however, this patient has consumed phenytoin and lamotrigine for about 13 years so these drugs can cause dyscrasias [36].

Solitary plasmacytomas are highly radiosensitive lesions. Radiation therapy, radical extensive surgery, or a combination of both is recommended as primary treatment. Radical radiotherapy comprising of 40–50 Gy has shown 80% of local disease control [9]. So the treatment used most commonly for both types of plasmacytoma is radiation therapy. Although chemotherapy is generally not used, treatment by local radiation and chemotherapy may delay converting it to multiple myeloma [37].

Surgery is rarely necessary but may be required in situations where plasmacytoma involvement of the bone causes skeletal instability and high risk of fracture. In these cases, radiation therapy may be delayed until after surgery. All patients with plasmacytomas require follow-up for at least the first five years after treatment has been completed. The course of solitary plasmacytoma of bone is relatively benign and the 5-year survival rate of it is 60%; however, it falls to 5.7% when progression to multiple lesions occurs [30].

The patient in the current case demonstrated partial response to radiation (40 Gy in 20 fractions) and chemotherapy (cyclophosphamide, hydroxydaunorubicin, and prednisone).

The disease remains stable and nonprogressive at this time. He is scheduled for at least 5-year follow-up appointments.

5. Conclusion

In this paper, we reported a male patient with a large destructive lesion in the posterior of mandible. It presented as an expansile multilocular radiolucent lesion, clinically and radiographically resembling an odontogenic cyst/tumor but it was solitary plasmacytoma.

Consent

Written informed consent was obtained from the patient for publication and presenting of this case and any accompanying images.

Competing Interests

The authors declare that there is no conflict of interests regarding the publication of this article.

References

[1] S. Matsumura, M. Kishino, T. Ishida, and S. Furukawa, "Radiographic findings for solitary plasmacytoma of the bone in the anterior wall of the maxillary sinus: a case report," *Oral surgery, oral medicine, oral pathology, oral radiology, and endodontics*, vol. 89, no. 5, pp. 651–657, 2000.

[2] J. J. Pisano, R. Coupland, S.-Y. Chen, and A. S. Miller, "Plasmacytoma of the oral cavity and jaws: a clinicopathologic study of 13 cases," *Oral Surgery, Oral Medicine, Oral Pathology, Oral Radiology, and Endodontology*, vol. 83, no. 2, pp. 265–271, 1997.

[3] N. Sharma, A. Singh, A. Pandey, and V. Verma, "Solitary plasmacytoma of the mandible: a rare case report," *National Journal of Maxillofacial Surgery*, vol. 6, no. 1, pp. 76–79, 2015.

[4] V. Sychra, D. Eßer, H. Kosmehl, and M. Herold, "Unusual manifestation of a multiple myeloma in the hyoid bone," *Dentomaxillofacial Radiology*, vol. 42, no. 3, Article ID 27101530, 2013.

[5] S. Kalayoglu-Besisik, I. Yonal, F. Hindilerden, M. Agan, and D. Sargin, "Plasmacytoma of the nasolacrimal duct simulating dacryocystitis: an uncommon presentation for extramedullary relapse of multiple myeloma," *Case Reports in Oncology*, vol. 5, no. 1, pp. 119–124, 2012.

[6] L. M. Gonzalez-Perez and J. J. Borrero-Martin, "An elderly man with a gingival mass that spontaneously regressed," *Oral Surgery, Oral Medicine, Oral Pathology and Oral Radiology*, vol. 121, no. 4, pp. 348–352, 2016.

[7] M. Ozsahin, R. W. Tsang, P. Poortmans et al., "Outcomes and patterns of failure in solitary plasmacytoma: a multicenter rare cancer network study of 258 patients," *International Journal Of Radiation Oncology, Biology, Physics*, vol. 64, no. 1, pp. 210–217, 2006.

[8] C. Alexiou, R. J. Kau, H. Dietzfelbinger et al., "Extramedullary plasmacytoma: tumor occurrence and therapeutic concepts," *Cancer*, vol. 85, pp. 2305–2314, 2000.

[9] B. Rodríguez-Caballero, S. Sanchez-Santolino, B. García-Montesinos-Perea, M.-F. Garcia-Reija, J. Gómez-Román, and R. Saiz-Bustillo, "Mandibular solitary plasmocytoma of the jaw: a case report," *Medicina Oral, Patologia Oral y Cirugia Bucal*, vol. 16, no. 5, pp. e647–e650, 2011.

[10] L. N. Souza, L. C. Farias, L. A. N. Santos, R. A. Mesquita, H. Martelli Jr., and A. M. B. De-Paula, "Asymptomatic expansile lesion of the posterior mandible," *Oral Surgery, Oral Medicine, Oral Pathology, Oral Radiology, and Endodontology*, vol. 103, no. 1, pp. 4–7, 2007.

[11] G. Bachar, D. Goldstein, D. Brown et al., "Solitary extramedullary plasmacytoma of the head and neck—Long-term outcome analysis of 68 cases," *Head and Neck*, vol. 30, no. 8, pp. 1012–1019, 2008.

[12] S. Reddy, A. Naag, and B. Kashyap, "Odontogenic myxoma: report of two cases," *National Journal of Maxillofacial Surgery*, vol. 1, no. 2, pp. 183–186, 2010.

[13] S. F. Khan, P. Agrawal, and J. Sur, "A rare case report of myxoid fibroma of maxilla," *Quantitative Imaging in Medicine and Surgery*, vol. 5, no. 5, pp. 778–782, 2015.

[14] H. Rashid and A. Bashir, "Surgical and prosthetic management of maxillary odontogenic myxoma," *European Journal of Dentistry*, vol. 9, no. 2, pp. 277–283, 2015.

[15] R. K. Manne, V. S. Kumar, P. V. Sarath, L. Anumula, S. Mundlapudi, and R. Tanikonda, "Odontogenic myxoma of the mandible," *Case Reports in Dentistry*, vol. 2012, Article ID 214704, 4 pages, 2012.

[16] R. Subramaiam, S. Narashiman, M. Narasimhan, V. Giri, and S. Kumar, "Odontogenic myxoma of the maxilla: a rare case report," *Journal of Clinical and Diagnostic Research*, vol. 9, no. 5, pp. ZD29–ZD31, 2015.

[17] E. N. M. Simon, M. A. W. Merkx, E. Vuhahula, D. Ngassapa, and P. J. W. Stoelinga, "A 4-year prospective study on epidemiology and clinicopathological presentation of odontogenic tumors in Tanzania," *Oral Surgery, Oral Medicine, Oral Pathology, Oral Radiology and Endodontology*, vol. 99, no. 5, pp. 598–602, 2005.

[18] R. R. Throndson and S. B. Sexton, "A mandibular central lesion with unusually rapid growth," *Oral Surgery, Oral Medicine, Oral Pathology, Oral Radiology and Endodontology*, vol. 98, no. 1, pp. 4–9, 2004.

[19] M. R. Darling and T. D. Daley, "Radiolucent lesion of the anterior mandible," *Oral Surgery, Oral Medicine, Oral Pathology, Oral Radiology and Endodontology*, vol. 99, no. 5, pp. 529–531, 2005.

[20] M. P. Chae, N. R. Smoll, D. J. Hunter-Smith, and W. M. Rozen, "Establishing the natural history and growth rate of ameloblastoma with implications for management: systematic review and meta-analysis," *PLoS ONE*, vol. 10, no. 2, Article ID e0117241, 2015.

[21] J. Mahadesh, D. K. Rayapati, P. M. Maligi, and P. Ramachandra, "Unicystic ameloblastoma with diverse mural proliferation—a hybrid lesion," *Imaging Science in Dentistry*, vol. 41, no. 1, pp. 29–33, 2011.

[22] J. De Lange and H. P. Van Den Akker, "Clinical and radiological features of central giant-cell lesions of the jaw," *Oral Surgery, Oral Medicine, Oral Pathology, Oral Radiology and Endodontology*, vol. 99, no. 4, pp. 464–470, 2005.

[23] L. Avril, T. Lombardi, A. Ailianou et al., "Radiolucent lesions of the mandible: a pattern-based approach to diagnosis," *Insights into Imaging*, vol. 5, no. 1, pp. 85–101, 2014.

[24] H. Myoung, S.-P. Hong, S.-D. Hong et al., "Odontogenic keratocyst: review of 256 cases for recurrence and clinicopathologic parameters," *Oral Surgery, Oral Medicine, Oral Pathology, Oral Radiology, and Endodontics*, vol. 91, no. 3, pp. 328–333, 2001.

[25] C. E. Poggio, "Plasmacytoma of the mandible associated with a dental implant failure: a clinical report," *Clinical Oral Implants Research*, vol. 18, no. 4, pp. 540–543, 2007.

[26] R. Ozdemir, O. Kayiran, M. Oruc, O. Karaaslan, U. Koçer, and D. Ogun, "Plasmacytoma of the hard palate," *Journal of Craniofacial Surgery*, vol. 16, no. 1, pp. 164–169, 2005.

[27] E. M. Canger, P. Celenk, A. Alkan, and O. Günhan, "Mandibular involvement of solitary plasmocytoma: a case report," *Medicina Oral, Patología Oral y Cirugía Bucal*, vol. 12, no. 1, pp. E7–E9, 2007.

[28] J. J. Pisano, R. Coupland, S.-Y. Chen, and A. S. Miller, "Plasmacytoma of the oral cavity and jaws: a clinicopathologic study of 13 cases," *Oral Surgery, Oral Medicine, Oral Pathology, Oral Radiology, and Endodontics*, vol. 83, no. 2, pp. 265–271, 1997.

[29] S. Y. An, C. H. An, K. S. Choi, and M. S. Heo, "Multiple myeloma presenting as plasmacytoma of the jaws showing prominent bone formation during chemotherapy," *Dentomaxillofacial Radiology*, vol. 42, no. 4, Article ID 20110143, 2013.

[30] J. A. Jeong, G. E. Seo, J. H. Song, and S. J. Park, "Solitary plasma cell myeloma on anterior maxilla: a case report," *Journal of Korean Association of Maxillofacial Plastic and Reconstructive Surgeons*, vol. 32, pp. 77–80, 2010.

[31] R. W. McKenna, R. A. Kyle, W. M. Kuehl, T. M. Grogan, N. L. Harris, and R. W. Coupland, "Plasma cell neoplasms," in *WHO Classification of Tumours of Haematopoietic and Lymphoid Tissues*, S. H. Swerdlow, E. Campo, N. L. Harris et al., Eds., pp. 200–213, IARC, Lyon, France, 2008.

[32] H. Kaur, S. Parhar, S. Kaura et al., "A large painless swelling of the posterior mandible," *Oral Surgery, Oral Medicine, Oral Pathology and Oral Radiology*, vol. 115, no. 2, pp. 152–156, 2013.

[33] J. H. Yoon, J. I. Yook, H. J. Kim, I. H. Cha, W. I. Yang, and J. Kim, "Solitary plasmacytoma of the mandible in a renal transplant recipient," *International Journal of Oral and Maxillofacial Surgery*, vol. 32, no. 6, pp. 664–666, 2003.

[34] E. Coşkun, Ö. Başlarlı, A. Aktaş, H. Tüz, and Ö. Günhan, "Multiple myeloma presenting as paresthesia," *Oral Surgery, Oral Medicine, Oral Pathology and Oral Radiology*, vol. 119, no. 3, p. e150, 2015.

[35] Á. M. Miranda, S. M. Amaral, F. R. Pires, C. de Noronha Santos Netto, C. C. Queiroz, and J. de Moraes Pereira, "Multiple myeloma: primary oral presentation of 3 aggressive cases," *Oral Surgery, Oral Medicine, Oral Pathology and Oral Radiology*, vol. 120, no. 2, article no. e22, 2015.

[36] S. C. Blackbum, A. D. Oliart, L. A. Garca Rodríguez, and S. Peréz Gutthann, "Antiepileptics and blood dyscrasias: a cohort study," *Pharmacotherapy*, vol. 18, no. 6, pp. 1277–1283, 1998.

[37] S. Marotta and P. Di Micco, "Solitary plasmacytoma of the jaw," *Journal of Blood Medicine*, vol. 1, pp. 33–36, 2010.

6

Prosthetic Management of a Child with Hypohidrotic Ectodermal Dysplasia: 6-Year Follow-Up

Antonione Santos Bezerra Pinto,[1] **Moara e Silva Conceição Pinto,**[2]
Cinthya Melo do Val,[3] **Leonam Costa Oliveira,**[4] **Cristhyane Costa de Aquino,**[5]
and Daniel Fernando Pereira Vasconcelos[2]

[1]*Department of Morphology, Faculty of Medicine, Federal University of Ceará, Fortaleza, CE, Brazil*
[2]*Department of Histology and Embryology, Faculty of Biomedicine, Federal University of Piauí, Parnaíba, PI, Brazil*
[3]*Department of Genetic and Applied Toxicology, Lutheran University of Brazil, Canoas, RS, Brazil*
[4]*Department of Medical Skills, Faculty of Medicine, Federal University of Piauí, Parnaíba, PI, Brazil*
[5]*Laboratory of the Biology of Tissue Healing, Ontogeny and Nutrition, Department of Morphology and Institute of Biomedicine, School of Medicine, Federal University of Ceará, Fortaleza, CE, Brazil*

Correspondence should be addressed to Antonione Santos Bezerra Pinto; antonione182@hotmail.com

Academic Editor: Asja Celebić

Ectodermal dysplasia (ED) is a genetically heterogeneous condition resulting from clinical anomalies of structures derived from the ectoderm, such as the hair, nails, sweat glands, and teeth. This clinical report presents the case of a child diagnosed with hypohidrotic ED at 2 years of age; clinical and imaging evaluation was performed with 6-year follow-up, and we present details of the prosthetic dental care, with a 12-month follow-up. The patient's masticatory capacity had improved, leading to the child gaining 4 kg. In conclusion, prosthetic management was noninvasive and appeared to lead to developmental benefits for the patient.

1. Introduction

Ectodermal dysplasia (ED) comprises a large group of clinical and genetically heterogeneous diseases affecting the ectoderm-derived structures, such as the hair, nails, sweat glands, and teeth [1]. The prevalence is estimated between 1,6 and 22 per 100,000 persons [2].

The most common forms of ED are the X-linked hypohidrotic (Christ-Siemens-Touraine syndrome) and hidrotic (Clouston syndrome) types. The former presents with hypodontia or anodontia, hypotrichosis, and hypohidrosis or anhidrosis, while the latter is more severe, involving nail dystrophy, hypotrichosis, and palmoplantar keratoderma [3, 4].

Prosthetic dental treatment for ED is necessary to improve chewing, facial aesthetics, speech, nutrition, and social integration, the last of which can influence the patient's emotional health [5]. For these reasons, the technique is widely discussed in the literature. The therapy must be adapted to each case and varies from simple restorations to prostheses and implants [6–9].

Herein, we report the case of a child with hypohidrotic ED (HED) who underwent imaging and prosthodontic treatment and was followed up for 6 years; we also examine the influence of the procedure on the child's development, consider his ability to contribute to clinical management at an early age, and discuss tailoring oral rehabilitation to the idiosyncrasies of each patient's facial bone with similar facial anomalies.

2. Clinical Report

The patient began visiting the dentist at 2 years of age. At this time, his mother complained that several teeth had not erupted.

The mother described several episodes of hyperthermia, lack of sweating, crying with few tears, constant water intake,

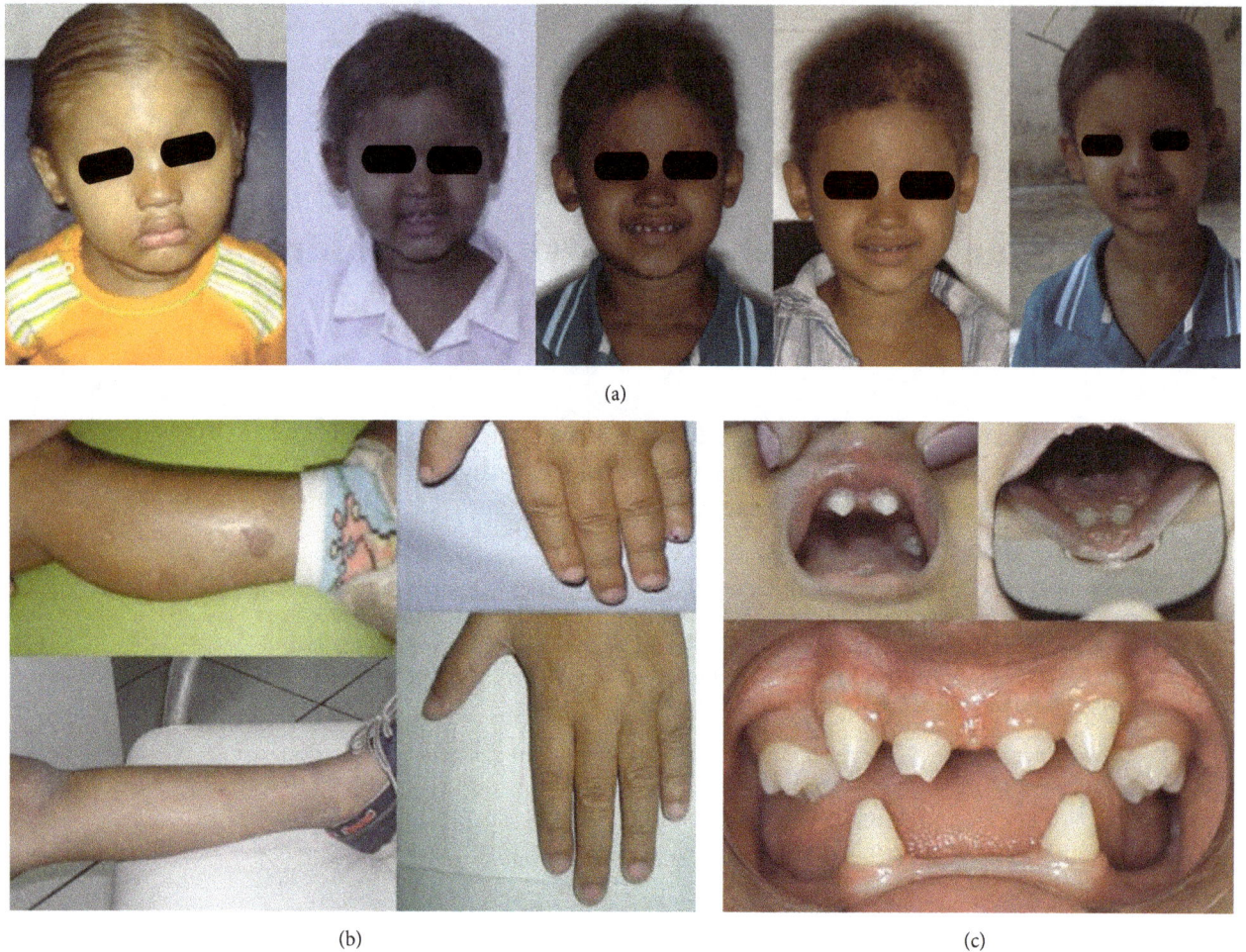

FIGURE 1: (a) Patient's visage at 2, 3, 4, 5, and 6 years of age with sparse hair, frontal bossing, saddle nose, and everted prominent lips. (b) Bright, dry skin on the leg; normal nails. (c) Intraoral examination showing variation in the timing and shape of the teeth, hypodontia, and ogival palate.

and frequent bathing. During viral infections, the mother had observed gelatinous, yellow-brown secretions from the respiratory tract. No anomalies were reported concerning the child's neurological development. He had been attending pediatric appointments, but the condition had never been suspected.

After anamnesis, wherein the boy's medical history was recalled by his mother, both extra- and intraoral examinations were performed (Figure 1); on this basis, the child was diagnosed with HED.

Initial dental treatment was based on maintaining oral health, which involved instructing both the boy and his mother in oral hygiene in order to preserve the teeth against oral diseases such as caries and periodontal disease. The mother was further instructed to seek the advice of a medical geneticist who would confirm the diagnosis of HED, request additional tests, and contribute to the patient's treatment.

From the age of 3 to 6 years, the child periodically attended clinical and imaging exams (Figures 1 and 2) to assess bone development and identify when to begin oral rehabilitation.

When the patient was 6 years old, a cephalometric analysis was carried out (Figure 2(b)) revealing that he had a convex profile, as well as a Class I skeletal malocclusion. Using the Eklof and Ringertz index and a carpal radiograph (Figure 2(d)), we determined that the patient's bone age matched his chronological age. What is more, cone-beam computed tomography (CBCT) revealed both hypertrophy in the tonsils and mandibular micrognathia (Figures 2(e) and 2(f)).

The patient was of school age and was willing to cooperate with treatment, especially since the characteristic phenotype of the syndrome, and in particular the dental condition, was affecting him emotionally—he felt different from his classmates.

Informed consent was given by the boy's mother, and the treatment consisted of restorations of the upper and lower teeth and the installation of a lower removable partial denture (Figure 4) when the boy was 7 years old.

An impression was taken using alginate (Figure 3(a)) (Jeltrate® Plus™; Dentsply) to obtain study cast models (Durone IV Salmon®; Dentsply). From these, diagnostic wax-up of

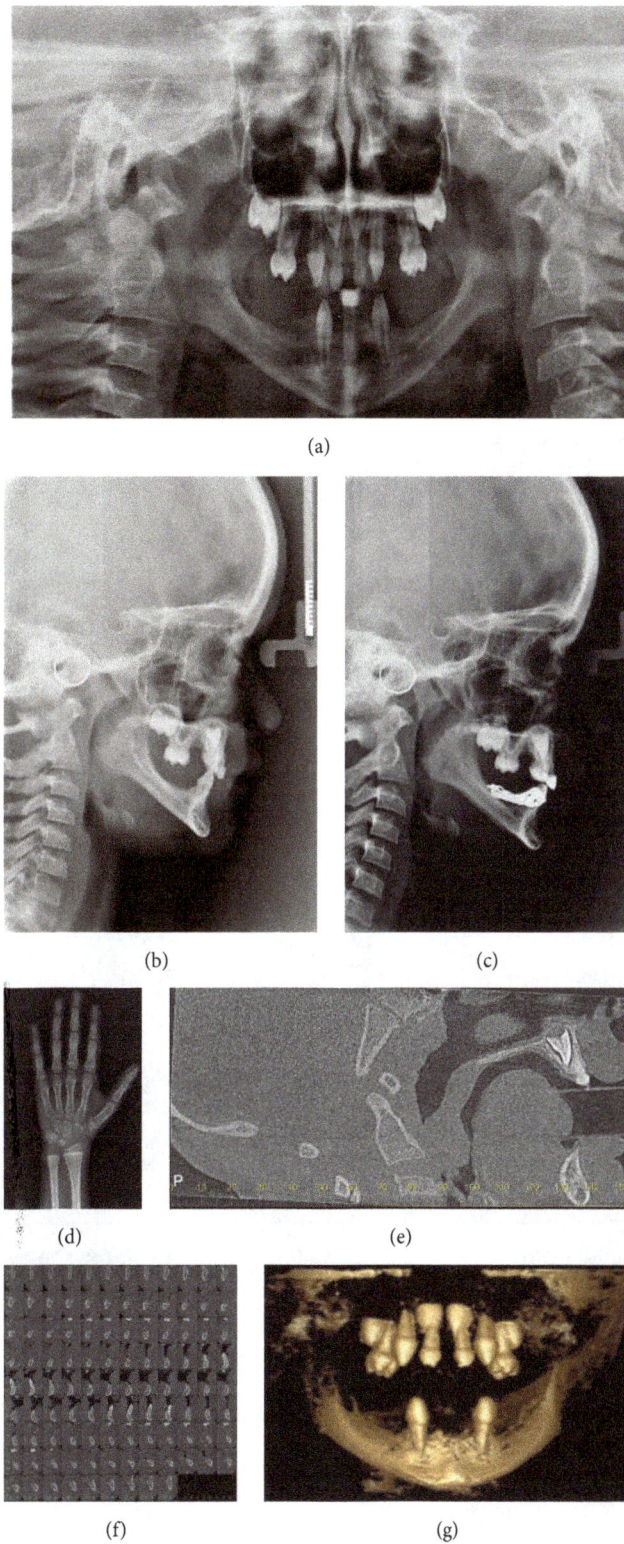

FIGURE 2: (a) Panoramic radiograph. (b) Lateral cephalogram showing decreased mandibular length and mandibular anterior facial height. (c) Lateral cephalogram taken 6 months after the patient began prosthetic rehabilitation. The image shows the growth pattern between the bone bases. (d) Carpal radiograph at 6 years of age matching the chronological age. (e) Computed tomography (CT) sagittal cut evidencing the presence of hypertrophic tonsils, consistent with recurrent infections of the lower respiratory tract. (f) Cross-sectional CT images showing reduced height and thickness of the alveolar bone, as well as mandibular micrognathia. (g) 3D reconstruction.

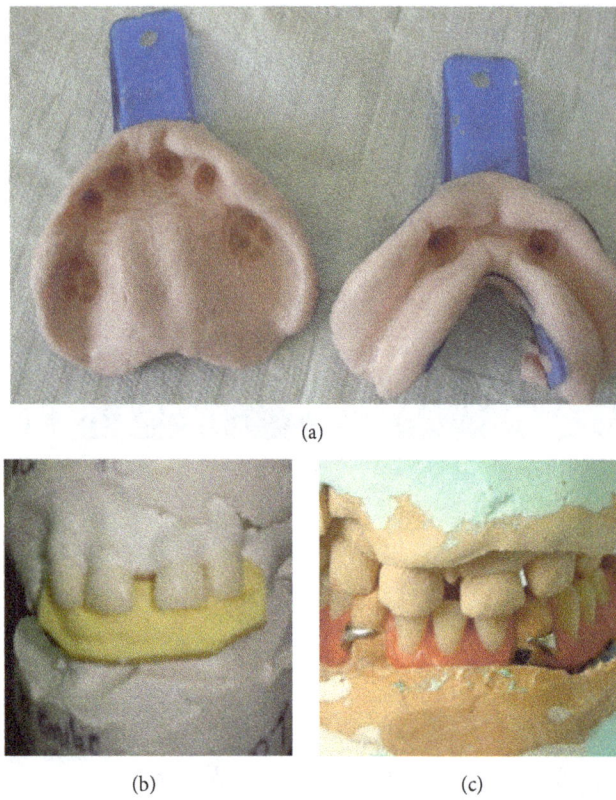

FIGURE 3: Stages of prosthetic rehabilitation. (a) Upper and lower impression. (b) Template for maxillary tooth restorations. (c) Mandibular partial dentures.

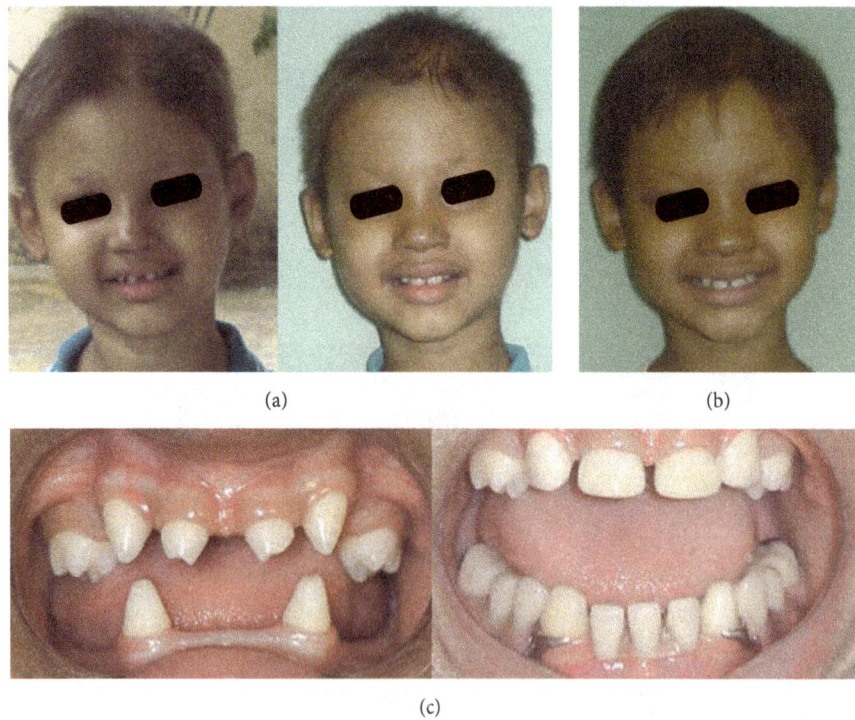

FIGURE 4: Patient before and after treatment. (a) Initial and final facial aspect. (b) 12 months after the installation of the prosthesis. (c) Oral aspects.

the upper anterior teeth was created to facilitate planning of the lower prosthesis.

A further impression of the diagnostic wax-up was made, using addition silicon (Adsil®; Vigodent) to construct a template that would guide restorations of the deciduous teeth (Figure 3(b)). The maxillary conoid teeth were reconstructed by increasing their dimensions, but maintaining the spaces characteristic of the deciduous dentition. The restorations were made using composite resin AO.5 (Opallis®; FGM) so as to be white and opaque.

The lower partial denture (Figure 3(c)) was supported by the mandibular primary canines, which received increments of resin A3 (IPS Empress® Direct™; Ivoclar Vivadent), so as to resemble the premolars. The appropriate tooth color was then selected (tooth color 60; SPG pop) and the gum was characterized (number 15; Tomaz Gomes System, VIPI).

At the installation of the prosthesis, both the patient and his mother were instructed regarding prosthesis placement, removal, and hygiene.

Adjustments were made 48 hours after installation. The prosthesis showed good retention, and the patient adapted well to it. Then, the next visit was scheduled at 6 months for follow-up and the patient's mother was advised to arrange additional visits in the case of complications.

Six months after installation of the prosthesis, the periodontal condition of the teeth, occlusion, functional adaptation, and cephalometrics were evaluated (Figure 2(c)). Clinical evaluation was repeated over six months when the patient was 8 years old (Figure 4(b)) and new adjustments in prosthesis were performed.

According to his mother, the child's chewing ability had improved and he was able to enjoy foods that he could not chew before, such as meat, cheese, and fibrous vegetables. This resulted in a gain of 4 kg—from 16 kg to 20 kg—during the first 6 months of adaptation.

Both the family and the teacher noticed the behavioral differences, and the classmates approved the child's new appearance, which suggested impact on his socialization.

It must be noted that the patient's mother, as his legal guardian, read and signed an informed consent form authorizing the use of data, images, and all information relating to the dental patient follow-up for use in publications and/or scientific events.

3. Discussion

Important dental defects are associated with the syndrome. During childhood particularly, this condition is a major cause of frustration that impacts the intellectual and psychological maturity of the patient [5, 6].

Many children require extensive treatment; however, treatment cost should be evaluated. All changes in the dental arches, including alveolar bone growth in response to tooth eruption, should be monitored to ensure appropriate adjustments are made. Long-term treatment is an active process that must be constantly adapted to the child's development and growth [10].

In the present case, after the prosthetic rehabilitation, the child experienced a wider variety of foods. The relationship between the upper and lower jaws, esthetics, and self-esteem were all improved. Children with these prostheses should perform standard oral hygiene and take care of the devices by themselves.

ED treatment using removable partial dentures is indicated for children and adults [6, 7]. Nonetheless, the use of partial dentures has been described in a 2-year-old HED patient; such early rehabilitation prevents growth abnormalities and improves socialization [7].

The installation of implants in adult ED patients has been widely reported as a treatment option with high success rate and the associated benefits of rehabilitation [8]. Nonetheless, the high cost, possible failure of osseointegration, and need for complete bone growth are disadvantages, particularly if dental implants are placed before dental and skeletal maturation [9].

In this case, dental implants were not indicated, because CBCT (Figures 2(e) and 2(f)) revealed both maxillary and mandibular micrognathism caused by the absence of teeth. The cephalometric analysis (Figures 2(b) and 2(c)) indicated that the patient should be followed up to assess bone growth after placement of the prosthesis.

After prosthetic rehabilitation, masticatory function improves, as in the present case, where the patient was able to eat meat, fish, fibrous vegetables, and cheese. In general, dentures are well accepted by parents and patients, and the psychological benefits after oral rehabilitation are many [5–7]. The authors are unanimous in recommending early prosthetic treatment in patients with this syndrome, especially when the child already has a social life, as is the case with children of school age.

4. Conclusion

A removable partial denture and restoration were a noninvasive, reversible, cost-effective, viable, and efficient treatment for a child with hypodontia and HED. Moreover, the treatment appeared to lead to marked developmental benefits for the patient.

Competing Interests

The authors have no potential competing interests to disclose.

References

[1] M. L. Mikkola, "Molecular aspects of hypohidrotic ectodermal dysplasia," *American Journal of Medical Genetics, Part A*, vol. 149, no. 9, pp. 2031–2036, 2009.

[2] M. Nguyen-Nielsen, S. Skovbo, D. Svaneby, L. Pedersen, and J. Fryzek, "The prevalence of X-linked hypohidrotic ectodermal dysplasia (XLHED) in Denmark, 1995–2010," *European Journal of Medical Genetics*, vol. 56, no. 5, pp. 236–242, 2013.

[3] S. N. de Aquino, L. M. R. Paranaíba, M. S. O. Swerts, D. R. B. Martelli, L. M. de Barros, and H. M. Júnior, "Orofacial features of hypohidrotic ectodermal dysplasia," *Head and Neck Pathology*, vol. 6, no. 4, pp. 460–466, 2012.

[4] A. Kutkowska-Kaźmierczak, K. Niepokój, K. Wertheim-Tysarowska et al., "Phenotypic variability in gap junction syndromic skin disorders: experience from KID and Clouston syndromes' clinical diagnostics," *Journal of Applied Genetics*, vol. 56, no. 3, pp. 329–337, 2015.

[5] N. A. Alencar, K. R. Reis, A. G. Antonio, and L. C. Maia, "Influence of oral rehabilitation on the oral health-related quality of life of a child with ectodermal dysplasia," *Journal of Dentistry for Children*, vol. 82, no. 1, pp. 36–40, 2015.

[6] M. V. Carvalho, J. R. S. de Sousa, F. P. C. de Melo et al., "Hypohidrotic and hidrotic ectodermal dysplasia: a report of two cases," *Dermatology Online Journal*, vol. 19, no. 7, article 18985, 2013.

[7] M. A. Derbanne, M. C. Sitbon, M. M. Landru, and A. Naveau, "Case report: early prosthetic treatment in children with ectodermal dysplasia," *European Archives of Paediatric Dentistry*, vol. 11, no. 6, pp. 301–305, 2010.

[8] G. Kearns, A. Sharma, D. Perrott, B. Schmidt, L. Kaban, and K. Vargervik, "Placement of endosseous implants in children and adolescents with hereditary ectodermal dysplasia," *Oral Surgery, Oral Medicine, Oral Pathology, Oral Radiology and Endodontics*, vol. 88, no. 1, pp. 5–10, 1999.

[9] I. P. Sweeney, J. W. Ferguson, A. A. Heggie, and J. O. Lucas, "Treatment outcomes for adolescent ectodermal dysplasia patients treated with dental implants," *International Journal of Paediatric Dentistry*, vol. 15, no. 4, pp. 241–248, 2005.

[10] C. Dellavia, F. Catti, C. Sforza, D. G. Tommasi, and V. F. Ferrario, "Craniofacial growth in ectodermal dysplasia. An 8 year longitudinal evaluation of Italian subjects," *The Angle Orthodontist*, vol. 80, no. 4, pp. 733–739, 2010.

Successful Fitting of a Complete Maxillary Denture in a Patient with Severe Alzheimer's Disease Complicated by Oral Dyskinesia

Hiromitsu Morita,[1,2] **Akie Hashimoto,**[2] **Ryosuke Inoue,**[2] **Shohei Yoshimoto,**[2] **Masahiro Yoneda,**[1] **and Takao Hirofuji**[1]

[1]*Section of General Dentistry, Department of General Dentistry, Fukuoka Dental College, Fukuoka 814-0193, Japan*
[2]*Special Patient Oral Care Unit, Kyushu University Hospital, Fukuoka 812-8582, Japan*

Correspondence should be addressed to Hiromitsu Morita; morita@college.fdcnet.ac.jp

Academic Editor: Emmanuel Nicolas

There is an increasing population of elderly patients suffering from Alzheimer's disease (AD), the most common form of dementia. In dentistry, a critical problem associated with these patients is the use of a new denture, as AD patients often refuse dental management and are disturbed by minor changes in their oral environment. Some AD patients have further complications associated with oral dyskinesia, a movement disorder that can make dental management difficult, including the stability of a complete denture. In this case, we successfully fitted a complete maxillary denture using modified bilateral balanced occlusion after multiple tooth extractions under intravenous sedation in a 66-year-old woman with severe AD complicated by oral dyskinesia. Following treatment, her appetite and food intake greatly improved. Providing a well-fitting complete denture applied by modified bilateral balanced occlusion, which removes lateral interference using zero-degree artificial teeth for movement disorder of the jaw in patients with severe AD complicated by oral dyskinesia, helps improve oral function.

1. Introduction

Alzheimer's disease (AD) is the most common form of dementia, and patients with severe AD experience problems associated with cognitive function such as aphasia, apraxia, agnosia, and disorientation, making daily social activities difficult [1–3]. Worldwide, 47.5 million people suffered from dementia in 2015, and there are 7.7 million new cases every year [4]. The communication ability of patients with severe AD is poor, and dental management for them is critically restricted [1–3]. It is therefore difficult for such patients to receive both dental treatment and periodic dental follow-up, including oral care. A further difficulty is that some patients are disturbed by minor changes in their oral environment, such as a new denture, and struggle to adapt to the change [1]. Patients with severe AD often experience oral dyskinesia, which makes it more difficult not only to manage dental treatment but also to stabilize dentures [1–3].

Here we report a patient with severe AD, possibly showing signs of agnosia rather than impairment in adaptation, whose eating disorder, caused by severe periodontitis and oral dyskinesia, greatly improved following multiple tooth extractions under intravenous sedation (IVS) and the making and placement of a new, functional, stabilized, and well-fitting complete maxillary denture with bilateral balanced occlusion using zero-degree artificial teeth.

2. Case Presentation

A 66-year-old woman with severe AD complicated by oral dyskinesia was referred for dental treatment by her neurologist. She was unable to eat any solid food because of limited mobility of her maxillary teeth as a result of severe periodontitis. Because of her oral condition and subsequent lack of food, her body weight had decreased by ~5 kg within 2 months. Her husband was concerned for her health and hoped that her oral function would improve with the extraction of her diseased teeth and replacement with a removable denture. Written informed consent was obtained from the patient's husband for publication of this case report following the Ethical Guidelines of Kyushu University Hospital.

Her medical history revealed that she developed severe AD in 2004. Her medical condition suddenly worsened in 2006, resulting in severe cognitive impairment. Since 2011, she has been medicated with NMDA inhibitors and cholinesterase inhibitors. She has continued to receive regular medical treatment.

Her dental history revealed that she routinely visited a local dental office for oral care and maintenance until July 2012. Her family dentist recommended extraction of all her remaining maxillary teeth and asked her husband to consent to extractions under IVS in hospital because of the difficulty of conducting the dental procedure while she was awake. The patient's neurologist wrote a referral for her, and her husband brought her to our department, the Special Patient Oral Care Unit, Kyushu University Hospital, in October 2012. When she presented at our department, she exhibited typical features of AD, such as aphasia, gait apraxia, and disorientation. Her height and weight were 151 cm and 46 kg, respectively. Her serum albumin was 3.8 g/dL. She could not walk by herself and needed her husband's assistance. Her cognitive function and activities of daily living using the functional independence measure [5] were 26 points (maximum possible score: 126, minimum possible score: 18). She frequently vocalized meaningless words and could not speak any meaningful words or understand any of our instructions. As she could not sit still, it was impossible to take X-ray images of her teeth. We were able to see and touch inside her mouth only when her husband held her face and opened her mouth gently in semi-Fowler's position. If we tried to insert any instrument into her mouth by ourselves, she brushed our hands away. With her husband's help, we were able to briefly assess her oral condition and established the necessity for multiple extractions of her remaining maxillary teeth and fabrication of a complete denture. We initially planned to take impression before extraction to maintain her original maxilla-mandibular horizontal relationship under IVS. However, this was not possible as the horizontal position had collapsed from severe lateral mobility of the metal bridge between 13 and 17. To avoid accidents and the need for restraint and to maintain the patient's dignity during dental treatment, we decided to use IVS for oral examination and dental management, with the approval of her husband. In addition, her medical doctor checked her general health and approved the use of IVS.

On the first day of her dental treatment, we planned to undertake a complete examination, tooth scaling, multiple tooth extractions, and an impression for her denture under IVS. The IVS procedure involved initial administration of 4 mg midazolam, and once the patient was drowsy, we added propofol for maintenance. Under IVS, we first took X-rays and checked the probing depth and mobility of the remaining teeth. We observed severe periodontitis of all maxillary teeth (12, 13, 15, 17, 21, 22, and 23) and moderate periodontitis of all mandibular teeth (Figure 1). We scaled the teeth

and subsequently extracted the maxillary teeth. All sockets were sutured using bioabsorbable thread. Using alginate in a custom impression tray, we took impressions of the maxillary arch and the opposing mandibular teeth for a complete maxillary denture. We finished the dental treatment after confirming that there was no bleeding from the sockets. The duration of the dental treatment was 57 min, and the duration of the anesthesia was 1 h and 20 min. In total, 49 mg of propofol was used. There were no perioperative complications.

To help stop bleeding and as an imitation trial of the complete denture, we made a temporary base plate that covered her maxilla with tray resin and a plaster model, which duplicated for her teeth impression for the denture until recovery from IVS. After recovery from IVS, we tried fitting the base plate and relined with tissue conditioner. Surprisingly, she easily accepted it. Following this success, we sought to fabricate a new complete denture, as requested by her husband.

One day after extraction, there was no bleeding inside the patient's mouth, and she was still wearing the base plate without any signs of refusal. We removed the temporary base plate, checked to ensure that there was indeed no bleeding, washed her sockets with saline, and then refitted the base plate to her maxilla. We provided her husband with instructions for care, which included removing and washing the base plate after every meal and before the patient went to sleep. This was done as training before use of the complete denture.

One week after the extractions, we attempted to take a bite using Willis's method in semi-Fowler's position, opening the patient's mouth with her husband's help. Maxilla-mandibular horizontal position was achieved by moving the patient's chin forward using our hands. After a trial fitting, we fabricated her initial denture. To avoid instability caused by lateral cuspal interference because of her oral dyskinesia, we used zero-degree artificial teeth (Figure 2(a)). On inserting the new complete maxillary denture, we found that the mucosal surface of the denture was ill-fitting, because the impression had been taken immediately after multiple tooth extractions. To improve the fit, we relined the denture using low-flow tissue conditioner, COE-COMFORT™ (GC, Tokyo, Japan) and held her jaw gently for a while in semi-Fowler's position because of her oral dyskinesia. When we tried fitting the new denture, she initially hesitated to wear it; however, she accepted it soon after it was relined, similar as to when she wore the base plate to stop bleeding. After occlusal adjustment of the denture using articulating paper to remove lateral cuspal interference when she was awake, we instructed her husband on how to manage the denture, including insertion, removal, and cleaning, and the patient went home wearing the denture.

One week later, she visited our department for a denture adjustment. Her husband told us that she had not complained or indicated that the denture caused any pain or discomfort and had not tried to remove the denture once inserted. Her husband reported that she was able to eat soft solid food such as grilled fish, and her appetite had increased. She visited our unit 2 days per week for a denture adjustment and relining over several weeks. Three months after the extractions, the sockets were almost completely healed and bone had recovered. We performed dynamic impressions for

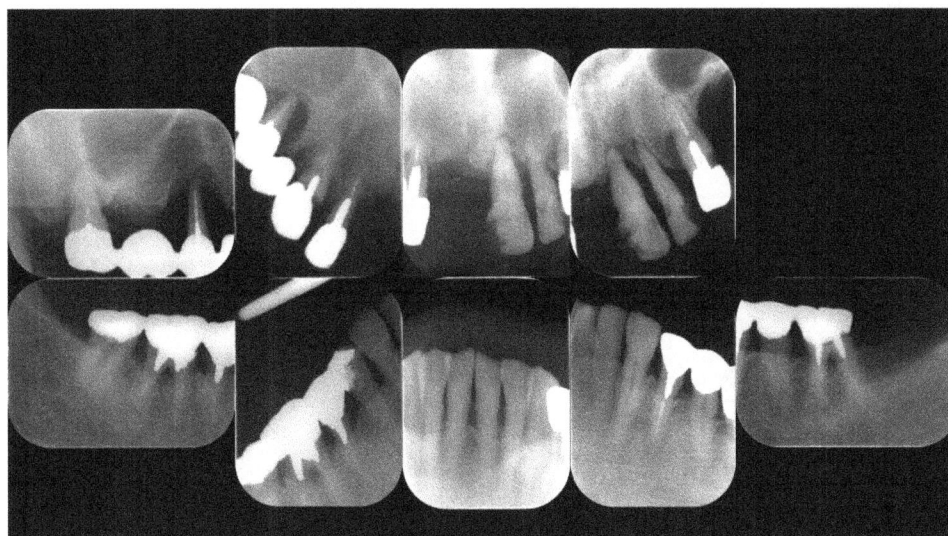

(a)

Mobility	2		2		2	2		2	3	2				
Probing depth	③⑧⑨		⑧⑨⑨		②2②	22③		③③③	③④④	④④④				
	③③⑨		⑧⑤⑨		2④2	2④3		3⑧3	3⑤④	④⑦④				
	17	16	15	14	13	12	11	21	22	23	24	25	26	27
	47	46	45	44	43	42	41	31	32	33	34	35	36	37
Probing depth	④④④	④④④	④④④	④④③	④④③	④③③	③③③	③③③	③③③	③③③	③③④	④③④	④④③	
	④④④	④④④	④④④	④④④	④④③	③③③	③3③	③3③	③③③	③③③	④④④	④④④	④④④	
Mobility	0	0	0	0	0	0	0	0	0	0	0	0	0	

(b)

FIGURE 1: (a) X-ray images and (b) periodontal chart at initial dental visit. Circle on number indicates bleeding on probing.

a week using the same tissue conditioner and temporarily kept her denture for relining, choosing an indirect procedure in the dental laboratory to avoid a poor result because of her oral dyskinesia and to avoid accidental swallowing of the reline materials. After relining and occlusal adjustment of the denture, she was again happy to wear the denture (Figure 2(b)).

The patient has since visited the department for oral hygiene management and denture adjustment, including partial direct rebasing around the sockets several times. Currently, she routinely receives oral examinations and hygiene management. She can eat almost all foods such as vegetables, meat, and fish, and her body weight has increased by 5 kg (now up to 51 kg) and her serum albumin level has also improved (4.3 mg/dL). From discussion with the patient's husband's and examining a visual analogue scale drawn by him, it is apparent that her appetite and food intake have greatly improved (Figure 2(c)).

3. Discussion

We successfully performed multiple tooth extractions under IVS and fabricated a stable complete maxillary denture using zero-degree artificial teeth for a patient with severe AD

complicated by oral dyskinesia. The treatment appears to have improved both the patient's oral function and her appetite and she has gained weight.

Following multiple tooth extractions, and being considerate of the patient's dignity and at the request of the patient's husband, we initially fitted a base plate. When we observed that she easily accepted the base plate and showed no signs of discomfort or stress, we took this as a sign that a complete denture may be possible. As it was requested by the patient's husband, we began the process of making and fitting a new complete denture.

We initially referred to the report by Fujisawa et al. in which they described successful multiple tooth extractions using IVS and the fitting of a new complete denture in a patient with severe AD [6]. We safely performed dental treatments such as probing, scaling, tooth extraction, and denture impressions under IVS as outlined in previous reports and reviews [1–4, 6–8] to minimize the risk of adverse effects.

An additional problem for our patient was that she suffered from oral dyskinesia, a jaw movement disorder, which is a complication of severe AD. This condition makes it more difficult to stabilize a complete denture. After referring to reports about the fabrication of prostheses for patients

(a)

(b)

Min: minimum
Max: maximum

(c)

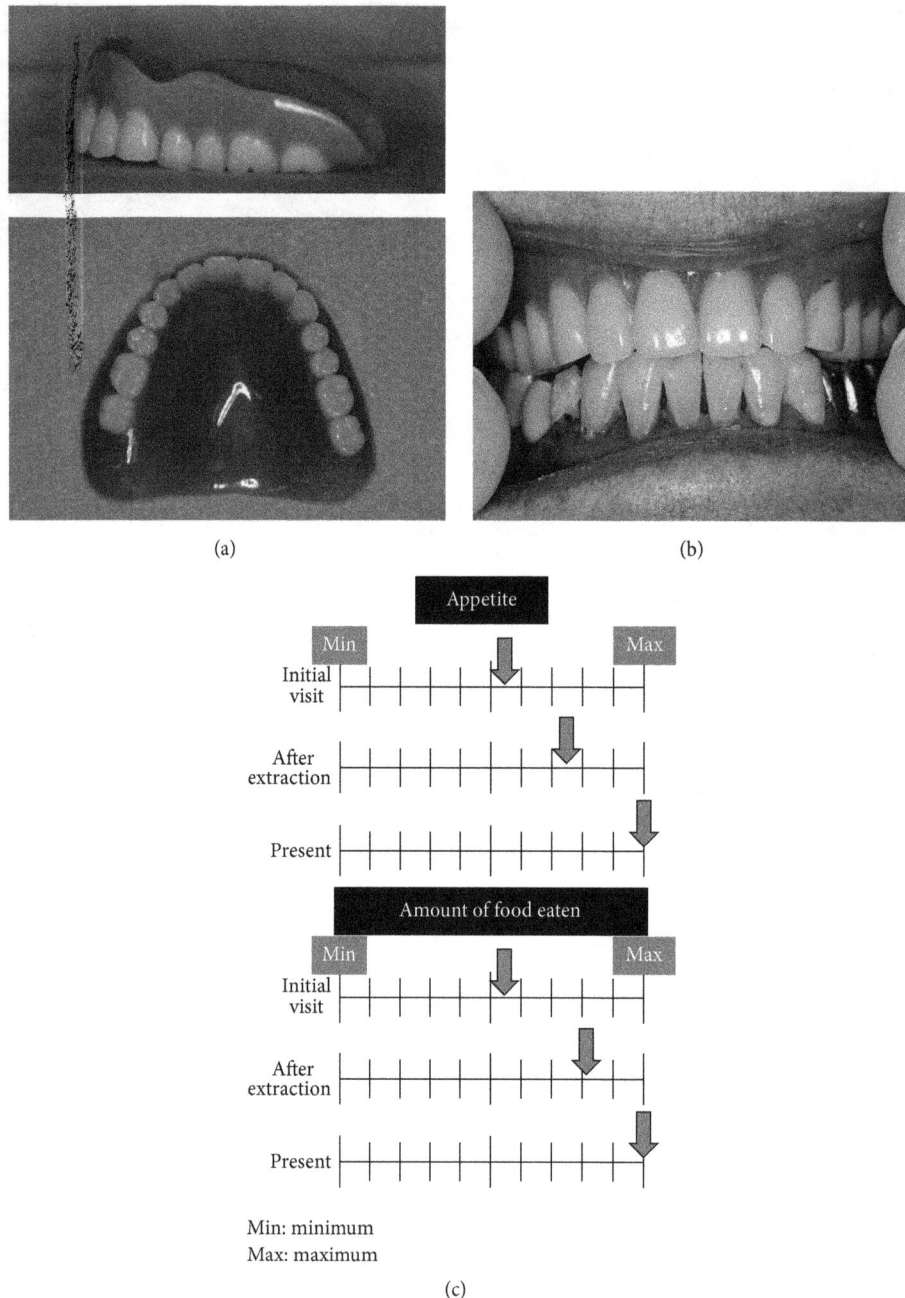

FIGURE 2: (a) Lateral and occlusal views of the complete maxillary denture. (b) Frontal view of the complete maxillary denture. (c) Visual analogue scale of appetite and amount of food eaten at the time of the initial visit, after extraction, and posttreatment, drawn by the patient's husband.

with Parkinson's disease complicated by oral dyskinesia, we applied modified bilateral balanced occlusion using zero-degree artificial teeth to avoid interference by the molar cusps during lateral movement [9, 10]. We succeeded in stabilizing the complete maxillary denture in this case. Accordingly, we consider that using zero-degree artificial teeth in complete dentures for patients with oral dyskinesia is useful. As a result of the dental management described above, and with the help of her husband, the patient's appetite and food intake have greatly improved and she has gained weight.

Interestingly, from our clinical observations, it appears that the patient forgot that she was wearing a denture after the fitting of the new complete maxillary denture, possibly suggestive of agnosia. Although it is known that minor changes in the oral environment, such as the fitting of a new denture, can cause distress to AD patients because of their impaired ability to adapt, the patient in this case easily accepted the new denture.

It is our suggestion that fabricating a painless, well-fitting complete denture using modified bilateral occlusion with zero-degree artificial teeth in patients with severe AD with oral dyskinesia may help improve the food intake in such patients.

Competing Interests

The authors declare that they have no competing interests.

Authors' Contributions

Hiromitsu Morita and Akie Hashimoto contributed equally.

Acknowledgments

The authors thank members of the Department of Dental Anesthesiology, Kyushu University Hospital for clinical collaboration with intravenous sedation. This study was partly supported by a Grant-in-Aid for Research in Control of Aging from the Ministry of Education, Culture, Sports, Science and Technology of Japan to Hiromitsu Morita (no. 16K11713).

References

[1] H. Kocaelli, M. Yaltirik, L. I. Yargic, and H. Özbas, "Alzheimer's disease and dental management," *Oral Surgery, Oral Medicine, Oral Pathology, Oral Radiology, and Endodontology*, vol. 93, no. 5, pp. 521–524, 2002.

[2] J. W. Little, "Dental management of patients with Altzheimer's disease," *General Dentistry*, vol. 53, pp. 289–296, 2005.

[3] E. M. Ghezzi and J. A. Ship, "Dementia and oral health," *Oral Surgery, Oral Medicine, Oral Pathology, Oral Radiology, and Endodontics*, vol. 89, no. 1, pp. 2–5, 2000.

[4] World Health Organization, *Dementia Fact Sheet*, World Health Organization, Geneva, Switzerland, 2016, http://www.who.int/mediacentre/factsheets/fs362/en/.

[5] J. M. Lincare, A. W. Heinemann, B. D. Wright et al., "The structure and stability of the functional independence measure," *Archives of Physical Medicine and Rehabilitation*, vol. 75, pp. 127–132, 1994.

[6] T. Fujisawa, A. Yokoyama, M. Muramatsu et al., "Fitting complete dentures after multiple tooth extraction in a patient with severe dementia," *Special Care in Dentistry*, vol. 27, no. 5, pp. 187–190, 2007.

[7] J. M. Chalmers, "Behavior management and communication strategies for dental professionals when caring for patients with dementia," *Special Care in Dentistry*, vol. 20, no. 4, pp. 147–154, 2000.

[8] M. T. Galli and R. G. Henry, "Using intravenous sedation to manage adults with neurological impairment," *Special Care in Dentistry*, vol. 19, no. 6, pp. 275–280, 1999.

[9] P. J. Blanchet, P. H. Rompré, G. J. Lavigne, and C. Lamarche, "Oral dyskinesia: a clinical overview," *International Journal of Prosthodontics*, vol. 18, no. 1, pp. 10–19, 2005.

[10] S. Neha, B. Vidya, D. Savitha et al., "Prosthodontic considerations in the management of Parkinson's disease: a review," *Unique Journal of Medical and Dental Sciences*, vol. 2, pp. 163–167, 2014.

Oral Rehabilitation and Management for Secondary Sjögren's Syndrome in a Child

Tatiana Kelly da Silva Fidalgo,[1,2] **Carla Nogueira,**[3]
Marcia Rejane Thomas Canabarro Andrade,[4]
Andrea Graciene Lopez Ramos Valente,[3] **and Patricia Nivoloni Tannure**[3]

[1]*Universidade do Estado do Rio de Janeiro, Boulevard Vinte e Oito de Setembro, 175 Vila Isabel, 21941-913 Rio de Janeiro RJ, Brazil*
[2]*Universidade Salgado de Oliveira, Pólo Niterói, Rua Marechal Deodoro, 263 Centro, 24030-060 Niterói, RJ, Brazil*
[3]*Universidade Veiga de Almeida, Rua Ibituruna 108, Tijuca, 20271-020 Rio de Janeiro, RJ, Brazil*
[4]*Department of Specific Formation, School of Dentistry, Universidade Federal Fluminense,*
 Rua Dr. Silvio Henrique Braune 22, 28625-650 Nova Friburgo, RJ, Brazil

Correspondence should be addressed to Marcia Rejane Thomas Canabarro Andrade; marciathomas13@gmail.com

Academic Editor: Pia L. Jornet

The aim of this paper is to describe a rare case report of a pediatric patient with secondary Sjögren's syndrome (SSS). A 12-year-old female child was referred to the Pediatric Dentistry Clinic with the chief complaint of tooth pain, dry mouth, and tooth sensibility. The patient was submitted to orthodontic treatment prior to syndrome diagnosis. The clinical treatment consisted of the interruption of orthodontic treatment and restoring the oral condition with dental treatment and the use of artificial saliva in an innovative apparatus. Dental therapy involved the control of dental caries, periodontal disease, and opportunistic fungal infections and the use of fluoride-rich solutions. The present clinical case describes clinical and laboratory aspects of SSS in pediatric patients. The management of the oral findings promoted an improvement in the oral health status and quality of life of the child.

1. Introduction

Sjögren's syndrome (SS) is a chronic autoimmune disease of the exocrine glands characterized by focal lymphocytic infiltration and destruction of these glands [1]. SS may occur alone, as primary SS, or may accompany other autoimmune disorders as secondary Sjögren's syndrome (SSS) [2, 3]. SS typically occurs when xerostomia and xerophthalmia are present. The prevalence in the general population is about 0.5% to 3% [4]. Females are more affected, especially in the fourth and fifth decades of life. Children and young adults are rarely affected. Although it is not an inherited disease, there is evidence of a genetic influence. Keratoconjunctivitis sicca and xerostomia characterize the main clinical symptoms. Neurologic complications are probably underestimated and have been reported in 8% to 70% of Sjögren syndrome patients [1, 5, 6].

Primary disease is rare in childhood [7]. Parotid swelling was the most common symptom reported, such as dry eyes and xerostomia. Serological analysis showed positivity to rheumatoid factor in most of the cases and elevated positivity to antinuclear antibodies was also observed [8–10]. Oral alterations of SS include salivary gland dysfunction (diminished salivary flow), dental caries, stomatitis, and candidiasis, each of which negatively impacts the quality of life [10]. Saliva plays an important role in maintaining homeostasis in the oral cavity, preventing diseases in the hard and soft tissues [11–13]. Hyposalivation is generally accompanied by rapid progression of caries and the presence of candidiasis, consisting of major worsening of dental health [14, 15].

Therefore, this report describes a rare case of SSS that affected a 12-year-old girl submitted to an orthodontic treatment prior to the diagnosis. The case describes severe

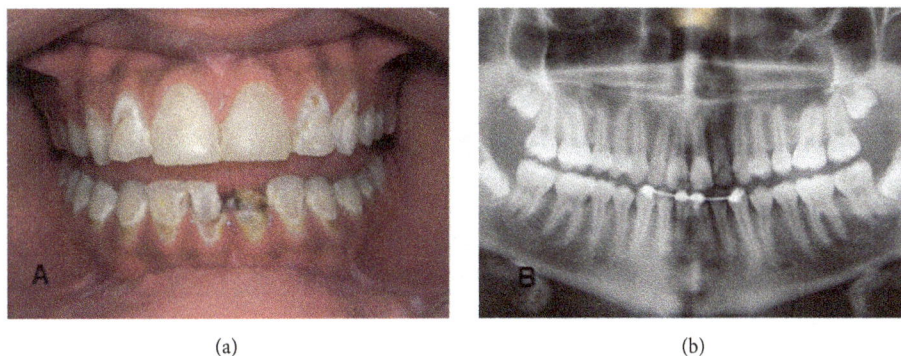

FIGURE 1: (a) The initial clinical appearance demonstrating carious lesions on buccal regions; (b) radiographic examination showing the fixed lingual orthodontic appliance for treatment contention and carious lesions.

tooth destruction with oral rehabilitation and hyposalivation management.

2. Case Report

A 12-year-old female patient was referred to the Pediatric Dentistry Clinic, complaining of dry mouth, tooth sensibility, and dental pain. The patient reported three episodes of parotid gland enlargement. Her medical history included rheumatoid arthritis diagnosed 6 months before consultation. Regarding family history, her mother reported that both she and her sister presented symptoms of autoimmune diseases. In the current case report, the diagnosis of Sjögren's syndrome was confirmed by anti-Ro/anti-La antibodies, magnetic resonance imaging of the parotid and sublingual salivary glands, and also parotid contrast sialography. The patient was monitored by a doctor in regular appointments for the control of Sjögren's syndrome and rheumatoid arthritis and the treatment consisted of corticoid therapy.

An extraoral investigation showed dry lips and no glandular enlargement. During the intraoral exam (Figure 1(a)), extensive caries, gingival inflammation, accumulation of biofilm, poor hygiene, and deficient tooth brushing were observed. The presence of a fixed lingual orthodontic appliance between elements 33 and 43 (Figure 1(b)) was noted. The intraoral examination also confirmed the dryness of the mucous membranes, reduced salivary flow, dry lips, and touch sensitivity response to clinical instruments. Salivary flow, which showed a severely reduced rate at rest (0.05 mL/min), confirmed the findings of the parotid sialography test.

The patient was instructed to use alcohol-free mouthwash and to replace her toothpaste and toothbrush with others with the following characteristics: fluoride toothpaste with low abrasion and a toothbrush with a small head and straight, soft bristles. In order to moisturize the lips, the patient was advised to use cocoa butter lipstick.

It was possible to observe caries lesions in both clinical (Figure 1(a)) and radiographic (Figure 1(b)) images. Elements 31 and 41 received endodontic treatment and restorations with composite resin until the definitive prosthetic rehabilitation. Teeth 13, 12, 11, 21, and 23 presented deficient proximal

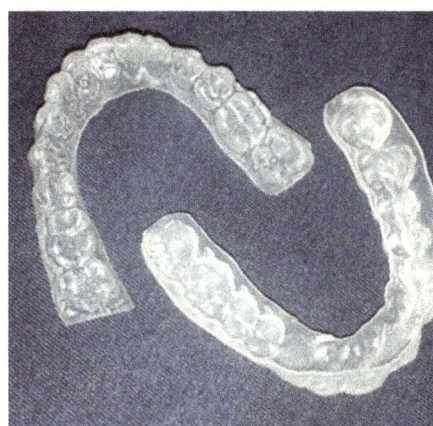

FIGURE 2: Tray for artificial saliva.

restorations and were restored. Premolars and molars 17, 25, 27, and 35 were restored due to caries lesions. Pulp capping was performed on element 37 with glass ionomer cement. The vestibular regions of 12, 13 22, 23, 35, 34, 32, 42, 43, and 44 presented structural loss and were restored. Teeth 46 and 47 received resin-based fissure sealants. Duraphat® fluoride varnish was applied in white spot vestibular lesions. This was effective in remineralizing teeth and controlling hypersensitivity.

To alleviate the xerostomia and manage the hyposalivation, artificial saliva was manipulated. We prepared a tray identical to those used in tooth whitening to be filled with artificial saliva (Figure 2) overnight. This procedure provided better hydration of the tissues of the oral cavity, in particular the oral mucosa, as shown in Figure 3.

3. Discussion

The preexistence of rheumatoid arthritis led to the classification of the patient as a case of SSS. Furthermore, the diagnosis was confirmed based on the most recent guidelines [16, 17]. In addition, the revised rules proposed by the Euro-American Group Consensus Criteria for the Classification of Sjögren's Syndrome were followed [17], which introduced more clearly

(a)

(b)   (c)

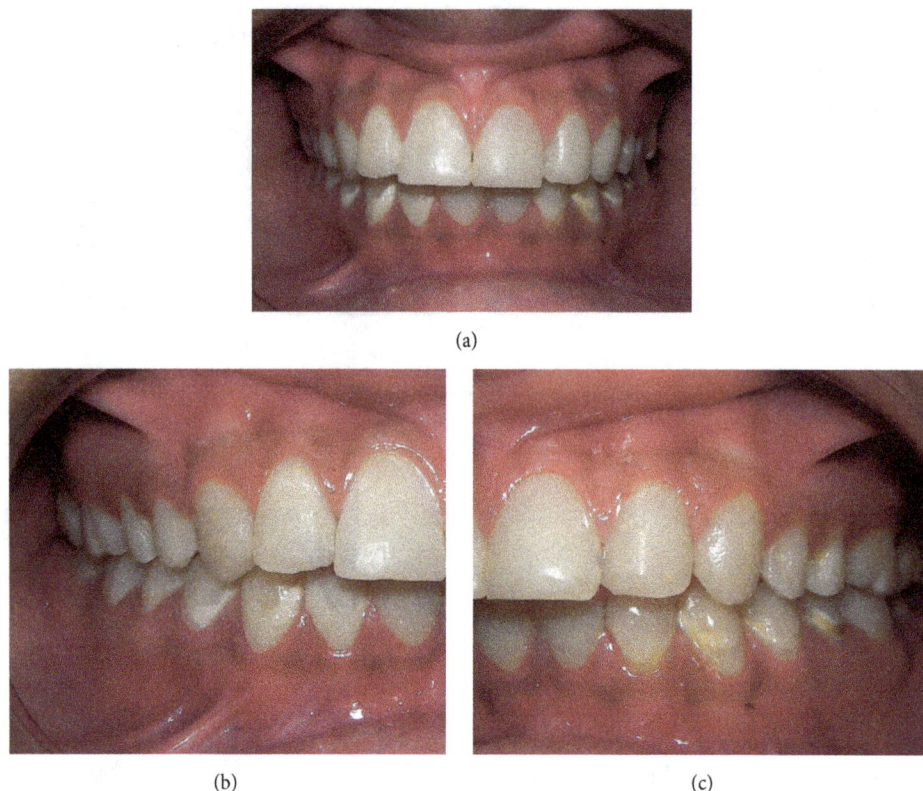

FIGURE 3: The clinical aspect after the restorative treatment (a). (b) and (c) are right and left sides, respectively.

defined rules to classify patients between primary and secondary types.

In the current case report, the patient reported autoimmune diseases in her family history. SSS presents in association with other autoimmune diseases [17]. In primary Sjögren's syndrome, clinical manifestations are limited to exocrine gland dysfunction while the secondary subtype of the disease involves the presence of other autoimmune diseases [18, 19]. Recurrent parotid gland enlargement often shows up as the first symptom of the disease in pediatric cases, followed by xerophthalmia and xerostomia. The occurrence of SSS in children and adolescents is not common and is often undiagnosed due to the limited applicability of the diagnostic criteria in pediatric patients [9, 17–19].

Decreased salivary secretion can lead to major changes in the oral mucosa, difficulty in swallowing and speaking, a sensation of burning in the mouth, and an increase in dental caries, but also to greater susceptibility to developing periodontal diseases [15]. Periodontal alterations were not present in the patient in the case reported here, perhaps due to her young age. The patient's condition was aggravated by poor oral hygiene that, combined with the use of an orthodontic appliance prior to the diagnosis of SSS, facilitated the occurrence of multiple carious lesions, which led to the need for endodontic procedures in several teeth.

The treatment of xerostomia in these patients is basically supportive therapy, with the aim of stimulating saliva production. In treating the oral symptoms of patients with respect to xerostomia, the use of artificial saliva and chewing

gum without sugar is often indicated [20]. Also, the use of pilocarpine, a parasympathomimetic drug with effects similar to acetylcholine, is able to increase the production of secretions from exocrine glands in the body [21, 22]. Pilocarpine is usually used in the treatment of patients with hyposalivation that may occur as a side effect of radiation therapy for the head and neck for the treatment of cancer, but its use should also be indicated in some other special cases [21]. In the current case report, the patient was monitored by a doctor who controlled the disease using corticoid therapy and did not recommend pilocarpine, but an increase of water consumption. Low-level laser therapy has been proven to be an alternative to reducing the xerostomia, pain, and facial edema [23]. Artificial saliva is often used due to its minimal restrictions. Despite the widespread use of artificial saliva to treat hyposalivation and xerostomia [24], there are no alternatives to resolving this diminished flow rate during the night, when it is drastically reduced. Thus, we opted to produce a tray similar to a tooth-whitening tray for the application of artificial saliva for the maintenance of oral hydration, since the clearance of artificial saliva conventionally used as mouth rinse is fast and the tray was able to keep the artificial saliva surrounding the tissues. This alternative method allowed hydrating the hard and soft tissues not only during the day, but also for much of the night for a long time. This method has been proven to be satisfactory and is recommended, since it promotes prolonged contact of the artificial saliva with oral tissues, providing greater patient comfort and aiding in the control of new lesions. The patient was also instructed to brush her teeth with nonabrasive toothpaste and fluoride varnish was applied to white spot vestibular lesions in order to remineralize them and control the hypersensitivity. The inferior first molars received resin-based fissure sealants to prevent dental caries. Additionally, the patient presented a fixed lingual orthodontic appliance that increased the biofilm accumulation and the risk of caries. The contention was removed and the anterior teeth were submitted to restorative treatment. A knowledge of the systemic condition is essential to avoid treatments that bring about more losses than benefits, such as the use of orthodontic appliances. Therefore, dentists must indicate individually the treatments of each patient.

4. Conclusion

The dental therapeutic approach involved the control of caries, periodontal disease, and opportunistic fungal infections, oral hygiene instruction, the use of fluoride-rich solutions, the use of artificial saliva in a tray, and regular follow-up at short intervals. This approach proved to be effective in recovering the oral health and self-confidence and consequently improved the quality of life of the patient.

Competing Interests

The authors declare that there are no competing interests regarding the publication of this paper.

References

[1] B. Qin, J. Wang, Z. Yang et al., "Epidemiology of primary Sjögren's syndrome: a systematic review and meta-analysis," *Annals of the Rheumatic Diseases*, vol. 74, no. 11, pp. 1983–1989, 2015.

[2] C. Salliot, J.-E. Gottenberg, D. Bengoufa, F. Desmoulins, C. Miceli-Richard, and X. Mariette, "Anticentromere antibodies identify patients with Sjögren's syndrome and autoimmune overlap syndrome," *Journal of Rheumatology*, vol. 34, no. 11, pp. 2253–2258, 2007.

[3] O. Meyer, "Evaluating inflammatory joint disease: how and when can autoantibodies help?" *Joint Bone Spine*, vol. 70, no. 6, pp. 433–447, 2003.

[4] R. I. Fox and P. Michelson, "Approaches to the treatment of Sjögren's syndrome," *The Journal of Rheumatology. Supplement*, vol. 61, pp. 15–21, 2000.

[5] M. Ramos-Casals, R. Solans, J. Rosas et al., "Primary Sjögren syndrome in Spain: clinical and immunologic expression in 1010 patients," *Medicine*, vol. 87, no. 4, pp. 210–219, 2008.

[6] L. Michel, F. Toulgoat, H. Desal et al., "Atypical neurologic complications in patients with primary Sjögren's syndrome: report of 4 cases," *Seminars in Arthritis & Rheumatism*, vol. 40, no. 4, pp. 338–342, 2011.

[7] M. Civilibal, N. Canpolat, A. Yurt et al., "A child with primary Sjögren syndrome and a review of the literature," *Clinical Pediatrics*, vol. 46, no. 8, pp. 738–742, 2007.

[8] S. C. Shiboski, C. H. Shiboski, L. A. Criswell et al., "American College of rheumatology classification criteria for Sjögren's syndrome: a data-driven, expert consensus approach in the Sjögren's International Collaborative Clinical Alliance cohort," *Arthritis Care and Research*, vol. 64, no. 4, pp. 475–487, 2012.

[9] S. J. Bowman, "Collaborative research into outcome measures in Sjogren's syndrome. Update on disease assessment," *Acta Rheumatologica Scandinavica. Supplementum*, vol. 116, pp. 23–27, 2002.

[10] T. R. de Souza, I. H. M. Silva, A. T. Carvalho et al., "Juvenile Sjögren syndrome: distinctive age, unique findings," *Pediatric Dentistry*, vol. 34, no. 5, pp. 427–430, 2012.

[11] T. K. S. Fidalgo, L. B. Freitas-Fernandes, F. C. L. Almeida, A. P. Valente, and I. P. R. Souza, "Longitudinal evaluation of salivary profile from children with dental caries before and after treatment," *Metabolomics*, vol. 11, no. 3, pp. 583–593, 2015.

[12] T. K. S. Fidalgo, L. B. Freitas-Fernandes, R. Angeli et al., "Salivary metabolite signatures of children with and without dental caries lesions," *Metabolomics*, vol. 9, no. 3, pp. 657–666, 2013.

[13] T. K. D. S. Fidalgo, L. B. Freitas-Fernandes, M. Ammari, C. T. Mattos, I. P. R. De Souza, and L. C. Maia, "The relationship between unspecific s-IgA and dental caries: a systematic review and meta-analysis," *Journal of Dentistry*, vol. 42, no. 11, pp. 1372–1381, 2014.

[14] A. M. L. Pedersen, A. Bardow, and B. Nauntofte, "Salivary changes and dental caries as potential oral markers of autoimmune salivary gland dysfunction in primary Sjögren's syndrome," *BMC Clinical Pathology*, vol. 5, no. 1, article 4, 2005.

[15] N. Ravald and T. List, "Caries and periodontal conditions in patients with primary Sjögren's syndrome," *Swedish Dental Journal*, vol. 22, no. 3, pp. 97–103, 1998.

[16] H. Locht, R. Pelck, and R. Manthorpe, "Clinical manifestations correlated to the prevalence of autoantibodies in a large ($n = 321$) cohort of patients with primary Sjögren's syndrome: a comparison of patients initially diagnosed according to the Copenhagen classification criteria with the American-European consensus criteria," *Autoimmunity Reviews*, vol. 4, no. 5, pp. 276–281, 2005.

[17] C. Vitali, S. Bombardieri, R. Jonsson et al., "Classification criteria for Sjögren's syndrome: a revised version of the European criteria proposed by the American-European Consensus Group," *Annals of the Rheumatic Diseases*, vol. 61, no. 6, pp. 554–558, 2002.

[18] T. E. Daniels, "Sjögren's syndrome: clinical spectrum and current diagnostic controversies," *Advances in Dental Research*, vol. 10, no. 1, pp. 3–8, 1996.

[19] N. G. Nikitakis, H. Rivera, C. Lariccia, J. C. Papadimitriou, and J. J. Sauk, "Primary Sjögren syndrome in childhood: report of a case and review of the literature," *Oral Surgery, Oral Medicine, Oral Pathology, Oral Radiology, and Endodontics*, vol. 96, no. 1, pp. 42–47, 2003.

[20] A. Pinto, "Management of xerostomia and other complications of Sjögren's syndrome," *Oral and Maxillofacial Surgery Clinics of North America*, vol. 26, no. 1, pp. 63–73, 2014.

[21] M. Ramos-Casals, A. G. Tzioufas, J. H. Stone, A. Sisó, and X. Bosch, "Treatment of primary Sjögren syndrome: a systematic review," *Journal of the American Medical Association*, vol. 304, no. 4, pp. 452–460, 2010.

[22] P. Brito-Zerón, A. Sisó-Almirall, A. Bové, B. A. Kostov, and M. Ramos-Casals, "Primary Sjögren syndrome: an update on current pharmacotherapy options and future directions," *Expert Opinion on Pharmacotherapy*, vol. 14, no. 3, pp. 279–289, 2013.

[23] A. Simões, M. D. Platero, L. Campos, A. C. Aranha, C. De Paula Eduardo, and J. Nicolau, "Laser as a therapy for dry mouth

symptoms in a patient with Sjögren's syndrome: a case report," *Special Care in Dentistry*, vol. 29, no. 3, pp. 134–137, 2009.

[24] F. Dost and C. S. Farah, "Stimulating the discussion on saliva substitutes: a clinical perspective," *Australian Dental Journal*, vol. 58, no. 1, pp. 11–17, 2013.

A Rare Malignant Peripheral Nerve Sheath Tumor of the Maxilla Mimicking a Periapical Lesion

José Alcides Arruda,[1] **Pamella Álvares,**[1] **Luciano Silva,**[1]
Alexandrino Pereira dos Santos Neto,[1] **Cleomar Donizeth Rodrigues,**[2] **Antônio Caubi,**[1]
Marcia Silveira,[1] **Sandra Sayão,**[1] **and Ana Paula Sobral**[1]

[1]*Faculdade de Odontologia de Pernambuco, Universidade de Pernambuco, Avenida General Newton Cavalcante,*
1650 Aldeia dos Camarás, 54.753-020 Camaragibe, PE, Brazil
[2]*Faculdades Integradas da União Educacional do Planalto Central, SIGA Área Especial para Indústria, n° 2, Setor Leste,*
72.445-020, Gama, DG, Brazil

Correspondence should be addressed to José Alcides Arruda; alcides_almeida@hotmail.com

Academic Editor: Evanthia Chrysomali

Malignant peripheral nerve sheath tumor is a malignant neoplasm that is rarely found in the oral cavity. About 50% of this tumor occurs in patients with neurofibromatosis type I and comprises approximately 10% of all soft tissue sarcomas of head and neck region. Intraosseous malignant peripheral nerve sheath tumor of the maxilla is rare. This article is the first to address malignant peripheral nerve sheath tumor of the maxilla presenting as a periapical radiolucency on nonvital endodontically treated teeth in the English medical literature. Surgical approaches to malignant soft tissue tumor vary based on the extent of the disease, age of the patient, and pathological findings. A rare case of intraosseous malignant peripheral nerve sheath tumor is reported in a 16-year-old woman. The patient presented clinically with a pain involving the upper left incisors region and with defined unilocular periapical radiolucency lesion involved between the upper left incisors. An incisional biopsy was made. Histological and immunohistochemical examination were positive for S-100 protein and glial fibrillary acidic protein showed that the lesion was an intraosseous malignant peripheral nerve sheath tumor of the maxilla. Nine years after the surgery, no regional recurrence was observed.

1. Introduction

Malignant peripheral nerve sheath tumor (MPNST) is a malignant neoplasm that is rarely found in the oral cavity. About 50% of this tumor occurs in patients with neurofibromatosis type 1 (NF-1) and comprises approximately 10% of all soft tissue sarcomas of both head and neck region [1]. Its incidence in the oral region is extremely low, roughly 0,001% [2]. Its occurrence in head and neck regions involves soft and hard tissues [3]. However, intraosseous maxillary MPNST presenting as a periapical lesion is exceptionally unusual. This tumor type occurs in peripheral nerves and may exhibit differentiation in nerve sheath elements such as Schwann cells and perineural cells, as well as fibroblasts [1]. The differential diagnosis of this neoplasm may be facilitated by additional information obtained from immunohistochemistry findings [2].

This article reports the unusual clinical case of intraosseous MPNST with no association with NF-1, presenting as a periapical lesion on nonvital endodontically treated teeth.

2. Case Presentation

A 16-year-old female was referred with pain involving the upper left incisors region. Patient history revealed endodontic treatment of the maxillary upper left incisors with necrotic pulp and periapical radiolucency six months earlier. A few months after the treatment, she experienced discomfort pain. Extraoral examination revealed an integrate mucosa with normal appearance, whereas, intraorally, the upper left lateral incisor presented chromatic alterations and mobility in the region. A periapical radiograph showed the presence of a defined radiolucency lesion between the upper left incisors of the endodontically treated teeth with a size of 2.5 × 1.0 cm in a high diameter (Figure 1). An incisional biopsy was made using local anesthesia and sent to the Oral Pathology Laboratory. The specimen was fixed in 10% neutral formalin and routinely prepared for light microscopy; the sections were stained with hematoxylin and eosin. Histological examination showed malignant neoplasm fragments consisting of fusiform cells with comma-shaped nuclei, originating from cell bundles exhibiting one of two forms: a round shape with large nuclei (occasionally palisading) or hyalinized strands and/or islets (Figures 2(a) and 2(b)). Immunohistochemistry analysis was performed using streptavidin-biotin technique with monoclonal antibodies; the cells were positive for both the S-100 protein and the glial fibrillary acidic protein (GFAP) (Figures 2(c) and 2(d)). The immunohistochemical expression of protein S-100 was weak at less than 50% of the tumor cells (Figure 2(c)), and a diagnosis of MPNST of the maxilla was made. The patient was referred to the Oncology Department and was subjected to surgical excision of the upper left lateral incisor as well as the total removal of the remaining lesion and adjuvant chemotherapy. The examination of the surgical part had not exhibited banks committed and it was staged as low grade of malignancy. The research of metastasis through the exams for images revealed no secondary tumors. The conduct of not using radiotherapy was a decision of the Clinical Oncology team. The patient was rehabilitated with an adhesive prosthesis in the region of the removal tooth (Figure 3). In the last exam, cone beam computerized tomography (CBCT) imaging examination revealed the absence of the upper left lateral incisor, a loss of bone matter, and the absence of vestibular and lingual cortices in the inferior and central thirds of the alveolar ridge (vide reconstructions: panoramic in Figure 3(a) and axial in Figure 3(b)). The tomography revealed normal trabeculation of adjacent bone tissue and preservation of the upper third of the alveolar ridge. The upper left central incisor exhibited a filled canal and a hypodense periapical area, suggestive of an inflammatory periapical lesion or a bone repair lesion after endodontic treatment. The absence of alveolar lamina dura and the loss of radicular matter in the mesiobuccal face were consistent with external root resorption and/or surgical resection (vide reconstructions: coronal in Figure 3(c) and upper left lateral incisor tooth in Figure 3(d) (sagittal)). The patient was tumor-free at the nine-year follow-up consultation.

3. Discussion

This paper describes an unusual case of intraosseous maxillary MPNST mimicking a periapical lesion in order to call attention of clinicians to the fact that several different diseases are able to mimic endodontic periapical lesions. The available literature shows that there are no reports of this tumor presenting as periapical lesion in the upper left incisors. It also shows the complexity of a diagnosis of rare bone

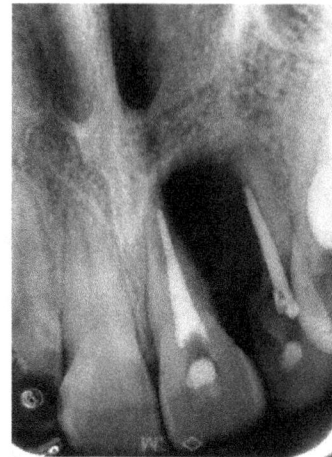

FIGURE 1: Periapical radiograph showing radiopaque image of the roots of teeth 21 and 22, which are compatible with root canal filling material, obtained from a radiolucent image of the blurred boundaries in the region of the upper incisors.

tumors when based on clinical and radiographic features only. Besides, MPNST onset occurs in a peripheral nerve that may exhibit differentiation of nerve sheath elements, which is more common in the proximal extremities and stem of the nerve [4]. Although uncommon, occurrence in cranial nerves usually targets the fiftieth cranial nerve pair [1].

Patient history, clinical examinations, pulp sensitivity tests, and endodontic treatment follow-up are essential for the diagnosis of inflammatory periapical lesions. The presence of periapical images and dental resorption are characteristic of endodontic and/or odontogenic origin lesions. Soft tissue tumor diagnoses are extremely difficult, and diagnosis of MPNST is particularly difficult because it lacks diagnostic criteria. Although no consensus exists regarding the classification of sarcomas as a type of MPNST, the reported lesion could be placed in this category because its onset occurred in a peripheral nerve or neurofibroma, and it fulfilled one of the three established diagnosis criteria, which include (1) the tumor originating in a peripheral nerve that does not exhibit lines of aberrant or heterologous differentiation; (2) the tumor originating from a preexisting benign nerve sheath tumor, usually a neurofibroma; or (3) the tumor exhibiting characteristics that are commonly observed in tumors originating from the aforementioned situations or malignant Schwann cell tumors [2, 3]. The present case fulfills the diagnostic criterion of MPNST onset occurring in a peripheral nerve.

Despite imaging features of MPNST being nonspecific and noncharacteristic, the role of radiologic diagnosis is to ensure that MPNST are preoperatively suggested as a diagnosis and are differentiated from malignant lesions through a series of specific imaging findings. It is important to highlight the aggressiveness of the lesion by a radiographic examination, once it is required to analyze bone destruction, extra bone invasion, structure of the lesion, and root resorption [5].

Radiographic findings of intraosseous MPNST may show a great variation, from unilocular to multilocular, with or

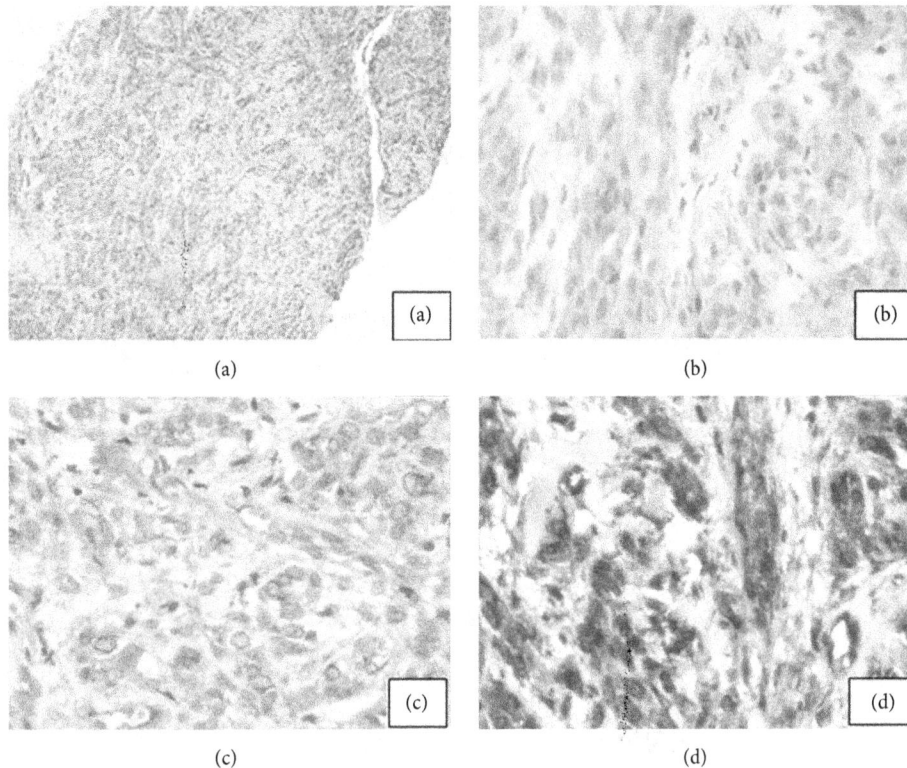

FIGURE 2: (a) Cell bundle arrangements with rounded, large nuclei that sometimes contain palisades, strands, and/or hyalinized islands. Hematoxylin and eosin (HE) staining, 40x. (b) Spindle cells with comma-shaped nuclei. HE staining, 100x. (c) Cells positive for S-100 protein. IHC, 200x. (d) Cells positive for glial fibrillary acidic protein (GFAP). IHC, 200x.

without well-defined borders of the lesion, and cortical expansion. Periapical radiographs of the presenting case of intraosseous MPNST showed a unilocular periapical lesion with a defined border and external dental resorption in the lateral region and apical region of upper left incisors. This radiographic appearance was suggestive of a periapical lesion of cyst, once external root resorption does not occur exclusively of malignancies, as what may occur for orthodontic movement, neoplasia, being more common in case of inflammatory origin, such as periapical lesion [5].

Establishing a diagnosis requires immunohistochemistry technique because MPNST may be similar to fibrosarcoma. And a plethora of other bone tumors are included in differential diagnoses such as central giant cell lesion, fibrous dysplasia, ameloblastoma, myxoma, haemangioma, neurofibroma, leiomyoma, sarcoma, or simply periapical lesions [1]. It is also essential to include S-100 protein for suspected neural tumors, since it is positive in all neural tumors [6]. And the use of GFAP refers to filament proteins type III intermediate and it is the essential component of the cytoskeleton in astrocytes of all vertebrates [7]. However, the latter exhibits irregularly shaped cells. These tumors also exhibit characteristics such as regular Schwann cells, with dense and hypodense fascicles creating a marbleized effect and myxoid areas; elongated, asymmetric cone-shaped cells with irregular, palisading, and comma- or buckle-shaped nuclei; spiral structures; peculiar hyperplastic perivascular

alterations; and, occasionally, heterologous elements (cartilage, bone, and muscle, which are present in 10–15% of tumors). These tumors may exhibit a greater degree of cellular differentiation, pleomorphism, and mitotic activity [3].

Malignant peripheral nerve sheath tumors were most commonly located on the extremities (45%), then trunk (34%), and head and neck region (19%) [8]. In head and neck region, they occur most frequently in both nasopharynx and the nasal cavity [9]. The absence of such reports confirms the difficulty of performing differential diagnoses of periapical pathologies because tumors can mimic an inflammatory periapical lesion. The recommended treatment option for MPNST is surgical excision. However, it is a difficult procedure due to poor anatomical accessibility and its probability of recurrence varies approximately between 40 and 65% in head and neck region and approximately between 40 and 68% elsewhere [4]. Surgical approaches to malignant soft tissue tumor vary based on the extent of the disease, age of the patient, and pathological findings. Yet, surgical excision with wide margins is the first treatment choice for the majority of patients. Radiation and/or chemotherapy may also be used due to the high recurrence rates or in the case of an incomplete lesion excision. Adjuvant radiation and/or chemotherapy treatment must always be considered and guided by the clinical stage [10, 11]. Nonetheless, in the case reported, the patient opted for surgical excision in conjunction with chemotherapy. The patient responded well

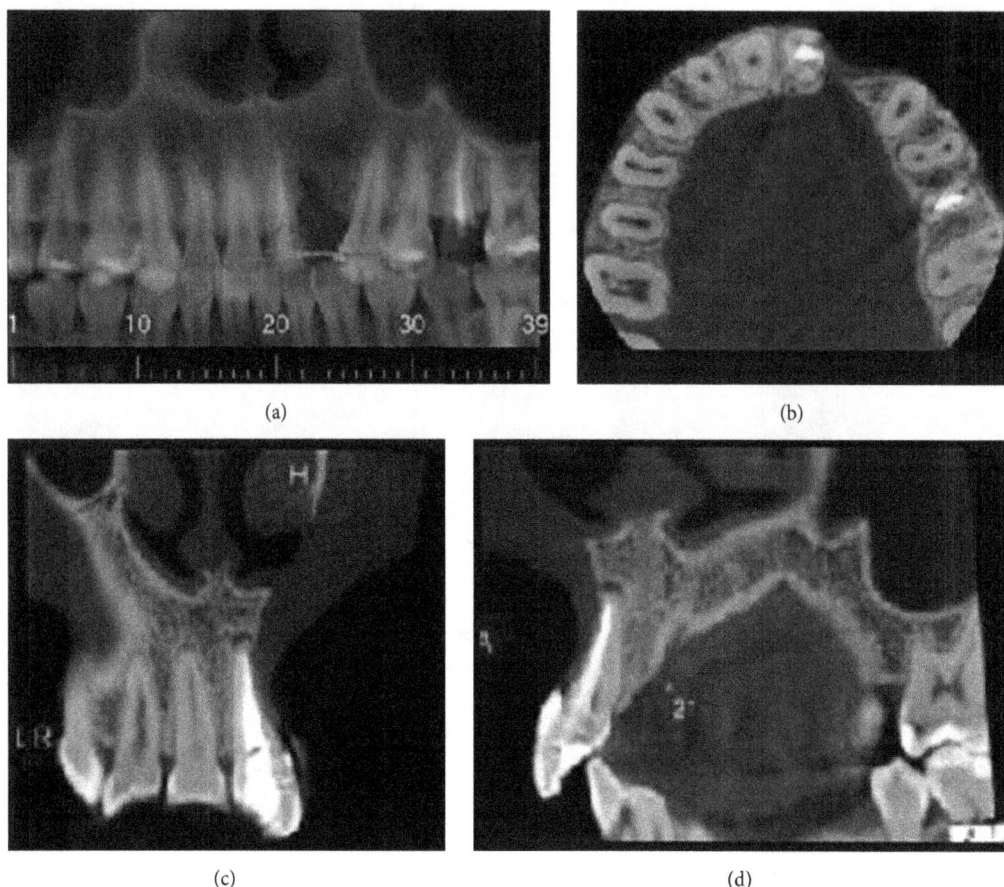

(a)

(b)

(c)

(d)

FIGURE 3: (a) CT panoramic reconstruction of maxilla. (b) CT axial reconstruction of the jaw. (c) CT coronal reconstruction of anterior region of maxilla. (d) CT sagittal reconstruction of tooth 11 region.

to the treatment and was disease-free at the nine-year control follow-up evaluation.

To establish the diagnoses of MPNST, it requires immunohistochemistry technique. Radiographically, maxillary intraosseous MPNST is difficult to differentiate from other bone lesions. The differential diagnosis of the case presented in this article included periapical inflammatory lesions, such as periapical granuloma or cyst. The root resorption is not a usual finding of the above lesions. Root resorption can be seen in central giant cell granuloma or an odontogenic neoplasm such as ameloblastoma or in malignant tumors. Nine years after the surgery, no regional recurrence was observed.

Competing Interests

The authors declare that there is no conflict of interests regarding the publication of this paper.

References

[1] I.-M. Schaefer and C. D. M. Fletcher, "Malignant peripheral nerve sheath tumor (MPNST) arising in diffuse-type neurofibroma: clinicopathologic characterization in a series of 9 cases,"

The American Journal of Surgical Pathology, vol. 39, no. 9, pp. 1234–1241, 2015.

[2] C. Zou, K. D. Smith, J. Liu et al., "Clinical, pathological, and molecular variables predictive of malignant peripheral nerve sheath tumor outcome," *Annals of Surgery*, vol. 249, no. 6, pp. 1014–1022, 2009.

[3] J. M. Baehring, R. A. Betensky, and T. T. Batchelor, "Malignant peripheral nerve sheath tumor: the clinical spectrum and outcome of treatment," *Neurology*, vol. 61, no. 5, pp. 696–698, 2003.

[4] W. V. B. S. Ramalingam, S. Nair, and G. Mandal, "Malignant peripheral nerve sheath tumor of the oral cavity," *Journal of Oral and Maxillofacial Surgery*, vol. 70, no. 10, pp. e581–e585, 2012.

[5] A. Consolaro and L. Z. Furquim, "Extreme root resorption associated with induced tooth movement: a protocol for clinical management," *Dental Press Journal of Orthodontics*, vol. 19, no. 5, pp. 19–26, 2014.

[6] E. Chrysomali, S. I. Papanicolaou, N. P. Dekker, and J. A. Regezi, "Benign neural tumors of the oral cavity: a comparative immunohistochemical study," *Oral Surgery, Oral Medicine, Oral Pathology, Oral Radiology, and Endodontics*, vol. 84, no. 4, pp. 381–390, 1997.

[7] E. G. Sukhorukova, D. É. Kruzhevskiĭ, and O. S. Alekseeva, "Glial fibrillary acidic protein: the component of intermediate

filaments in the vertebrate brain astrocytes," *Zhurnal Evoliut-sionnoĭ Biokhimii i Fiziologii*, vol. 51, no. 1, pp. 3–10, 2015.

[8] A. N. Meshikhes, M. A. Duhaileb, and S. S. Amr, "Malignant peripheral nerve sheath tumor with extensive osteosarcomatous and chondrosarcomatous differentiation: a case report," *International Journal of Surgery Case Reports*, vol. 25, pp. 188–191, 2016.

[9] C.-C. H. Stucky, K. N. Johnson, R. J. Gray et al., "Malignant peripheral nerve sheath tumors (MPNST): the Mayo Clinic experience," *Annals of Surgical Oncology*, vol. 19, no. 3, pp. 878–885, 2012.

[10] M. Kar, S. V. Deo, N. K. Shukla et al., "Malignant peripheral nerve sheath tumors (MPNST)—clinicopathological study and treatment outcome of twenty-four cases," *World Journal of Surgical Oncology*, vol. 4, article 55, 2006.

[11] A. Ziadi and I. Saliba, "Malignant peripheral nerve sheath tumor of intracranial nerve: a case series review," *Auris Nasus Larynx*, vol. 37, no. 5, pp. 539–545, 2010.

10

Esthetic Rehabilitation of Anterior Teeth with Copy-Milled Restorations: A Report of Two Cases

Sapna Rani,[1] **Jyoti Devi,**[2] **Chandan Jain,**[2] **Parul Mutneja,**[2] **and Mahesh Verma**[2]

[1]*Department of Prosthodontics, ITS Dental College, Ghaziabad, India*
[2]*Department of Prosthodontics, MAIDS, Delhi, India*

Correspondence should be addressed to Sapna Rani; drsapnadaksh@gmail.com

Academic Editor: Mine Dündar

Digitalization has become part and parcel of contemporary prosthodontics with the probability of most of the procedures being based on the digital techniques in the near future. This digital revolution started in the latter half of the 20th century by converting analog objects/signals into digital bits and bytes. Recent developments in all-ceramic materials and systems of computer-aided designing and computer-aided manufacturing (CAD/CAM), copy milling, and so forth offer excellent esthetics and superb biocompatibility. Copy milling system for ceramics enables milling of the zirconia cores of all-ceramic restorations precisely and also if this system is properly used the procedure for fabricating all-ceramic restorations can be substantially simplified. This case report presents fabrication of all-ceramic Maryland Bridge and post-core with a copy milling system for esthetics and preservation of integrity of tooth. For both of the patients, the use of biologic, all-ceramic, copy-milled restorations resulted in clinical success and recovered function and esthetics.

1. Introduction

Digitization has become an integral part and parcel of contemporary dentistry. New era has shifted to digital dentistry at each step beginning from patient education till final restoration. Initially, an impression was thought to be made of either alginate or rubber base impression material but introduction of computer and laser technology has enabled capture of digital impressions [1]. The digital dentistry provides endless treatment options with enhanced approach, minimum time, and reduced chances of error [2]. Early 1980s paved the way for computer-aided design/computer-aided manufacturing (CAD/CAM) technology. The advantages of this technology are decreasing laboratory work, automation by machine, and production of similar multiple restorations while the disadvantages include technique sensitivity and expensive unit. To overcome disadvantages copy milling was introduced due to its economic set-up and reduced human error [3, 4].

In past time CAD/CAM and copy milling were supposed to be the same but this is not true. CAD/CAM stands for computer-aided designing and computer-aided milling while copy milling is manually designed and computer machined restorations. The information for CAM phase comes from scanning wax/composite coping or framework. Besides the lower cost factor for these types of milling machines, this method of milling allows the dental technician to correct any discrepancies found in the tooth preparation by compensating during waxing of the pattern.

Copy milling is based on pantographic principle that is used to duplicate keys at hardware shops. Using exact mechanical-tactile model surveying and analogous milling [5], it is considered to be highly precise. First, a coping or framework is manually fabricated in wax or composite, and then the pattern is placed into the pantographic machine. The copying arm of the machine traces the wax pattern while the cutting arm, which has a carbide cutter, mills a selected presintered zirconia block. The final shape is 20% to 25% larger to account for shrinkage during the sintering step. The zirconia block has a density barcode label, so the copy mill machine can be adjusted properly to allow for shrinkage during the sintering phase. With the proper use of this system, the procedure for fabricating restorations can be substantially simplified. The simplicity of use of copy milling system, in comparison with complicated software in CAD/CAM technology, makes it a common system for laboratory applications [4]. Zirconia has been widely used as a biomaterial by CAD/CAM technology and also copy milling technique.

Zirconia as a biomaterial was introduced in 1998; yttrium-oxide is added to zirconia in order to stabilize the tetragonal form at room temperature. In today's generation, excellent esthetics and biocompatibility of yttria oxide zirconia based all-ceramic material meet all demands of an ideal prosthetic and restorative material. Yttrium stabilized zirconia has high flexural strength and fracture toughness. Yttrium-oxide partially stabilized zirconia (Y-TZP) has adequate chemical and dimensional stability and its radiopacity makes it easier to distinguish marginal integrity and caries [6]. Due to absence of metal, finishing line at the level of gingiva provides optimal esthetics. In 1990s first copy milling system came into the market, that is, Celay/Cerec, but later on different CAD/CAM systems developed their copy milling units.

Patients not only are becoming more demanding with regard to esthetics but also are often opting for more conservative and less invasive procedures (i.e., more tooth preservation). Successful restoration of dentition depends on three fundamental principles: mechanical preparation to achieve retention and resistance, hence ensuring longevity; aesthetic factors such as minimizing the appearance of margins and display of metal; and the biological consequences of achieving the first two factors which concern the health and ultimate durability of the tooth and periodontium.

The purpose of this clinical report is to present functional and esthetic restoration techniques through the use of copy milling all-ceramic restorations to meet biologic and functional requirements of patients.

2. Case Reports

2.1. Case 1. A young male patient reported to the Department of Prosthodontics with missing left central incisor (Figure 1(A)). On intraoral examination, wear facets were present on the teeth due to the habit of using abrasive tooth powder for brushing. Treatment options available for the patient were porcelain fused to metal (PFM) fixed dental prosthesis (FDP), all-ceramic FDP, and PFM or zirconia Maryland Bridge or implant placement followed by PFM or all-ceramic crown. Although overjet and overbite were not ideal for fabrication of Maryland Bridge, patient insisted on a conservative option which would require lesser amount of tooth preparation. He was unwilling to go for implant therapy because of financial constraints. After taking consent from the patient, rehabilitation of central incisor was planned with all-ceramic copy-milled zirconia Maryland Bridge framework and porcelain layering with a compatible ceramic.

Procedure. Tooth preparation was done on right central incisor and left lateral incisor for Maryland Bridge. 1 mm of incisal enamel was left intact and light chamfer finish line was given 1 mm supragingivally. To provide mechanical retention form for the lingual wings, a box preparation was made on the lingual and interproximally leaving buccal line area contact. It was assessed that the occlusal clearance was minimal, so

the desired area was then reduced by 0.5 mm with butt-joint cavosurface walls.

Elastomeric single step impression was made using putty and light body silicone (Aquasil, Dentsply) and model was poured in die stone (Ultrarock, Kalabhai). Separating media were applied on the prepared tooth surfaces and pontic area. First wings of the framework were fabricated using pattern resin (GC Corp., Tokyo, Japan) and then pontic area was built up in increments using a small painting brush to give a desired shape and 2 mm of gingival clearance.

After framework has gained initial strength it was carefully retrieved from the model and the pattern was attached with sprue wax (Cercon Wax, Dentsply, Germany) to the respective holder (Figure 1(B)). Later whole assembly was sprayed with scan spray (Cercon, Dentsply, Germany) for copy milling (Figure 1(C)). After milling, zirconia Maryland Bridge framework was separated from blank with straight fissure bur and sintered in Cercon furnace at 1350°C for 6 hours (Cercon Heat, Dentsply, Germany).

Fit of the framework was checked with occlusal spray (Okklean, DFS) and clearance with the opposing arch was assessed. The pontic was then veneered on the labial and incisal surfaces with zirconia Layering Ceramic (Degudent, Dentsply) to give a life-like appearance (Figures 1(D) and 1(E)). After necessary occlusal adjustments, pretreatment of zirconia framework was done with 40 μm alumina, dried with alcohol, and teeth were treated with 37% orthophosphoric acid for 30 sec. Zirconia Maryland Bridge was cemented with adhesive cement (RelyX Unicem; 3M ESPE, St. Paul, Minn) according to manufacturer's instructions. Extra cement was removed with explorer and final restoration was found to have good esthetic and functional value.

2.2. Case 2. A 29-year-old male patient reported to the Department for Rehabilitation of right central incisor. On examination it was found that central incisor was endodontically treated and crown was dislodged (Figure 2(A)). Treatment options available for the patient were metal post and core supported by porcelain fused to metal crown, all-ceramic post with core build-up, and all-ceramic crown and completely milled all-ceramic post-core as one unit supported by all-ceramic crown. After consent from the patient, rehabilitation of central incisor was planned using copy-milled zirconia post and core supported by zirconia based all-ceramic FDP.

Procedure. Post space was prepared in the conventional manner [7], assuring that the pulpal axial line angle was rounded and not sharp. Small diameter autopolymerizing acrylic resin (DPI RR Cold Cure, Dental Products, India) dowel was fabricated to make impression of post space. Vaseline was applied in the post space with paper points so that dowel could be relined with pattern resin (GC Corp., Tokyo, Japan) and core build-up was done with the same pattern resin. Pattern was assessed so that there were no sharp angles internally or externally. The pattern was attached with sprue wax (Cercon Wax, Dentsply) to the respective holder (Figure 2(B)) and sprayed with scan spray (Cercon, Dentsply, Germany) for scanning for copy milling. After milling, zirconia post and core was separated from blank with straight fissure bur and

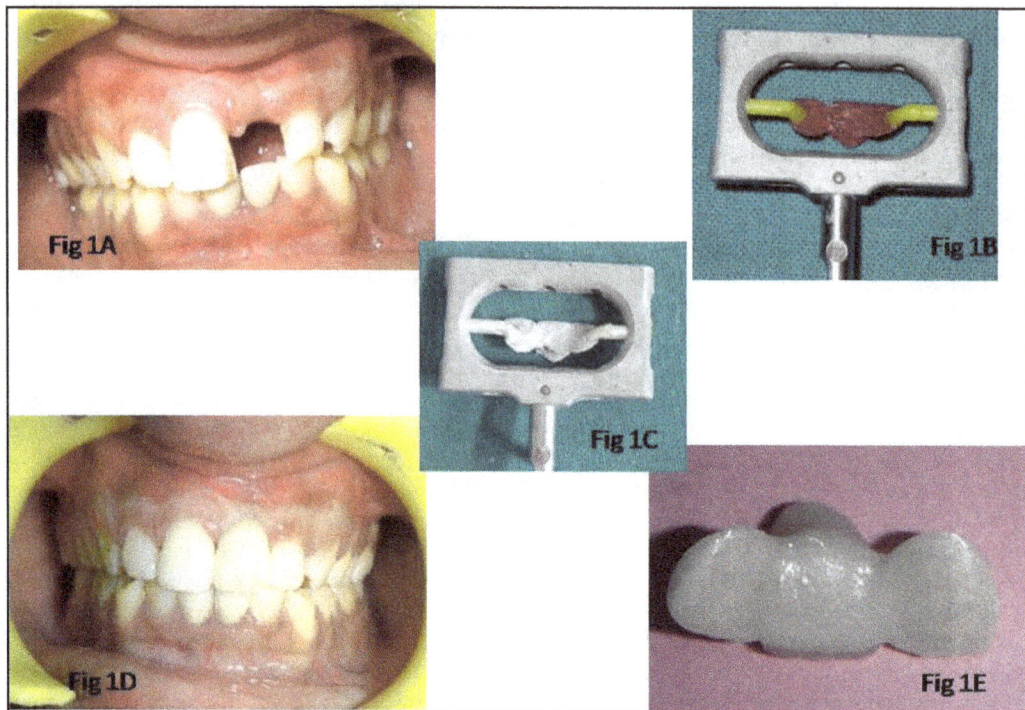

FIGURE 1: Missing central incisor restored with copy-milled all-ceramic Maryland Bridge. (A) Preoperative photograph showing missing left central incisor. (B) Pattern resin attached to scan holder. (C) Scan spray on pattern resin. (D) Maryland Bridge cemented. (E) Maryland Bridge framework veneered with ceramic.

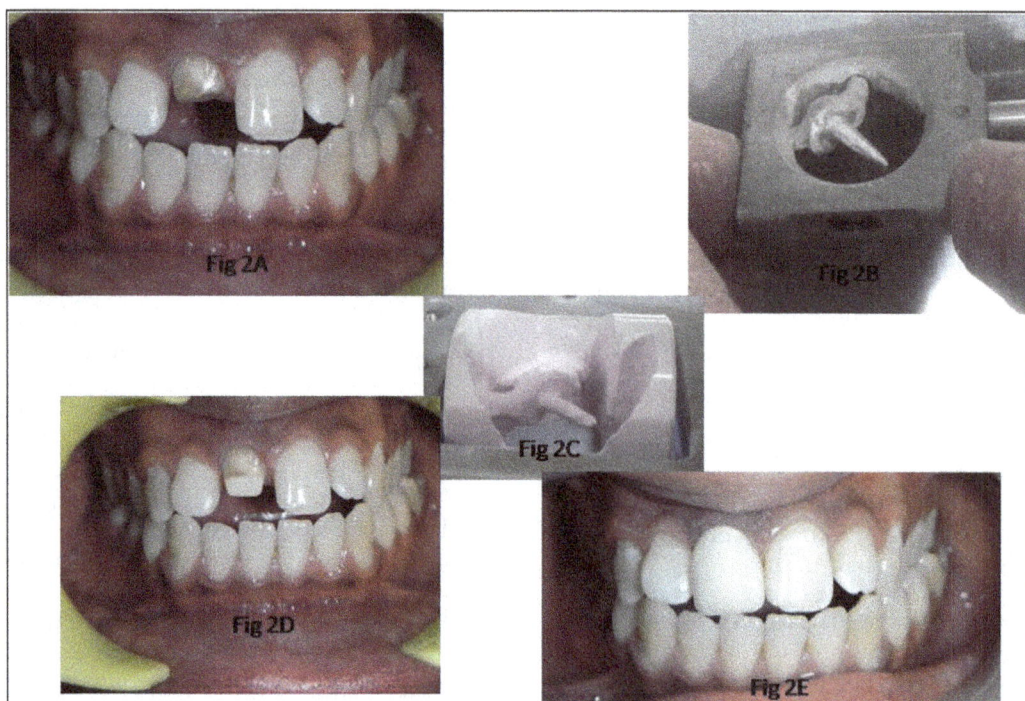

FIGURE 2: Fractured central incisor restored with copy-milled all-ceramic post and core. (A) Preoperative photograph showing fractured right central incisor. (B) Pattern attached to scan holder. (C) Zirconia framework after milling. (D) Zirconia framework cemented to central incisor. (E) All-ceramic fixed restoration.

sintered in Cercon furnace (Figure 2(C)). Fit of post and core was checked with occlusal spray (Okklean, DFS) and seated completely in the canal space. Post-core was cemented with adhesive cement (RelyX Unicem; 3M ESPE, St. Paul, Minn) according to manufacturer instructions (Figure 2(D)); margins of the preparation were refined for central incisor as necessary for all-ceramic restorations. A two-step putty wash polyvinylsiloxane impression of the prepared tooth was made and poured in type IV gypsum. The die was scanned in Cercon eye and zirconia coping was milled from Y-TZP machinable zirconia block and sintered. The milled unit was then veneered on the labial, incisal, and palatal surfaces with ceramic to give a life-like appearance. Zirconia all-ceramic full-coverage FDP (Cercon, Dentsply) was cemented with adhesive cement (RelyX Unicem; 3M ESPE, St. Paul, Minn) (Figure 2(E)). Extra cement was removed with scalpel and all exposed margins were finished. Final restoration was evaluated clinically and radiographically and appeared to give good esthetic and functional value.

3. Discussion

Contemporary dental practice provides endless options for preservation of oral health and for attaining natural esthetics. Digitization has influenced the dental fraternity with the use of computers and scanning methods which has reduced the time for fabrication of restoration. The burnout oven and casting machine have been replaced by model scanning and milling machines.

It is a conflicting topic of discussion that copy milling is at an edge over CAD/CAM. Some literature evaluated that copy milling all-ceramic restorations provided less marginal adaptation as compared to CAD/CAM restorations [8]; however others analyzed that copy milling system may produce more accurate zirconia restorations [9]. Copy-milled restorations in both cases showed good marginal adaptation. In the present case report stabilized zirconia is used for copy milling because of its properties and high survival rate. In dentistry, highest fracture toughness, a high Weibull modulus, and considerable flexural strength (900 Mpa to 1200 Mpa) and great esthetics have made zirconia ceramics a promising material for anterior as well as posterior restorations [10].

Cercon system was used to copy mill restorations in presented case reports and partially sintered zirconia blocks are used in this system. There is less wear of milling instruments in this system as compared to milling of sintered blocks which further minimizes chances of error due to wear of milling burs. Industrially fabricated zirconia blocks lead to increased fracture strength as compared to other ceramics if the shear component of the total load is substantial, as is typically found with anterior teeth. Stabilized zirconia had been chosen for the restoration keeping in mind wear pattern of patients existing dentition which directs the need for stronger material for restoration.

A missing tooth in anterior region is not only a physical loss but also an emotional deprivation for the patient. Restoring a single missing anterior tooth has been a challenge for the dentist as various aspects need to be considered (shade, morphology, gingival contours, and occlusion) [11]. Fixed

dental prosthesis may be an aggressive treatment plan when involving tooth preparation of adjacent abutments. Implant therapy is an expensive treatment option and moreover presence of wear facets on dentition is not indicated for implant therapy. The implication of Maryland Bridge prosthesis for the above-mentioned patient with proper treatment plan can serve as a shelter from ill effects related to edentulous space and invasive replacement procedures like fixed dental prosthesis and implants. Metal reinforced Maryland Bridge complicates shade matching because of the shade change that generally occurs on the abutments at cementation due to the cast-metal lingual retainers that impart a gray appearance in the incisal third. The technique described in this article had the advantages of good color match and reduced chances of debonding due to use of adhesive technique. It also allows preservation of tooth structure and makes periodontal assessment easier [12].

The choice of an appropriate restoration for fractured anterior tooth is guided by strength and esthetics. Zirconia copy-milled post and core was chosen for the presented patient as one-piece milled zirconia post and core showed sufficient mean load to failure values for anterior restorations [13]. High elastic modulus makes them less likely to fail adhesively during mastication and permits a more conservative root canal preparation, decreasing the chances of root fracture [14]. Problems encountered in the fabrication of post and core was attachment of sprue to the wax pattern and nonpassive fit of the one-piece milled zirconia post and cores. Nonpassive fit was due to zirconia particles attached to dowel part as scan spray powder particles are also scanned along with the post and core wax pattern and milled from block which requires trimming of post and core to fit in canal space.

4. Clinical Significance

Clinician decision should be based on available materials and patient's demands. Copy-milled restorations are a viable treatment option especially when meeting esthetic need of patient.

Competing Interests

The authors declare that they have no competing interests.

References

[1] M. Singh, M. Mohan, S. Choudhary, and R. Mittal, "Digitization in prosthodontics," *International Journal of Dental And Health Sciences*, vol. 1, no. 2, pp. 208–219, 2014.

[2] A. Moritz, *Oral Laser Application*, Quintessence, Chicago, Ill, USA, 2006.

[3] G. Davidowitz and P. G. Kotick, "The use of CAD/CAM in dentistry," *Dental Clinics of North America*, vol. 55, no. 3, pp. 559–570, 2011.

[4] M. Karl, F. Graef, M. Wichmann, and T. Krafft, "Passivity of fit of CAD/CAM and copy-milled frameworks, veneered frameworks, and anatomically contoured, zirconia ceramic, implant-supported fixed prostheses," *Journal of Prosthetic Dentistry*, vol. 107, no. 4, pp. 232–238, 2012.

[5] A. Reichert, D. Herkommer, and W. Müller, "Copy milling of zirconia," *Spectrum Dialogue*, vol. 60, pp. 40–56, 2007.

[6] M. Zahran, O. El-Mowafy, L. Tam, P. A. Watson, and Y. Finer, "Fracture strength and fatigue resistance of all-ceramic molar crowns manufactured with CAD/CAM technology," *Journal of Prosthodontics*, vol. 17, no. 5, pp. 370–377, 2008.

[7] S. Rani, J. Devi, and S. Gupta, "Innovative approach of rehabilitation of fractured anterior tooth with copy milled post and core," *International Journal of Dental Research*, vol. 6, no. 3, pp. 52–57, 2016.

[8] A. Alhavaz and L. Jamshidy, "Comparison of the marginal gap of zirconia-fabricated copings generated by CAD/CAM and Copy-Milling methods," *Dental Hypotheses*, vol. 6, no. 1, pp. 23–26, 2015.

[9] J. H. Park, T. K. Kwon, J. H. Yang et al., "A comparative study on the marginal fit of zirconia cores manufactured by CAD/CAM and copy milling methods," *Dentistry*, vol. 3, no. 2, pp. 1–4, 2012.

[10] M. Dayalan, A. Jairaj, K. R. Nagaraj, and R. C. Savadi, "An evaluation of fracture strength of zirconium oxide posts fabricated using CAD-CAM technology compared with prefabricated glass fibre posts," *Journal of Indian Prosthodontist Society*, vol. 10, no. 4, pp. 213–218, 2010.

[11] J. Jaiswal, F. N. Samadi, A. Sharma, and S. Saha, "Maryland Bridge: an interim prosthesis for tooth replacement- a case report," *Jounral Of Dentofacial Sciences*, vol. 2, no. 1, pp. 31–34, 2013.

[12] M. C. Thompson, K. M. Thompson, and M. Swain, "The all-ceramic, inlay supported fixed partial denture. Part 1. Ceramic inlay preparation design: a literature review," *Australian Dental Journal*, vol. 55, no. 2, pp. 120–127, 2010.

[13] F. T. Dilmener, C. Sipahi, and M. Dalkiz, "Resistance of three new esthetic post-and-core systems to compressive loading," *Journal of Prosthetic Dentistry*, vol. 95, no. 2, pp. 130–136, 2006.

[14] G. Freedman, G. Glassman, and K. Serota, "Endoesthetics. Part 1: intra-radicular rehabilitation," *Ontario dentist*, vol. 69, no. 9, pp. 28–31, 1992.

11

Minimally Invasive Laminate Veneers: Clinical Aspects in Treatment Planning and Cementation Procedures

R. K. Morita,[1] **M. F. Hayashida,**[2] **Y. M. Pupo,**[3] **G. Berger,**[3]
R. D. Reggiani,[4] **and E. A. G. Betiol**[3]

[1]*Graduate Pontifical Catholic University of Parana, Curitiba, PR, Brazil*
[2]*Department of Dentistry, School of Dentistry, University Tuiuti of Parana, Curitiba, PR, Brazil*
[3]*Department of Restorative Dentistry, Federal University of Parana, Curitiba, PR, Brazil*
[4]*Graduate Federal University of Parana, Curitiba, PR, Brazil*

Correspondence should be addressed to Y. M. Pupo; yasminemendes@hotmail.com

Academic Editor: Mine Dündar

When a definitive aesthetic treatment is determined, it is crucial to grant the patient's wish with the necessary dental treatment. Thus, conservative treatments that are the solution to aesthetic problems involving morphologic modifications and provide the result that the patient expects should always be the first therapeutic option. In this context, ceramic laminate veneers, also known as "contact lens," are capable of providing an extremely faithful reproduction of the natural teeth with great color stability and periodontal biocompatibility. Minimal or no preparation veneers are heavily advertised as the answer to our patients' cosmetic needs, which they can be if they are used correctly in the appropriate case. This report is about ultraconservative restorations to achieve functional and aesthetic rehabilitation through treatment planning. Thus, clinicians should be aware that the preparation for laminate veneers remains within enamel, to ensure the bond strength and avoid or minimize the occurrence of postoperative sensitivity.

1. Introduction

One of patients' greatest desires when seeking dental treatment is the aesthetic transformation of their smiles to include healthy and harmonious dentition. Because of this, conservative treatments that are able to modify the shape, size, and color of the teeth and that provide the result that the patient expects should always be the first therapeutic option [1–3].

Contrary to what many clinicians think, the concept of ceramic laminates without tooth surface wear is not new. Historically, during the 1930s, a California dentist Charles Leland Pincus [4] worked in the US film industry; he had the difficult and privileged task of aesthetically improving the smiles of stars such as Shirley Temple, Bob Hope, Montgomery Clift, Elizabeth Taylor, Barbara Stanwyck, Fred Astaire, James Dean, Walt Disney, Judy Garland, and many others. Pincus used thin ceramic veneers with an adhesive aid for the temporary fixation of full dentures. However, due to a lack of appropriate cement, the procedure lasted only a few hours.

During the 1980s, after the development of techniques for adhesive cementation, ultrathin laminates were relaunched. However, at the time, the practice did not spread as quickly as expected, due mainly to professionals' fears regarding the strength of the very thin porcelain veneers in resisting masticatory forces [5]. Due to increasing aesthetic demand and the possibility of joining laminated ceramic to the tooth structure (particularly enamel), a new concept was introduced: minimally invasive restorative dentistry, which causes little damage to dental structures [2].

In this context, laminate veneer, also known as contact lenses, emerged. This extremely aesthetic solution uses nothing more than thin ceramic fragments but presents excellent optical properties. It is considered one of the most conservative treatments for oral rehabilitation, as it requires minimal or no tooth preparation [6, 7]. With thicknesses ranging from 0.2 to 0.5 mm, ceramic laminate is capable of providing an extremely faithful reproduction of the natural teeth with great color stability [5]. Laminate veneer also offers

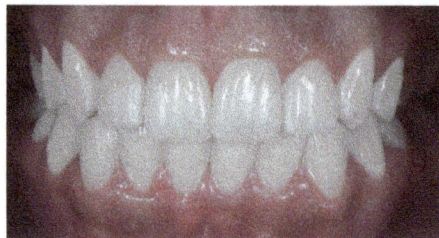

FIGURE 1: Intraoral view of the anterior maxillary teeth (Case 1).

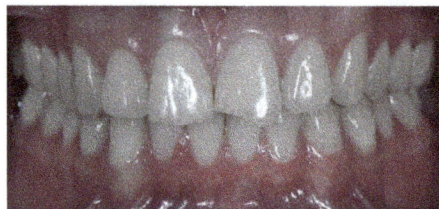

FIGURE 2: Intraoral view of the anterior maxillary teeth (Case 2).

biocompatibility with the periodontal and dental substrates [8, 9], and it may be used with minimal wear or even without preparation [10].

Patients undergoing this type of treatment require that the ceramic laminates offer clinical longevity. However, planning is a crucial step in successful aesthetic rehabilitation treatment. Planning each clinical case using a photographic protocol provides better predictability in the final outcome. In addition to photos and videos, wax-up/mock-up binomial important tools to establish correct values and to ensure the symmetry and proportion to the new smile [2, 11, 12]. Therefore, the purpose is to describe two clinical cases in a step-by-step process from the planning through the cementing phase, showing that it is possible for ultraconservative restorations to combine planning with technical and multidisciplinary treatment.

2. Case Presentations

Case 1. A female patient (23 years old) with high aesthetic requirements sought dental care in private practice, complaining about the color and size of her anterior teeth because talking does not reveal her upper incisors.

Case 2. A male patient (25 years old) sought dental care in private practice due to a fracture in his maxillary central incisors after hitting the bottom of a pool while diving.

3. Treatment Planning

Case 1. An intraoral clinical examination revealed that the anterior teeth had a small axial inclination and asymmetric gingival margins (Figure 1), and the patient elected to plan for the removal and refurbishment of the gingival tissues through periodontal plastic surgery techniques such as gingivoplasty or gingivectomy after first fabricating ceramic laminates.

In clinical practice, especially in prosthetic restorative procedures, there is often a need for prior corrections of the contours and the gingival anatomy due to the goals of achieving facial aesthetics and ensuring harmony between the gum tissue and the dental anatomy.

Case 2. An intraoral clinical examination revealed Class IV fracture in tooth 21 and small fractures in the incisal edge of tooth 11. The patient also presented with a diastema between the canines and the maxillary lateral incisors (Figure 2). A dental diastema is a space (or lack of contact) between two or more adjacent teeth. Diastemata are more frequent in the anterior maxilla, although they can occur in other regions of the mouth.

Regarding minimally invasive restorations, planning should not be restricted to the steps of forming and cementing. Other essential steps in the planning process for laminated ceramics include photographic and video analysis, Digital Smile Design (DSD), and mock-ups.

4. Photographic Protocol and Digital Planning

The photographic protocols were performed (Figure 3) to assist in the evaluation of various parameters that can influence the final result, such as smile height, amplitude of the buccal corridor, lip position, dental midline, and individual characteristics of each tooth.

With a photographic protocol, it was feasible to plan both cases using DSD. This process involves adding lines and digital designs to face photos in a specific sequence to better assess the aesthetic relationship between teeth, gums, smile, and face; this allows for a better understanding of the problems and can lead to possible solutions (Figures 4 and 5). For this study, the images were displayed on a computer using the Keynote slide show program (Apple, Cupertino, California, US), which allowed the patient to view the photos and participate in the planning. The virtual

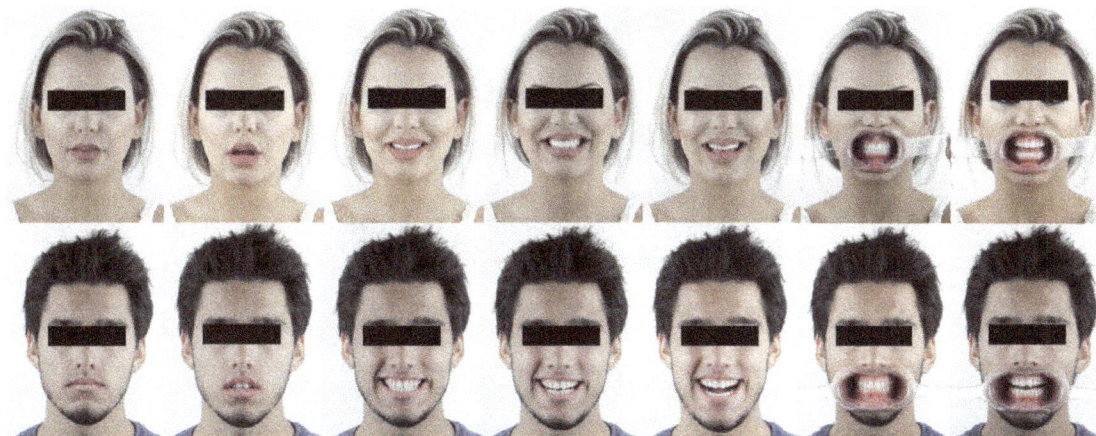

FIGURE 3: Photographic protocol for an aesthetic design and analysis of the patient's smile disharmonies.

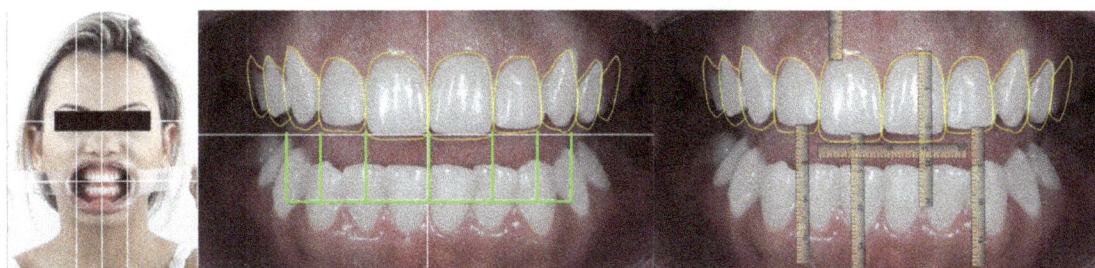

FIGURE 4: Digital Smile Design (DSD) protocol, Case 1. In this protocol, the ideal horizontal plane and vertical midline on the facial photograph were determined. After that, the cross to the intraoral photography to establish the vertical midline and occlusal plane was transferred. Furthermore, measurements of the distance were between the horizontal line and incisal edge on the photograph. Final teeth outline and gingival contour demonstrated the relationship between the preoperative situation and the final design.

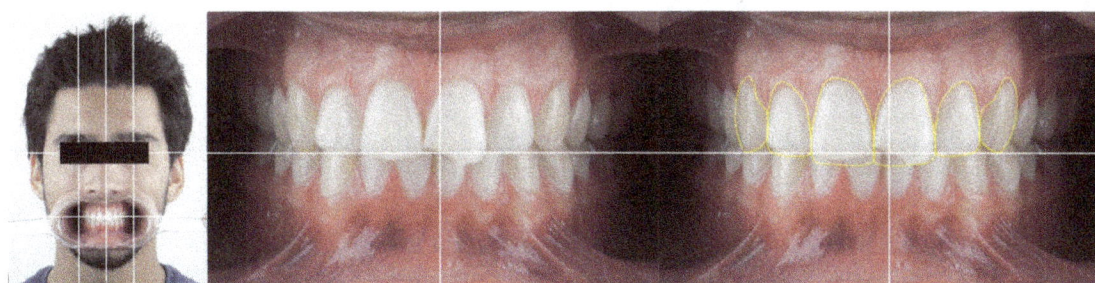

FIGURE 5: Digital Smile Design (DSD) protocol, Case 2.

planning tool also helped in the making of the diagnostic wax models.

5. Diagnostic Wax-Up

For the case study, DSD was used to create a diagnostic wax additive that shows the individual anatomical features of the teeth. Case 1 involved an increase in mesiodistal dimensions, the cervical alignment of the incisor edges, and buccal volumes of teeth 13–23 (Figure 6). Case 2 involved the reanatomization of fractured teeth and the closing of diastema (Figure 7). After defining this process and getting the patients'

approval, we conducted a test (mock-up) by placing wax directly over the patients' teeth without the need to erode the surfaces. In a mock-up, the patient can correct any of his/her dislikes [13].

Once the wax-up was completed, a silicone guide (Futura AD, DFL, Jacarepaguá, RJ, Brazil) was made and put under 2 atm of pressure to increase detail reproduction. This silicone guide was partially filled with a bis-acryl resin material (Protemp 4, 3M ESPE, St. Paul, MN, US) and placed in the patient's mouth (Figure 8). Before complete setting, a scalpel blade was used to define the correct gingival contour, respecting the manufacturer's recommendations. Gauze

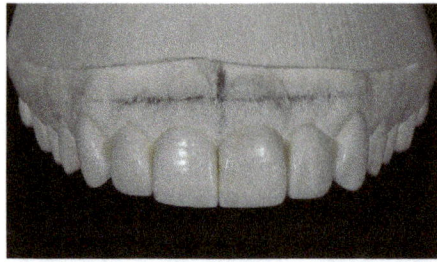

FIGURE 6: Diagnostic wax-up, Case 1.

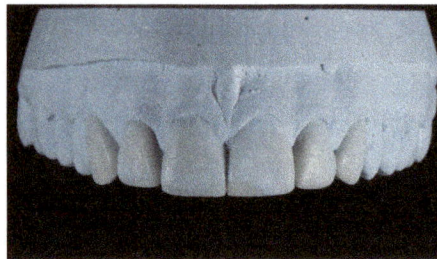

FIGURE 7: Diagnostic wax-up, Case 2.

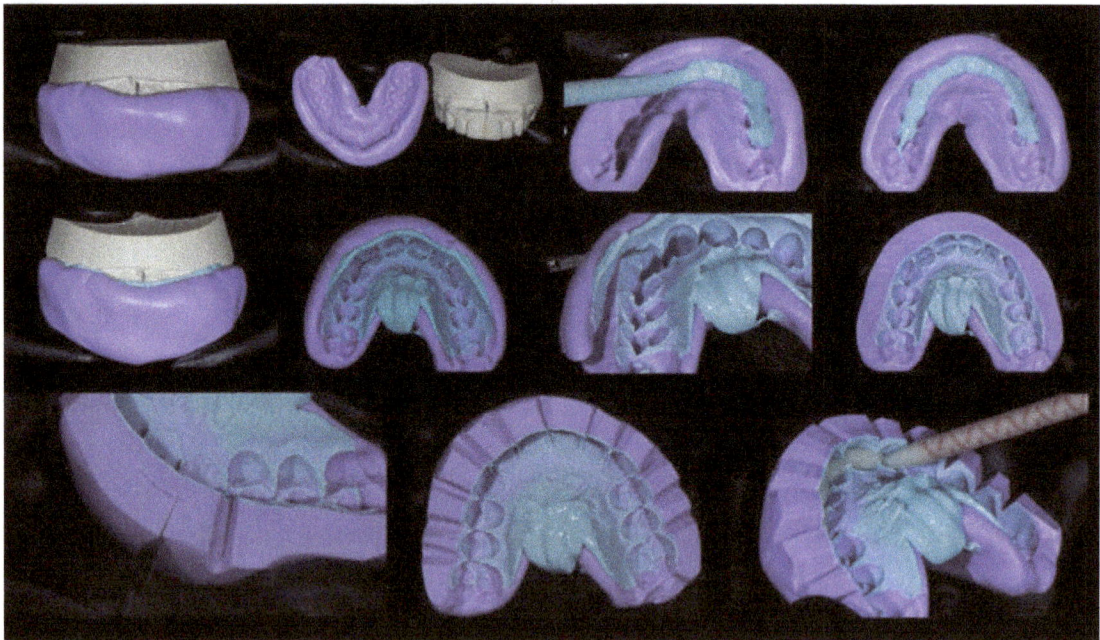

FIGURE 8: Step-by-step process for obtaining a matrix of addition silicone to make the mock-up and load it with the bis-acryl resin.

moistened with alcohol was used to create a polished and shiny appearance. In this way, it was possible to preview the end result of treatment (Figures 9 and 10).

6. Clinical and Laboratory Stages

6.1. Gingivoplasty. In Case 1, after the diagnostic wax-up was fabricated, gingivoplasty was performed on the predetermined elements. A period of 45 days was expected for perfect healing and maturation of the gingival tissue. In

this treatment, multidisciplinary dentistry, represented by the relationship between periodontics and prosthodontics, is not restricted only to the need to observe periodontal health for the completion of a restorative treatment; it also extends to the indication of gingivoplasty to improve the treatment's final result.

6.2. Color Choice. The color selection was made, while the teeth were hydrated at the beginning of the consultation.

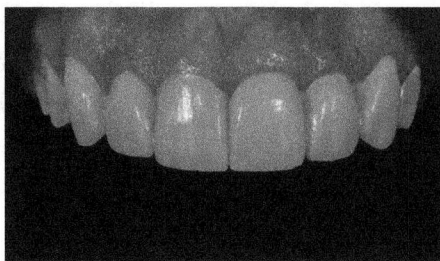

FIGURE 9: Mock-up without tooth preparation.

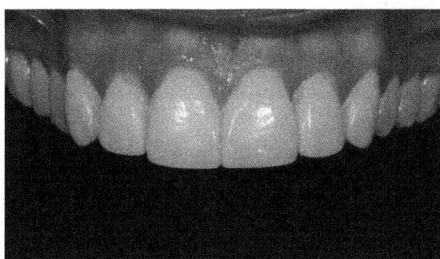

FIGURE 10: Mock-up after finishing with a scalpel blade.

Furthermore, a mapping of the colors was conducted to facilitate communication with the dental laboratory.

6.3. *Minimally Invasive Preparations.* In the case of the ultrathin ceramic restorations for the diastema closure, the insertion axis will begin in the cervical incisal direction, involving the mesial and distal surfaces [14]. Therefore, it is necessary to note areas of retention in the teeth before the molding step.

Minimally invasive preparations were performed using diamond burs and sanding discs, which were oriented with silicone guides (Zetalabor [Zhermack, Badia Polesine, Italy] and Coltène Speedex Putty [Coltène AG, Altstätten, Switzerland]) (Figures 11 and 12). During this phase, it was important to use the silicone matrix, obtained from the wax-up, to guide the amount of reduction in tooth preparation. This matrix may be constructed on the diagnostic wax study model or on the plaster model (which has provisional veneers). In these cases, the provisional veneers serve the same function as the dental wax.

6.4. *Impression Procedure.* In Case 1, the impression was carried out in two steps, with heavy and light addition silicone (Elite HD+, Zhermack) to obtain an accurate copy of the entire tooth and the gingival structures. Gingival retraction cord was used, as the terms of the preparations were all supragingival. In the first step, the dense addition silicone (Elite HD+, Zhermack) was manipulated and placed on the previously selected tray. It was placed in the patient's mouth, and internal relief was carried out simultaneous with the movements of the "strip and set." The second step involved the use of a small amount of the same silicone rubber that was applied to the dental preparations and the first mold. The

tray assembly and the dense silicone portion were placed into position on the light mixture and allowed to set.

In Case 2, the impression was performed in two steps with heavy and light bases of addition silicone (Virtual, Ivoclar Vivadent, Schaan, Liechtenstein) to obtain an accurate copy of the entire tooth and the gingival structure, following the same sequence as in Case 1. The retractor cord was not used, as the preparations were strictly supragingival. The lower jaw of each patient was molded with the same material that was used to form the antagonist of the upper jaw in the production model.

The feldspathic porcelain laminate veneers were manufactured with IPS d.SIGN (Ivoclar Vivadent) to maintain the teeth's naturalness (Figure 13).

7. Try-In/Shade Selection

To minimize the chances of errors during the cementation stage, such as possible fractures in the ceramics, two types of tests were done in the mouth: dry proof and damp proof using try-in paste (Case 1: Allcem Veneer with try-in paste, [FGM, Joinville, SC, Brazil]; Case 2: Variolink Veneer with try-in paste, Ivoclar Vivadent) (Figure 14). The veneers were tested on the preparations with the help of the try-in paste in the colors Trans (Case 1) and MV 0 (Case 2), which was deposited on the inner surfaces of all the veneers. The nonpolymerizable try-in paste is soluble in water and mimics the colors of resin cement after being light-cured, providing the professional with more confidence to carry out works with great aesthetic requirements. After removing the excess paste, a snapshot was taken to evaluate the color. At that time, the patient viewed and commented on the final color of the dental elements. Therefore, 30-second application of 37%

(a)

(b)   (c)   (d)   (e)

(f)

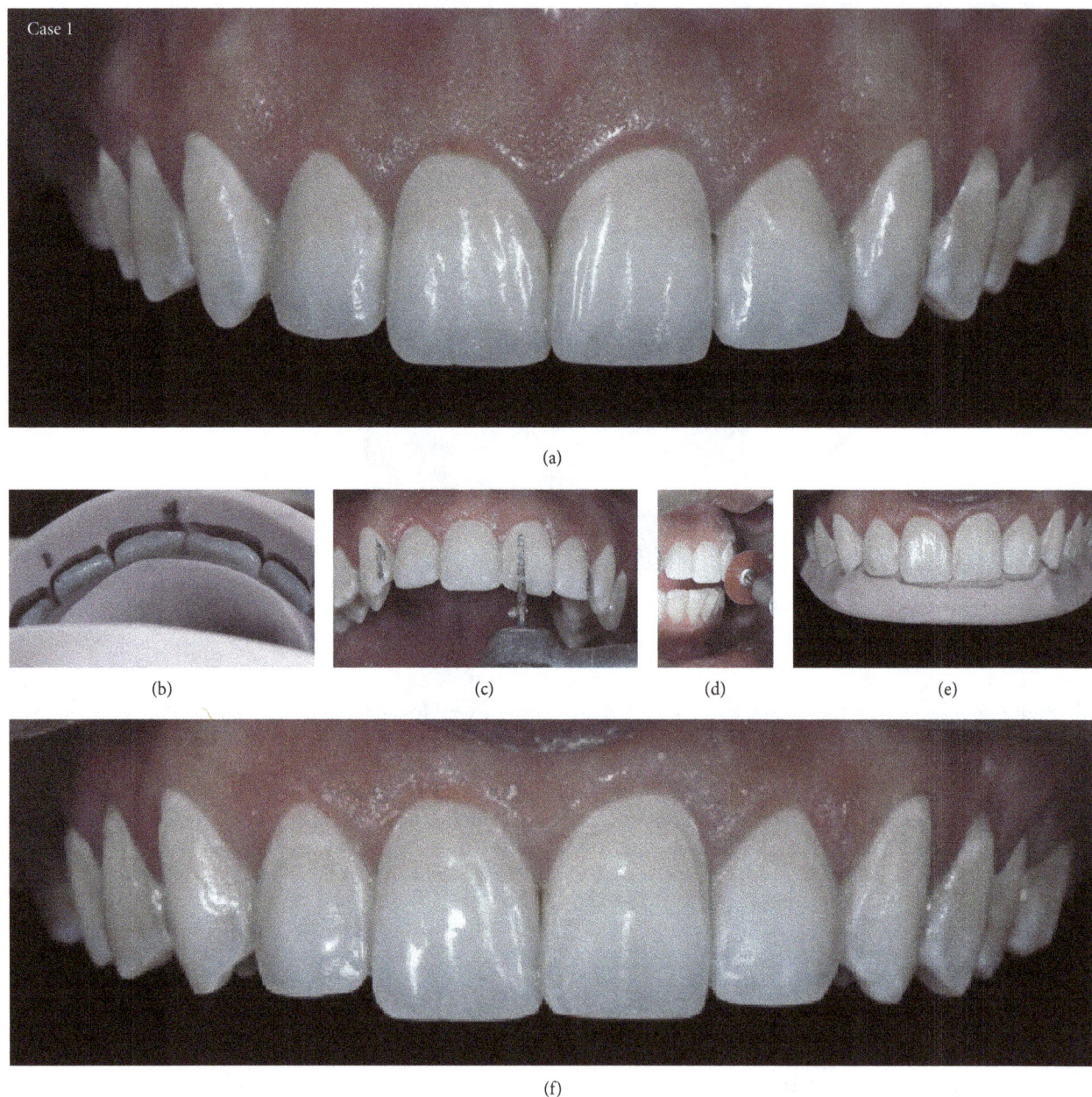

FIGURE 11: Case 1. (a) Initial view of the teeth before preparation. During treatment, the patient chose to extend the treatment to the bilateral second premolars. (b) Vestibular guide to assess the distance between the dental tissue and the correct placement indicated by the wax model, with information necessary to direct the professional in the decision of whether to wear down the sound tooth structure. (c) Palatal guide to aid the professional in determining the proper cervicoincisal size and the correct positioning of the incisal edge. (d)-(e) Minimally invasive preparations using a sanding disc and diamond burs. (f) Appearance immediately after minimally invasive preparation.

phosphoric acid is used only for cleaning, not for etching, and rinse with water and dry.

8. Cementation of Veneers

The cementation of the ceramic laminates is fundamental, as it will be the last step in the work; it should be done with extreme caution. It is important to remember that, unlike conventional crowns, which use dual-type resin cements, ceramic laminates should use a purely light-cured luting agent to prevent the color shifts that can occur due to chemical changes in the curing process. Furthermore, due to thin restorations such as contact lenses, which most allow photoactivation through them, there is no guarantee that the resin cement will be effectively cured.

For minimally invasive restorations, the choice was acid-sensitive ceramics, those that experience surface changes when conditioned with 10% hydrofluoric acid, because this process increases the adhesion between the restoration and the tooth.

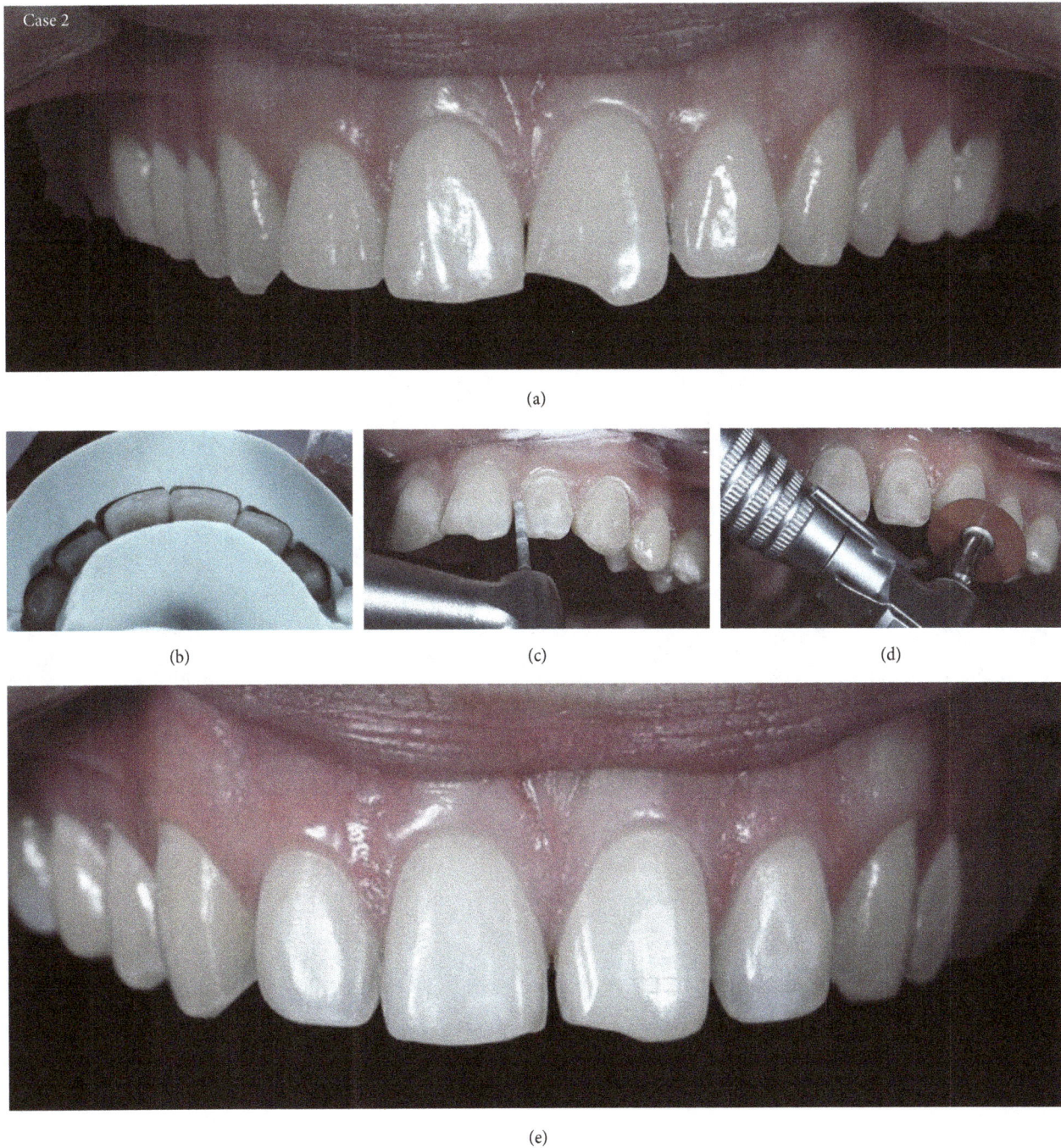

FIGURE 12: Case 2. (a) Initial view of the teeth before tooth preparation. (b) Enamel planning and demarcation of the end line of the future ceramic restoration with diamond burs. (c) Entrance exam guide to evaluate the distance between the dental tissue and the correct placement indicated by the wax model. (d) Removal of the retentive and incisal settlement areas with sandpaper discs. (e) Appearance immediately after minimally invasive preparation.

The essential difference in the internal etching processes of ceramics is the duration of hydrofluoric acid exposure [15]. The internal surface of the restoration was etched with 9% hydrofluoric acid (Ultradent Porcelain Etch, South Jordan, UT, USA) for 90 s (etching time for feldspathic glass ceramic) [16], washed under running water, and air-dried. Insoluble silica-fluoride salts as by-products precipitate on the surface were removed by cleaning the restorations by etching and rubbing the surface with 37% phosphoric acid (Nova DFL Industry and Trade SA, Rio de Janeiro, Brazil) for 1 minute before application of the silane [17, 18]. Silane coupling agent was applied (RelyX Ceramic Primer, 3M ESPE) for 1 minute,

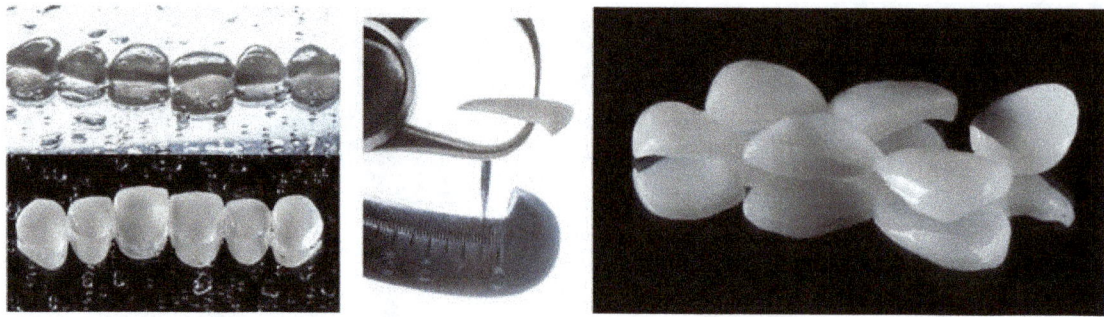

FIGURE 13: Ceramic laminate veneers.

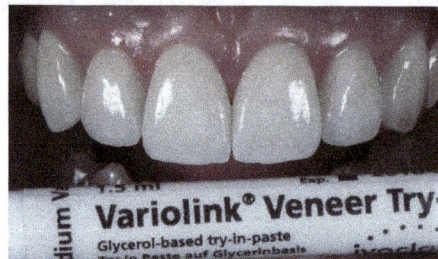

FIGURE 14: Case 2. Proofing of ceramic laminates with try-in paste (MV0, Variolink Veneer, Ivoclar Vivadent).

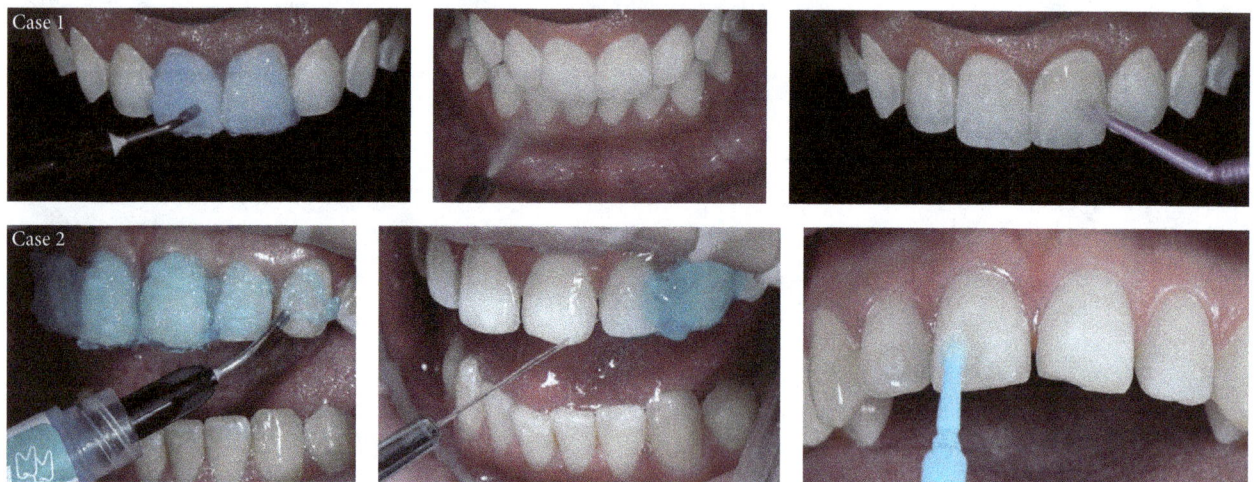

FIGURE 15: Etching with phosphoric acid at 37% for 30 seconds, followed by thorough washing for 20 seconds and the application of the adhesive system without being light-cured.

followed by a layer of adhesive (Case 1: Ambar, FGM; Case 2: Excite, Ivoclar Vivadent), and a gently air-dried. The adhesive should not be polymerized in this stage.

In the dental substrate, a total etching technique was carried out using 37% phosphoric acid for 30 seconds. The acid was subsequently removed with water before the total drying of the enamel surface and the application of a two-step adhesive system (Case 1: Ambar, FGM; Case 2: Excite, Ivoclar Vivadent) (Figure 15). The surface was gently air-dried to further remove the solvent and adhesive layer was unpolymerized.

The luting agents used in these cases (Case 1: Trans, Allcem Veneer, FGM; Case 2: MV 0, Variolink Veneer, Ivoclar Vivadent) were applied in the internal surface of the veneer,

and then the veneer was positioned with light and continuous digital pressure. It is important for cement extravasation to occur on all sides so that the entire inner surface is filled. The excess cement was removed with a brush, and the veneer was light-cured for 10 seconds. Resin cement residues were removed with manual tools and the veneer was once more light-cured at the facial and lingual sides for 90 seconds. (LED Bluephase, Ivoclar Vivadent) (Figure 16).

9. Finishing and Polishing

The finishing and polishing of the cement line were performed with flexible aluminum oxide disks (Sof-Lex XT Pop-On, 3M ESPE, St. Paul, MN, USA). The laminate ceramic

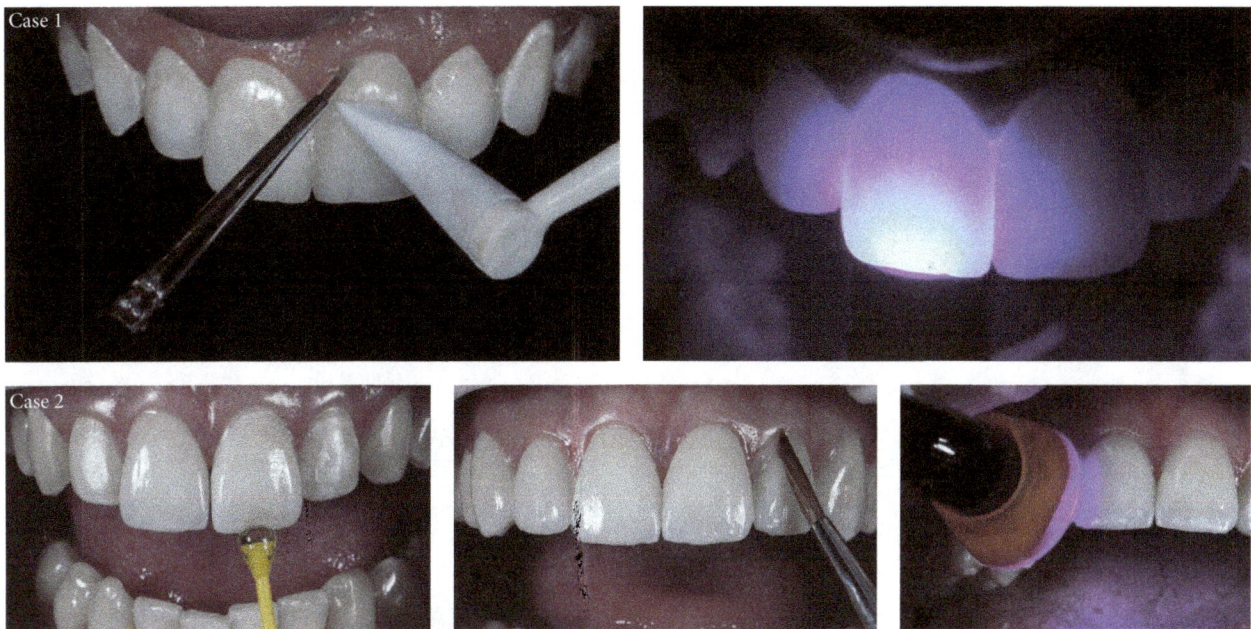

FIGURE 16: Removal of excess cement with a brush, followed by curing for 90 seconds on each side of the tooth.

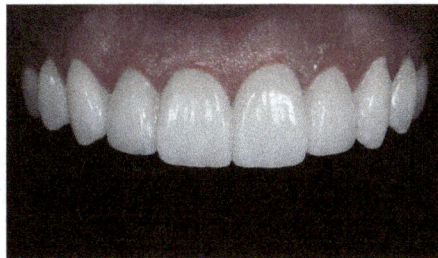

FIGURE 17: Case 1 immediately after cementation of the ceramic laminates.

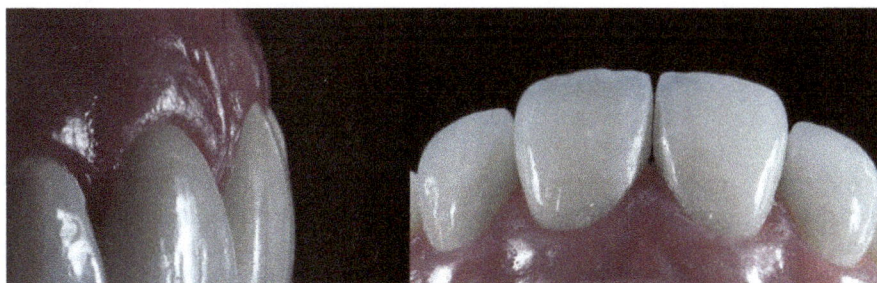

FIGURE 18: Case 2 immediately after cementation of the ceramic laminates. Ceramic-end-tooth transition with the resin cement, demonstrating periodontal health because the preparations are located at the supragingival level.

contact lens is a restoration that requires no finishing after cementation—only polishing with a scalpel and abrasive rubbers to remove excess cement. That is, the surface of the restoration is not changed by a glaze performed in a laboratory, thus ensuring the stability of the restoration over its years in the patient's mouth. The occlusion was assessed to make sure the anterior guidance and the lateral excursions were correct, while obtaining even occlusal contacts throughout the restorations. Finally, the patients were pleased with the aesthetics and function of the restorations. Furthermore, all prosthetic questions (stability, cement color, point of contact, and marginal adaptation), dentofacial harmony, and relationship dentolabial and maxillomandibular were conferred (Figures 17–20).

10. Discussion

Aesthetic rehabilitation with ceramic laminates is being increasingly used as a way to preserve tooth structure,

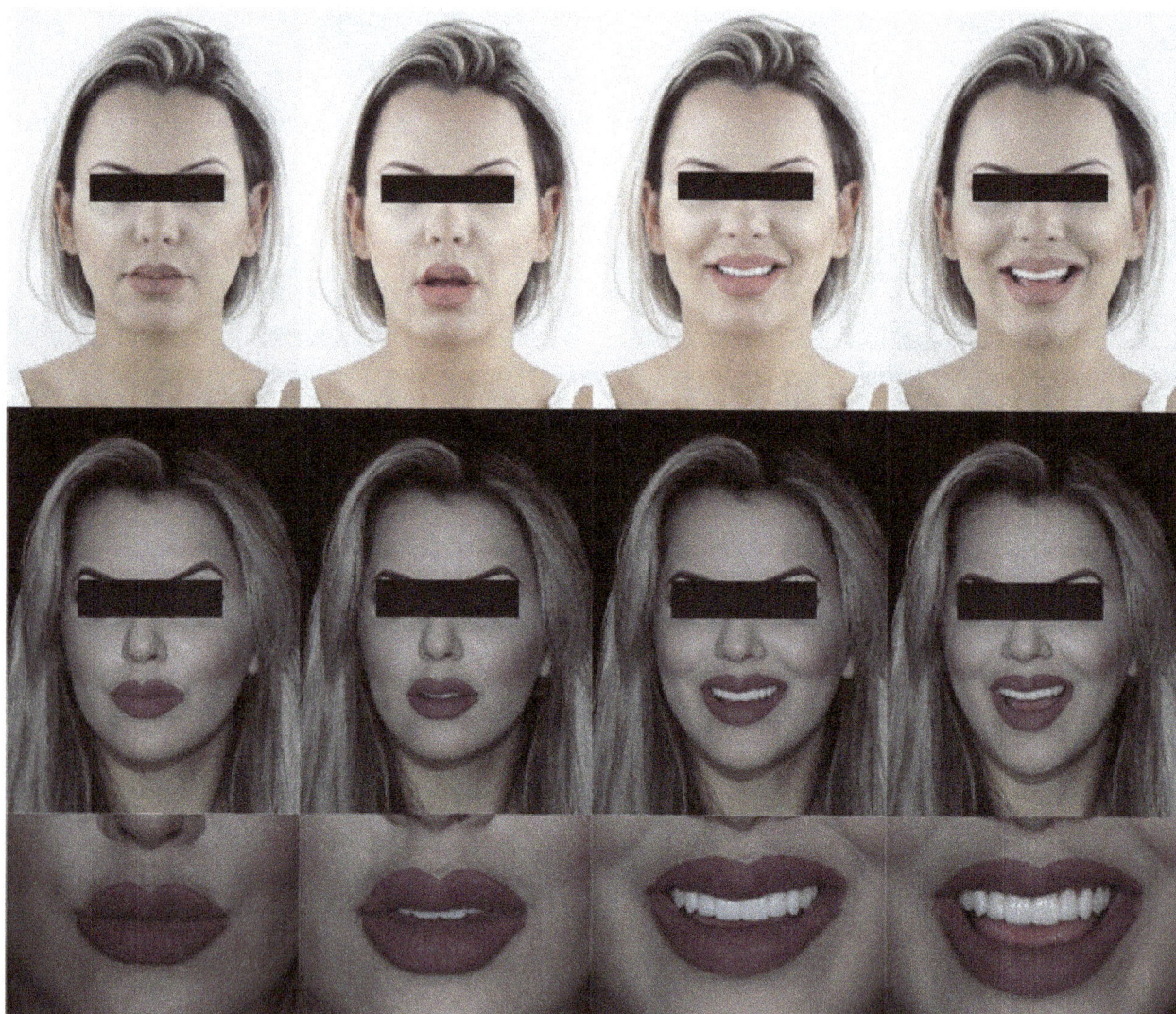

FIGURE 19: Case 1. Comparison between the initial planning and the finished case. The professional team obtained the patient's desired result by reestablishing dentofacial harmony.

especially in young patients. The diagnostic wax mock-up allows for individualized planning and a predictable outcome in cases where a certain shape and position are expected. These procedures require a refined knowledge of tooth anatomy and insight into each patient's personality [19]. The manufacture of this type of restoration has become feasible due to the development of adhesion mechanisms for dental structures. Enamel and dentin etching, combined with the use of primers, adhesives, and resin cements, provide security in this restorative procedure [20].

The first step is to assess the need for periodontal plastic surgery, gingival biotype, and obtain dimensions for the biologic width for each tooth involved in the treatment to determine whether an osteotomy would be needed [21]. By understanding the biologic width for each tooth we can prevent future problems with gingival health and restorations overhangs [22]. The periodontal probe is gently positioned into the gingival sulcus with light pressure to determine the probing depth and gingival biotype [21], which in *Case 1* was a thin tissue biotype. Furthermore, a mock-up was used to allow the surgeon to visualize the final gingival margin and guide the incision shape [21].

Another factor to be considered in the planning is the previous orthodontic treatment to minimize the amount of wear of the tooth structure and provide options for dental alignment problems. Aesthetics is often a primary concern among those seeking treatment through short orthodontic treatment and there are several other factors relating to this that need to be borne in mind when treating the adult patient [23]. However, adult patients desire the resolution of their cases quickly. In *Case 1*, the patient would not want to remake orthodontic treatment, because this was done in childhood and looking for immediate results.

The great advantages of consolidating membership in the enamel increase the indications of ceramic restorations with minimal or no preparation [24]. The majority of

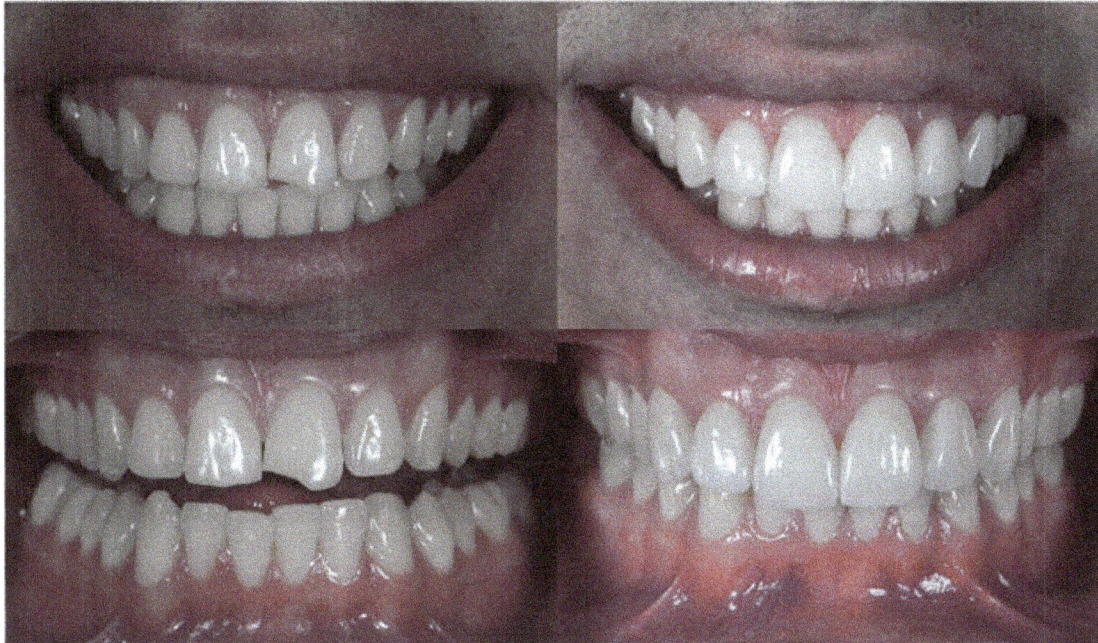

FIGURE 20: Case 2. The dentolabial and maxillomandibular relationships, before and after treatment.

cases restored with laminate veneers do not require tooth preparation but rather enamel recontouring [25]. Enamel recontouring is guided by three aspects: (1) need to increase volume to the teeth's facial surface, (2) color of the dental substrate, and (3) path of insertion for the ceramic restorations [25]. In *Case 2*, a minimal and calculated enamel proximal recontouring might be necessary to remove undercuts or to minimize the influence of the proximal height of contour (crest of convexity) [25]. Similarly, the treatment of porcelain with hydrofluoric acid and silane to create an adhesive interface serves as the basis for ceramic laminate veneers, thus developing a structural unit [26]. In this study, care was taken to use a conservative preparation of the enamel, using a silicone mock-up to control the amount of tooth wear necessary to provide a suitable ceramic thickness.

The decision regarding the most appropriate material for these types of situations always leads to questions, as dentists often have difficulty choosing between the use of direct composite resins and the production of ceramic laminates. Dental ceramics can both improve teeth's aesthetic appearance and reestablish their strength and function [10, 27]. When comparing ceramic veneers with composite resins, we can see that the ceramics offer substantial improvements in optical behavior, color stability, shape, surface smoothness, and mechanical and physical properties; ceramic veneers emulate the shape of the dental tissue to be replaced or repaired [28].

To achieve better clinical outcomes in the long term and improve the properties of restorative materials, various studies have been conducted. Improvements in the coefficient of thermal expansion and in the size and distribution of particles have led to abrasive ceramic restorations that are more

resistant to fracture, giving an improved prognosis and making the ceramic dental restorative material superior to composite resin [29].

The clincher, however, is that ceramics, both feldspathic and lithium disilicate-reinforced, have almost equal resistance after cementation. The explanation for this is the principle of the adhesive bond, which ensures resistance and bond strength through the transfer of one substrate to another. Thus, there is no advantage to using ceramic lithium disilicate-reinforced ceramics, as they will not result in more resilient restorations relative to pure ceramics, such as feldspar or fluorapatite [15]. By using adhesive feldspathic porcelain restorations, we can return the teeth's original strength [30].

Proper selection of luting material is critical to the clinical longevity of ceramic restorations. Using light-cured resin cements is recommended because they have a variety of colors and different degrees of opacity. In addition, the light-cured luting agent has greater color stability than the dual-curing luting agent [31]. Furthermore, the working time and the degree of flow for the dual-cured cements greatly hinder indications. By contrast, the light-cured luting agent provides a thin cementation line, along with high fluidity and excellent flow grade, facilitating the removal of excess cement [32].

The brush technique seems to be the best option for removing excess resin cement in the clinical routine due to this method's good results and technical simplicity; brushing promotes dental and periodontal health and increases the longevity of aesthetic results [33]. In these cases, cervical margin fall veneers were placed 1 mm above the cement enamel junction, to prevent the restorative material from being eliminated. This decision was based on the mechanical properties of the ceramic material, which exhibits a high modulus of elasticity and has almost nonexistent elastic deformation (these are also known as friability characteristics).

The margin placement of the restorations was located at the supragingival or equigingival (even with the tissue) for all restored teeth [34]. This choice was made to obtain periodontal health, as it reduces subgingival preparation, overcontoured plaque buildup, and difficulty of cleaning; it also facilitates the molding work, as it can be performed without a gingival retraction cord. In addition, the cervical end was located in the enamel, guaranteeing greater longevity of adhesion [35, 36], and the aesthetics were not compromised, as the resin cement mimics the ceramic-end-tooth transition.

The available literature shows that ceramic laminates have performed well over the years. Studies show results ranging from 5 to 20 years of clinical outcomes after the procedure [8, 9, 37, 38]. A functional balance and the correct adjustment of the contacts are also essential to avoid problems, especially fractures of the incisal edges; protrusive and lateral guides should be checked for proper system stability [39]. Successful anterior restorations can be achieved when using a detailed treatment plan and when considering both the aesthetic and the functional parameters [39, 40].

11. Conclusion

These clinical reports describe the laminate veneers as an excellent option for effective, conservative, and aesthetic treatment. Therefore, all of the treatment sequences are ruled by the same plan, taking into consideration the adhesive systems, ceramics, ceramic etching, light curing, resin cements, and the correct photographic protocol. As a result, the aesthetics and function expected by the patients were achieved. The use of ceramic veneers enabled a conservative and aesthetic successful rehabilitation treatment. Thus, for the clinical longevity of restorations with laminate veneers, it is necessary for professionals to carefully follow all clinical steps.

Competing Interests

The authors declare that they have no competing interests.

References

[1] U. C. Belser, P. Magne, and M. Magne, "Ceramic laminate veneers: continuous evolution of indications," *Journal of Esthetic Dentistry*, vol. 9, no. 4, pp. 197–207, 1997.

[2] G. M. Radz, "Minimum thickness anterior porcelain restorations," *Dental Clinics of North America*, vol. 55, no. 2, pp. 353–370, 2011.

[3] B. T. Rotoli, D. A. N. L. Lima, N. P. Pini, F. H. B. Aguiar, G. D. S. Pereira, and L. A. M. S. Paulillo, "Porcelain veneers as an alternative for esthetic treatment: clinical report," *Operative Dentistry*, vol. 38, no. 5, pp. 459–466, 2013.

[4] C. R. Pincus, "Building mouth personality," *Journal of the California Dental Association*, vol. 14, pp. 125–129, 1938.

[5] H. E. Strassler, "Minimally invasive porcelain veneers: indications for a conservative esthetic dentistry treatment modality," *General Dentistry*, vol. 55, no. 7, pp. 686–694, 2007.

[6] L. F. Da Cunha, L. O. Pedroche, C. C. Gonzaga, and A. Y. Furuse, "Esthetic, occlusal, and periodontal rehabilitation of anterior teeth with minimum thickness porcelain laminate veneers," *Journal of Prosthetic Dentistry*, vol. 112, no. 6, pp. 1315–1318, 2014.

[7] A. S. Nobrega, A. F. Silva Signoreli, J. V. Quinelli Mazzaro, R. A. Zavanelli, and A. C. Zavanell, "Minimally invasive preparations: contact lenses," *Journal of Advanced Clinical & Research Insights*, vol. 2, pp. 176–179, 2015.

[8] M. Fradeani, M. Redemagni, and M. Corrado, "Porcelain laminate veneers: 6- to 12-year clinical evaluation—A Retrospective Study," *International Journal of Periodontics and Restorative Dentistry*, vol. 25, no. 1, pp. 9–17, 2005.

[9] D. Layton and T. Walton, "An up to 16-year prospective study of 304 porcelain veneers," *International Journal of Prosthodontics*, vol. 20, no. 4, pp. 389–396, 2007.

[10] L. F. da Cunha, L. O. Pedroche, C. C. Gonzaga, and A. Y. Furuse, "Esthetic, occlusal, and periodontal rehabilitation of anterior teeth with minimum thickness porcelain laminate veneers," *Journal of Prosthetic Dentistry*, vol. 112, no. 6, pp. 1315–1318, 2014.

[11] C. Coachman and M. Calamita, "Digital smile design: a tool for treatment planning and communication in esthetic dentistry," *Quintessence Journal of Dental Technology*, vol. 35, pp. 103–111, 2012.

[12] C. Meereis, G. de Souza, L. Albino, F. Ogliari, E. Piva, and G. Lima, "Digital smile design for computer-assisted esthetic rehabilitation: two-year follow-up," *Operative Dentistry*, vol. 41, no. 1, pp. E13–E22, 2016.

[13] J. Gurrea and A. Bruguera, "Wax-up and mock-up. A guide for anterior periodontal and restorative treatments," *The International Journal of Esthetic Dentistry*, vol. 9, no. 2, pp. 146–162, 2014.

[14] B. LeSage, "Establishing a classification system and criteria for veneer preparations," *Compendium of Continuing Education in Dentistry*, vol. 34, no. 2, pp. 104–117, 2013.

[15] B. LeSage, "Revisiting the design of minimal and no-preparation veneers: a step-by-step technique," *Journal of the California Dental Association*, vol. 38, no. 8, pp. 561–569, 2010.

[16] J. H. Phark, N. Sartori, and S. Duarte, "Bonding to silica-based glass-ceramics: a review of current techniques and novel self-etching ceramic primers," in *QDT 2016*, S. Duarte, Ed., pp. 26–36, Quintessence Publishing, 1st edition, 2016.

[17] P. Magne and D. Cascione, "Influence of post-etching cleaning and connecting porcelain on the microtensile bond strength of composite resin to feldspathic porcelain," *Journal of Prosthetic Dentistry*, vol. 96, no. 5, pp. 354–361, 2006.

[18] Ş. Canay, N. Hersek, and A. Ertan, "Effect of different acid treatments on a porcelain surface," *Journal of Oral Rehabilitation*, vol. 28, no. 1, pp. 95–101, 2001.

[19] P. Magne, M. Magne, and U. Belser, "Natural and restorative oral esthetics part I: rationale and basic strategies for successful esthetic rehabilitations," *Journal of Esthetic Dentistry*, vol. 5, no. 4, pp. 161–173, 1993.

[20] A. Signore, V. Kaitsas, A. Tonoli, F. Angiero, A. Silvestrini-Biavati, and S. Benedicenti, "Sectional porcelain veneers for a maxillary midline diastema closure: a case report," *Quintessence International*, vol. 44, no. 3, pp. 201–206, 2013.

[21] I. C. Molina, G. C. Molina, C. A. M. Volpato, S. A. Jovanovic, and K. Stanley, "Ultrasonic devices for minimally invasive periodontal surgery and restorative dentistry," in *QDT 2016*, S. Duarte, Ed., pp. 197–208, Quintessence Publishing, 1st edition, 2016.

[22] J. Y. K. Kan, T. Morimoto, K. Rungcharassaeng, P. Roe, and D. H. Smith, "Gingival biotype assessment in the esthetic zone: visual versus direct measurement," *The International journal of periodontics & restorative dentistry*, vol. 30, no. 3, pp. 237–243, 2010.

[23] J. H. Noar, S. Sharma, D. Roberts-Harry, and T. Qureshi, "A discerning approach to simple aesthetic orthodontics," *British Dental Journal*, vol. 218, no. 3, pp. 157–166, 2015.

[24] B. A. Vanlıoğlu and Y. Kulak-Özkan, "Minimally invasive veneers: current state of the art," *Clinical, Cosmetic and Investigational Dentistry*, vol. 6, pp. 101–107, 2014.

[25] V. Clavijo, N. Sartori, J. H. Phark, and S. Duarte, "Novel Guidelines for bonded ceramic veneers: part 1. Is tooth preparation truly necessary?" in *QDT 2016*, S. Duarte, Ed., pp. 7–25, Quintessence Publishing, 1st edition, 2016.

[26] H. E. Strassler and D. Nathanson, "Clinical evaluation of etched porcelain veneers over a period of 18 to 42 months," *Journal of Esthetic Dentistry*, vol. 1, no. 1, pp. 21–28, 1989.

[27] M. Fradeani, G. Barducci, L. Bacherini, and M. Brennan, "Esthetic rehabilitation of a severely worn dentition with minimally invasive prosthetic procedures (MIPP)," *The International Journal of Periodontics & Restorative Dentistry*, vol. 32, no. 2, pp. 135–147, 2012.

[28] N. P. Pini, F. H. B. Aguiar, D. A. N. Leite Lima, J. R. Lovadino, R. S. Suga Terada, and R. C. Pascotto, "Advances in dental veneers: materials, applications, and techniques," *Clinical, Cosmetic and Investigational Dentistry*, vol. 4, pp. 9–16, 2012.

[29] T.-M. Lin, P.-R. Liu, L. C. Ramp, M. E. Essig, D. A. Givan, and Y.-H. Pan, "Fracture resistance and marginal discrepancy of porcelain laminate veneers influenced by preparation design and restorative material in vitro," *Journal of Dentistry*, vol. 40, no. 3, pp. 202–209, 2012.

[30] P. Magne and W. H. Douglas, "Porcelain veneers: dentin bonding optimization and biomimetic recovery of the crown," *International Journal of Prosthodontics*, vol. 12, no. 2, pp. 111–121, 1999.

[31] D. Nathanson and F. Banasr, "Color stability of resin cements—an in vitro study," *Practical Procedures & Aesthetic Dentistry*, vol. 14, no. 6, pp. 449–456, 2002.

[32] E. Öztürk, R. Hickel, Ş. Bolay, and N. Ilie, "Micromechanical properties of veneer luting resins after curing through ceramics," *Clinical Oral Investigations*, vol. 16, no. 1, pp. 139–146, 2012.

[33] M. H. Harasani, F. Isidor, and S. Kaaber, "Marginal fit of porcelain and indirect composite laminate veneers under in vitro conditions," *Scandinavian Journal of Dental Research*, vol. 99, no. 3, pp. 262–268, 1991.

[34] A. Shenoy, R. Babannavar, and N. Shenoy, "Periodontal considerations determining the design and location of margins in restorative dentistry," *Journal of Interdisciplinary Dentistry*, vol. 2, no. 1, pp. 3–10, 2012.

[35] E. Oztürk and S. Bolay, "Survival of porcelain laminate veneers with different degrees of dentin exposure: 2-year clinical results," *The Journal of Adhesive Dentistry*, vol. 16, no. 5, pp. 481–489, 2014.

[36] D. Re, F. Cerutti, G. Augusti, A. Cerutti, and D. Augusti, "Comparison of marginal fit of Lava CAD/CAM crown-copings with two finish lines," *The International Journal of Esthetic Dentistry*, vol. 9, no. 3, pp. 426–435, 2014.

[37] M. Peumans, J. De Munck, S. Fieuws, P. Lambrechts, G. Vanherle, and B. Van Meerbeek, "A prospective ten-year clinical trial of porcelain veneers," *Journal of Adhesive Dentistry*, vol. 6, no. 1, pp. 65–76, 2004.

[38] J. R. Calamia and C. S. Calamia, "Porcelain laminate veneers: reasons for 25 years of success," *Dental Clinics of North America*, vol. 51, no. 2, pp. 399–417, 2007.

[39] L. F. da Cunha, R. A. Prochnow, A. O. Costacurta, C. C. Gonzaga, and G. M. Correr, "Replacement of anterior composite resin restorations using conservative ceramics for occlusal and periodontal rehabilitation: an 18-month clinical follow-up," *Case Reports in Dentistry*, vol. 2016, Article ID 9728593, 7 pages, 2016.

[40] M. Miranda, K. Olivieri, F. Rigolin, and A. de Vasconcellos, "Esthetic challenges in rehabilitating the anterior maxilla: a case report," *Operative Dentistry*, vol. 41, no. 1, pp. 2–7, 2016.

12

Sclerotherapy of Intraoral Superficial Hemangioma

Resmije Ademi Abdyli,[1] **Yll Abdyli,**[2] **Feriall Perjuci,**[1] **Ali Gashi,**[1]
Zana Agani,[1] **and Jehona Ahmedi**[1]

[1]*Department of Oral Surgery, Medical Faculty, University of Prishtina, Dental Branch, 10000 Prishtina, Kosovo*
[2]*Medical Faculty, University of Prishtina, Dental Branch, 10000 Prishtina, Kosovo*

Correspondence should be addressed to Yll Abdyli; yllabdyli10@gmail.com

Academic Editor: Giuseppe Colella

Hemangioma is the clinical term for a benign vascular neoplasm due to proliferation of the endothelial lining of blood vessels. Their most frequent location is the body skin and oral mucosa. One of the treatment modalities for hemangiomas is intralesional injection of sclerosing agents which cause the damage of blood vessels followed by their obliteration. The objective of the study was to describe the facility of application and evaluate the efficiency of sclerotherapy with aethoxysklerol 1%. *Method.* The case presented with intraoral submucosal hemangioma of the cheek was treated by intralesional injection of aethoxysklerol 3% diluted in water for injections at a 4 : 1 ratio (0.75%) at the first appointment and 3 : 1 (1%) at the second appointment. The effect of sclerotherapy was evaluated on the following visits in time intervals of two weeks. *Results.* The hemangioma disappeared without complications after the second injection of aethoxysklerol 1%. The successful results of the study were comparable to the data of literature with variations according to the used sclerosant agent, its concentration, the number of injections, and the intervals between each session. *Conclusion.* Since sclerotherapy is a very effective, inexpensive, and easy-to-apply treatment, it should be the treatment of choice, especially for intraoral superficial hemangiomas.

1. Introduction

Hemangioma is a vascular neoplasm or a vascular anomaly due to proliferation of blood vessels. They occur anywhere in the body, but skin and oral mucosa in the region of the lips, tongue, and buccal mucosa are most commonly affected. Therefore, the dentist or oral surgeon should be informed about their clinical aspect, diagnosis, and therapy [1–3].

The clinical aspect of oral hemangiomas depends on their location and depth. Usually hemangiomas present as blood-filled asymptomatic swellings or red/bluish-purple discolorations, but their progressive growth can increase the likelihood of local traumatic injuries followed by unexpected bleeding [4–7]. The size of hemangiomas is variable, ranging from a few millimeters to several centimeters in the form of a macule, papule, nodule, or tumor, with elastic or fibrous consistency [8].

In order to obtain a definite diagnosis of vascular malformations (of suspected hemangioma), different clinical examination methods can be implemented, including digital compression and diascopy [6, 7] and other supplementary imaging tests such as ultrasonography with Doppler and MRI [9, 10].

Various modalities have been used in the treatment of hemangiomas, depending on their location, size and depth, evolution of injury, and involvement of adjacent structures [8, 10].

The gold standard for hemangioma treatment, especially for smaller circumscribed lesions and peripheral hemangiomas, is conventional surgical excision [3, 11]. However, complications that arise from conventional invasive surgical procedures such as excessive postoperative bleeding compelled the use of other different therapeutic alternatives including systemic corticosteroids, laser therapy, cauterization, cryotherapy, radiotherapy, and sclerotherapy [4, 12–14]. These modes of treatment can be applied individually or in concert.

The Objective. The Objective of the study was to describe the facility of the application of sclerosing agents and evaluate the

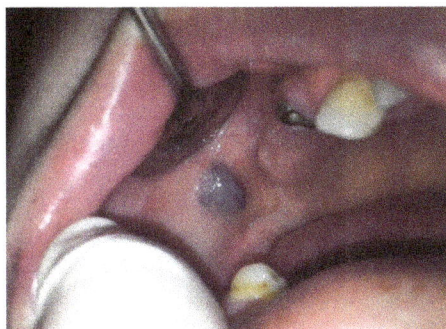

FIGURE 1: Submucosal hemangioma of the cheek at the right molar region.

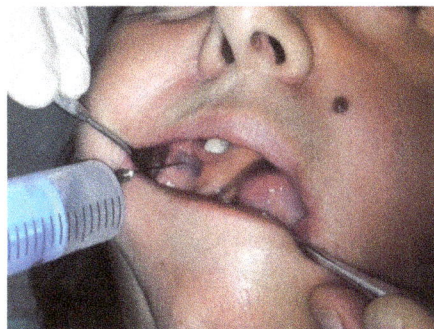

FIGURE 2: First intralesional injection of aethoxysklerol 0.75%.

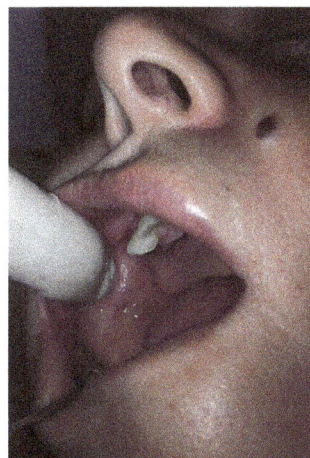

FIGURE 3: Second appointment after twelve days: regression of hemangioma.

effectiveness of sclerotherapy with aethoxysklerol 1% as one of the treatment options of oral superficial hemangioma.

2. Case Description and Treatment Method

A 53-year-old female was referred to the Department of Oral Surgery at UDCCK, Dental Branch of Medical Faculty, University of Prishtina, Kosovo, for surgical treatment of an intraoral submucosal lesion. According to patient's complaint, she had noticed an asymptomatic blue-colored lesion on the right side of the cheek about six months ago. Intraoral physical examination revealed an indolent, well defined purple colored lesion under intact mucosa of the cheek, soft on palpation with dimensions around 1.5×0.8 cm (Figure 1). Based on medical history and clinical examination, the lesion was diagnosed as submucosal hemangioma of the cheek.

Considering the superficial location of the lesion, the decision was, in lieu of surgical treatment, to opt for sclerotherapy with aethoxysklerol 1% applied on 3-4 (three to four) sessions) at intervals of 10–14 days, depending on the lesion's treatment progress. Taking into account the fact that we had only 3% aethoxysklerol at our disposal, this sclerosing agent was diluted with normal saline to desired concentration prior to intralesional injection.

Owing to the doubt that aethoxysklerol 1% can cause tissue damage at the injection site after intralesional injection, the available aethoxysklerol 3% was diluted with normal saline at a 1 : 4 ratio, obtaining 0.75% concentration of sclerosing agent. Slow injection of 1–1.5 mL aethoxysklerol 0.75% was performed without anesthesia into the lumen of the lesion (Figure 2). After injecting the agent, local hemostasis was performed by digital compression at the site of injection. The effect of therapy was evaluated on the following visits.

At the next visit, appointed after twelve days (Figure 3), the size of the lesion was reduced dramatically, necessitating only one other subsequent intralesional injection of 1 mL aethoxysklerol solution of 1% concentration, obtained by dilution of aethoxysklerol 3% at normal saline at a ratio of 3 : 1 (Figure 4).

During the following third visit (Figure 5), around two weeks later, intraoral examination revealed complete disappearance of the lesion, so the sclerosant therapy was terminated and the patient was appointed for the next visit after

one month. After almost two months, by a phone call, the patient notified us that the lesion had completely disappeared without any sign of recurrence.

3. Discussion

There are many treatment modalities reported in the literature for oral hemangiomas, such as intralesional and systemic corticosteroid treatment, surgical excision, thermocauterization, laser photocoagulation, and sclerotherapy [4, 12–14]. Each of the treatment modalities has its own risks and advantages.

Advantages of sclerotherapy to other hemangioma treatment modalities include it being very simple and safe to apply, affordable, and readily available, with most of this being due to not requiring special equipment for application and having no need for hospitalization of the patient.

Most importantly, it has shown high efficacy, offering partial or complete regression of the lesion without bleeding [4, 15–18]. Disadvantages of sclerotherapy include postoperative pain and burning sensation, potential anaphylactic reaction, tissue necrosis, and airway compromise [19].

Currently, sclerotherapy is largely employed because of its effectiveness and ability to conserve the surrounding tissues [20]. Sclerotherapy has been proven effective in the treatment

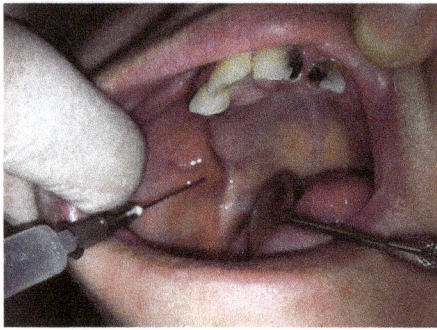

FIGURE 4: Second intralesional injection of aethoxysklerol 1%.

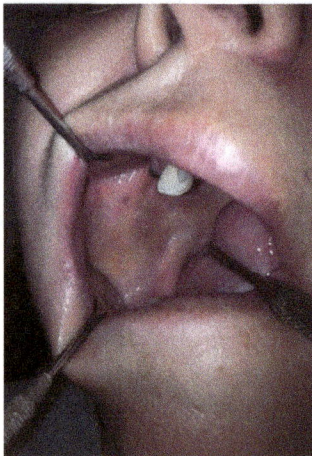

FIGURE 5: Third following visit: hemangioma disappeared without complications.

of benign vascular lesions, especially small lesions located on sites with esthetic impact, where surgery could leave unpleasant scarring [4, 15, 16, 21, 22].

Frequently used sclerosing agents are sodium morrhuate, sodium psylliate, hypertonic glucose solution, sodium tetradecyl sulfate, ethanolamine oleate, and polidocanol (aethoxysklerol 3%, 1% or 0.5%) [3, 4, 13, 15].

One of the sclerosing agents used for many years in the treatment of hemangioma and varicose veins is polidocanol (aethoxysklerol 3%, 1%, or 0.5%) [13, 15, 16, 18, 23–28].

Polidocanol (aethoxysklerol) and sodium tetradecyl sulfate (STS) are the best known detergent solutions which act by causing localized inflammatory reaction, obliterative thrombosis of hemangiomatous space, and subsequent fibrosis of the endothelial spaces, leading to the regression of the lesion [25–27]. These advantages of sclerosant use are the absence of pain on intravascular injection, a high level of efficacy and safety, and a very low occurrence rate of allergic reactions [28].

The quantity of injected sclerosing agents and the number of applications during the sclerotherapy treatment depend on the size and location of the lesion and involvement of adjacent structures, not forgetting to mention the obtained results, which should be evaluated before the administration of the next dose after an interval of 1 to 2 weeks [4, 14, 15, 26].

The treatment employed in the presented case was sclerotherapy with aethoxysklerol 1%. The concentration of the sclerosing agent (1%), number of treatment sessions (3-4), and intervals between each session (12 to 14 days) were planned based on our previous experience with hemangioma treatment by aethoxysklerol 1%. Due to the fact that we only had aethoxysklerol 3% at our disposal, the 3% solution was diluted in normal saline in a ratio of 1 : 4 obtaining aethoxysklerol 0.75% for intralesional injection on the first session. On the second session after twelve days, the agent was diluted 1 : 3 (1%) obtaining aethoxysklerol 1%. The results of sclerotherapy were followed and assessed after a certain time period (ten days–two weeks) from the sclerotherapy session. The case has proven that intralesional injection of the aethoxysklerol 0.75%–1% was very effective, inducing rapid regression of the lesion after the second intralesional injection; therefore, it was considered that two sessions of injections were sufficient for the treatment of this superficial hemangioma.

The results of the actual study were similar to the data of literature relating to sclerotherapy, with variations according to the type of sclerosing agent, its concentration, the number of injections, and the intervals between each treatment session [13, 14, 18, 24, 29, 30].

Winter et al. in 2000 also published their experience with polidocanol in 132 patients with cavernous hemangiomas, demonstrating a satisfactory response and requiring only one to three injections [18].

Another treatment option of oral hemangioma treatment is laser therapy based on the coagulative effect of superpulsed laser beams, leading to a virtually painless vaporization of tissue [31]. Lasers have indications for use in dentistry for incision, excision, and coagulation of intraoral soft tissue. They are well suited for surgical removal of intraoral hemangiomas because they offer a bloodless operational technique and avoid tissue damage. Advantages of laser therapy include minimal postoperative pain, minimally invasive surgery, and no need for sutures with no intraoperative or postoperative adverse effects [32, 33].

Laser treatment is currently used for thin, superficial lesions, ulcerated hemangiomas, and residual erythema and telangiectasias. Several lasers are used for hemangioma treatment, such as the pulsed dye laser (PDL), Nd:YAG laser, the KTP and the CO_2, and Erbium lasers [31–34].

The effective depth of penetration of PDL is minimal to a depth of around 1.2 mm; therefore, it is not very effective in treating deeper hemangiomas, which may continue to grow even if the superficial component recedes [34].

Nd:YAG laser is used for treating the deep component of hemangiomas of the oral cavity and requires very careful use by experienced physicians.

KTP lasers are also an option, especially for deeper, thicker lesions. The KTP laser is actually a type of Nd:YAG laser (1064 nm) that is modified when the 1064 nm light is passed through a KTP crystal. When the KTP laser is used with an intralesional bare fiber, the laser light is sent directly into the deep component of the hemangioma, delivering the maximum amount of laser energy to this section while limiting cutaneous damage [35]. This allows better lesion penetration than a PDL laser but it carries less risk of scarring than an Nd:YAG laser [36].

Currently, there are no optimal laser systems for hemangioma treatment [37].

Crisan et al. in 2010 confirmed that laser therapy in the treatment of vascular lesions was more effective than the sclerotherapy procedure [35], while Witman et al in 2006 revealed complications from PDL treatment of hemangiomas, including ulceration, pain, residual scarring components of hemangiomas, and in one instance life-threatening bleeding [38]. Therefore, laser and cryotherapy are not commonly used in treatment of haemangiomas due to scarring or hyperpigmentation, skin atrophy, and slight depression of the skin and due to high cost [39, 40].

The surgical treatment of oral hemangiomas, similar to other treatment modalities, has its own risks and advantages.

The advantage of the surgical treatment is that, unlike other forms of hemangioma treatment, it allows for a microscopic diagnosis. In addition, the complete surgical excision of these lesions offers the best chance of cure, but it is often accompanied with the risk of excessive postoperative bleeding and severe functional impairment of vital functions, such as swallowing, speech, and airway maintenance. Therefore, surgical intervention as a treatment modality for haemangioma is considered a last resort due to intraoperative bleeding, postoperative scarring, incomplete excision, recurrence, functional impairment, and surgical morbidity [15, 41].

4. Conclusion

Since sclerotherapy is a very effective, inexpensive, and easy-to-apply treatment modality, it should be regarded as the primary choice of treatment, especially for intraoral superficial hemangiomas.

Competing Interests

The authors declare that they have no competing interests.

References

[1] P. H. Corrêa, L. C. Caldeira Nunes, A. C. B. Rodrigues Johann, M. C. Ferreira de Aguiar, R. S. Gomez, and R. A. Mesquita, "Prevalence of oral hemangioma, vascular malformation and varix in a Brazilian population," *Brazilian Oral Research*, vol. 21, no. 1, pp. 40–45, 2007.

[2] A. A. de Lorimier, "Sclerotherapy for venous malformations," *Journal of Pediatric Surgery*, vol. 30, no. 2, pp. 188–194, 1995.

[3] C. L. Cardoso, L. M. P. da Silva Ramos Fernandes, J. F. Rocha, E. S. Gonçales, O. Ferreira Júnior, and L. A. de Assis Taveira, "Surgical approach of intraoral hemangioma," *Odontologia Clínico-Científica*, vol. 9, no. 2, pp. 177–180, 2010.

[4] A. C. B. Rodrigues Johann, M. C. Ferreira Aguiar, M. A. Vieira Do Carmo, R. S. Gomez, W. H. Castro, and R. A. Mesquita, "Sclerotherapy of benign oral vascular lesion with ethanolamine oleate: an open clinical trial with 30 lesions," *Oral Surgery, Oral Medicine, Oral Pathology, Oral Radiology and Endodontology*, vol. 100, no. 5, pp. 579–584, 2005.

[5] D. C. Gomes, R. S. Gomez, M. A. V. Carmo, W. H. Castro, and R. A. Gala-Garcia, "Mosque. Mucosal varicosities: case report treated with monoethanolamine oleate," *Medicina Oral, Patología Oral y Cirugía Bucal*, vol. 11, pp. E44–E46, 2006.

[6] H. Toledo, E. Castro, A. Castro, A. Soubhia, and F. B. Salvador Jr., "Hemangioma cavernoso de lábio inferior: caso clínico," *Revista Odontológica de Araçatuba*, vol. 25, no. 1, pp. 9–11, 2004.

[7] B. Prado, S. Trevisan, and D. Passarelli, "Estudo epidemiológico das lesões bucais no período de 5 anos," *Revista de Odontologia da Universidade de São Paulo*, vol. 22, no. 1, pp. 25–29, 2010.

[8] B. W. Neville, D. D. Damm, C. M. Allen, and J. E. Bouquot, "Patologia epitelial," in *Patologia Oral & Maxilofacial. Tradução de Danielle Resende Camisasa*, pp. 363–453, Elsevier, Rio de Janeiro, Brazil, 3rd edition, 2009.

[9] H. Yoshida, H. Yusa, and E. Ueno, "Use of doppler color flow imaging for differential diagnosis of vascular malformations. A preliminary report," *Journal of Oral and Maxillofacial Surgery*, vol. 53, no. 4, pp. 369–374, 1995.

[10] P. Redondo, "Vascular malformations (II). Diagnosis, pathology and treatment," *Actas Dermo-Sifiliograficas*, vol. 98, no. 4, pp. 219–235, 2007.

[11] J. N. McHeik, V. Renauld, G. Duport, P. Vergnes, and G. Levard, "Surgical treatment of haemangioma in infants," *British Journal of Plastic Surgery*, vol. 58, no. 8, pp. 1067–1072, 2005.

[12] M. Waner, J. Y. Suen, and S. Dinehart, "Treatment of hemangiomas of the head and neck," *Laryngoscope*, vol. 102, no. 10, pp. 1123–1132, 1992.

[13] S. Agarwal, "Treatment of oral hemangioma with 3% sodium tetradecyl sulfate: study of 20 cases," *Indian Journal of Otolaryngology and Head and Neck Surgery*, vol. 64, no. 3, pp. 205–207, 2012.

[14] B. Minkow, D. Laufer, and D. Gutman, "Treatment of oral hemangiomas with local sclerosing agents," *International Journal of Oral Surgery*, vol. 8, no. 1, pp. 18–21, 1979.

[15] H. Selim, A. Selim, A. Khachemoune, and S. A. F. A. Metwally, "Use of sclerosing agent in the management of oral and perioral hemangiomas: review and case reports," *Medical Science Monitor*, vol. 13, no. 9, pp. CS114–CS119, 2007.

[16] J. Seo, E. Utumi, C. Zambon, I. Pedron, and A. Rocha, "Escleroterapia de hemangioma labial," *Revistas de Odontologia*, vol. 17, no. 34, pp. 106–112, 2009.

[17] V. Jairath, S. Dayal, V. K. Jain et al., "Is sclerotherapy useful for cherry angiomas?" *Dermatologic Surgery*, vol. 40, no. 9, pp. 1022–1027, 2014.

[18] H. Winter, E. Dräger, and W. Sterry, "Sclerotherapy for treatment of hemangiomas," *Dermatologic Surgery*, vol. 26, no. 2, pp. 105–108, 2000.

[19] M. K. Parvathidevi, S. Koppal, T. Rukmangada, and A. R. Byatnal, "Management of haemangioma with sclerosing agent: a case report," *BMJ Case Reports*, vol. 2013, 2013.

[20] C. Bonet-Coloma, I. Mínguez-Martínez, C. Palma-Carrió, S. Galán-Gil, M. Peñarrocha-Diago, and J.-M. Mínguez-Sanz, "Clinical characteristics, treatment and outcome of 28 oral haemangiomas in pediatric patients," *Medicina Oral, Patologia Oral y Cirugia Bucal*, vol. 16, no. 1, pp. e19–e22, 2011.

[21] J. Hou, M. Wang, H. Tang, Y. Wang, and H. Huang, "Pingyangmycin sclerotherapy for infantile hemangiomas in oral and maxillofacial regions: an evaluation of 66 consecutive patients," *International Journal of Oral and Maxillofacial Surgery*, vol. 40, no. 11, pp. 1246–1251, 2011.

[22] I. Zanettini, R. N. Zanettini, and G. Gollo, "Sclerotherapy as an alternative treatment of oral vascular lesions," *Revista de Clínica e Pesquisa Odontológica*, vol. 2, pp. 119–126, 2005.

[23] G. M. Assis, S. Silva, P. Moraes, J. Amaral, and A. Germano, "Hemangioma de língua: relato de caso," *Revista de Cirurgia e Traumatologia Buco-Maxilo-Facial*, vol. 9, no. 2, pp. 59–66, 2009.

[24] C. Levy and L. Mandel, "Sclerotherapy of intraoral hemangioma," *The New York State Dental Journal*, vol. 78, no. 3, pp. 19–21, 2012.

[25] J. Van der Stricht, "The sclerosing therapy in congenital vascular defects," *International Angiology*, vol. 9, no. 3, pp. 224–227, 1990.

[26] T. Cadere, "Treatment of varices with ethoxysclerol," *Phebologie*, vol. 33, pp. 377–378, 1980.

[27] V. M. Lopez Perez, C. M. Hernandez Canete, and E. Rodriguez Moreno, "Sclerosing therapy in hemangiomas of the tongue," *Angiologia*, vol. 43, no. 6, pp. 228–230, 1991.

[28] R. A. Weiss, C. F. Feied, and M. A. Weiss, *Vein Diagnosis and Treatment*, McGraw-Hill, New York, NY, USA, 2001.

[29] S. Bhadoria, R. Saxena, and A. Lavania, "Management of haemangioma neck using sclerosing agent—a case report," *Journal of College of Medical Sciences-Nepal*, vol. 8, no. 1, pp. 56–59, 2012.

[30] S. I. M. L. Queiroz, G. M. de Assis, V. D. Silvestre, A. R. Germano, and J. S. P. da Silva, "Treatment of oral hemangioma with sclerotherapy: case report," *Jornal Vascular Brasileiro*, vol. 13, no. 3, 2014.

[31] J. T. Lambrecht, S. Stübinger, and Y. Hodei, "CO_2 laser therapy for intraoral hemangiomas," *Journal of Oral Laser Applications*, vol. 4, no. 2, pp. 89–96, 2004.

[32] J. T. Lambrecht, S. Stübinger, and Y. Hodel, "Treatment of intraoral hemangiomas with the CO_2 laser," *Schweizer Monatsschrift für Zahnmedizin*, vol. 114, no. 4, pp. 348–359, 2004.

[33] J. M. White, S. I. Chaudhry, J. J. Kudler, N. Sekandari, M. L. Schoelch, and S. Silverman Jr., "Nd:YAG and CO_2 laser therapy of oral mucosal lesions," *Journal of Clinical Laser Medicine and Surgery*, vol. 16, no. 6, pp. 299–304, 1998.

[34] R. Ashinoff and R. G. Geronemus, "Failure of the flashlamp-pumped pulsed dye laser to prevent progression to deep hemangioma," *Pediatric Dermatology*, vol. 10, no. 1, pp. 77–80, 1993.

[35] B. V. Crisan, M. Baciut, G. Baciut, R. S. Campian, and L. Crisan, "Laser treatment in oral and maxillofacial hemangioma and vascular malformations," *Timisoara Medica Journal*, vol. 60, no. 1, pp. 34–38, 2010.

[36] B. M. Achauer, B. Celikoz, and V. M. VanderKam, "Intralesional bare fiber laser treatment of hemangioma of infancy," *Plastic and Reconstructive Surgery*, vol. 101, no. 5, pp. 1212–1217, 1998.

[37] K. Batta, H. M. Goodyear, C. Moss, H. C. Williams, L. Hiller, and R. Waters, "Randomised controlled study of early pulsed dye laser treatment of uncomplicated childhood haemangiomas: results of a 1-year analysis," *The Lancet*, vol. 360, no. 9332, pp. 521–527, 2002.

[38] P. M. Witman, A. M. Wagner, K. Scherer, M. Waner, and I. J. Frieden, "Complications following pulsed dye laser treatment of superficial hemangiomas," *Lasers in Surgery and Medicine*, vol. 38, no. 2, pp. 116–123, 2006.

[39] I. Kaplan, S. Gassner, and Y. Shindel, "Carbon dioxide laser in head and neck surgery," *The American Journal of Surgery*, vol. 128, no. 4, pp. 543–544, 1974.

[40] T. Imai, N. Matsuo, T. Yamashita et al., "Two cases of haemangioma of the upper lip in infants—treatment using the Nd: YAG laser," *Aichi-Gakuin Dental Science*, vol. 4, pp. 35–44, 1991.

[41] J. Govrin-Yehudain, A. R. Moscona, N. Calderon, and B. Hirshowitz, "Treatment of hemangiomas by sclerosing agents: an experimental and clinical study," *Annals of Plastic Surgery*, vol. 18, no. 6, pp. 465–469, 1987.

13

Mandibular Canal Widening and Bell's Palsy:
Sequelae of Perineural Invasion in Oral Cancer

Gopinath Thilak Parepady Sundar,[1] Vishwanath Sherigar,[2] Sameep S. Shetty,[3] Shree Satya,[1] and Sourabh M. Gohil[1]

[1]Department of Oral and Maxillofacial Surgery, A.B. Shetty Memorial Institute of Dental Sciences, Mangalore, India
[2]K.S. Hegde Charitable Hospital, Mangalore, India
[3]Department of Oral and Maxillofacial Surgery, Manipal College of Dental Sciences, Manipal University, Manipal, India

Correspondence should be addressed to Sameep S. Shetty; sameep.shetty@manipal.edu

Academic Editor: Paolo Giacomo Arduino

Perineural invasion is an underrecognized route of metastatic spread along the nerve bundles within the nerve sheath into the surrounding tissues. It hinders the ability to establish local control as tumour cells can traverse along nerve tracts well beyond the extent of any local invasion rendering them inoperable and unresectable. Perineural invasion is a marker of poor prognosis. Oral submucous fibrosis with oral cancer constitutes a clinicopathologically distinct disease. Our case highlights an enigmatic presentation of oral submucous fibrosis and its coexistence with oral cancer presenting with unusual neurological disturbance of the inferior alveolar nerve and facial nerve and diffuse widening of the mandibular canal. The objective of this case report is to enumerate the significance of perineural invasion in determining the course of the disease and necessitate the need for future studies that can shed light on molecular mediators and pathogenesis of perineural spread.

1. Introduction

The mandibular canal widening is an unusual presentation related only to a few pathologic conditions affecting the lower jaw. Loss of cortical bone surrounding the mandibular canal appears as wide radiolucency on a radiograph, inferred as canal widening [1]. Generalized widening of the mandibular canal may indicate pathologies of neural tissue origin or those that secondarily invade the neural tissue [2, 3].

Perineural invasion (PNI) is considered as a distinct third mode of tumour metastasis for oral squamous cell carcinoma (OSCC) together with lymphatic and blood vessel invasion [4]. It can be detected by the histological presence of tumour cells inside the neural space or by imaging techniques [5]. The trigeminal and facial nerves are commonly infiltrated by the invading tumour cells, resulting in sensory as well as motor function disturbances in the head and neck region [6]. Ambiguous symptoms unrelated to primary site of origin often obfuscate the diagnosis. Clinicians need to be cognizant of multiple hidden causes of paraesthesia in the head and neck region that can have a local or a distant origin.

2. Case Report

A 48-year-old man with a swelling on the right side of his face below the lower lip reported to our Department of Oral and Maxillofacial Surgery. He presented with a six-month history of nonhealing ulcer in the right side of the buccal mucosa with an extraoral draining sinus and dysphagia for one month (Figure 1(a)).

In addition, he also presented with a two-month history of inability to close his right eye and deviation of the corner of the mouth to the left side followed by numbness in the lower lip and chin region. General health status of the patient and blood and urine analyses were unremarkable. Extraoral examination confirmed the classical signs of lower motor neuron type facial nerve palsy which included absence of wrinkles on the forehead, lagophthalmos of the right eye

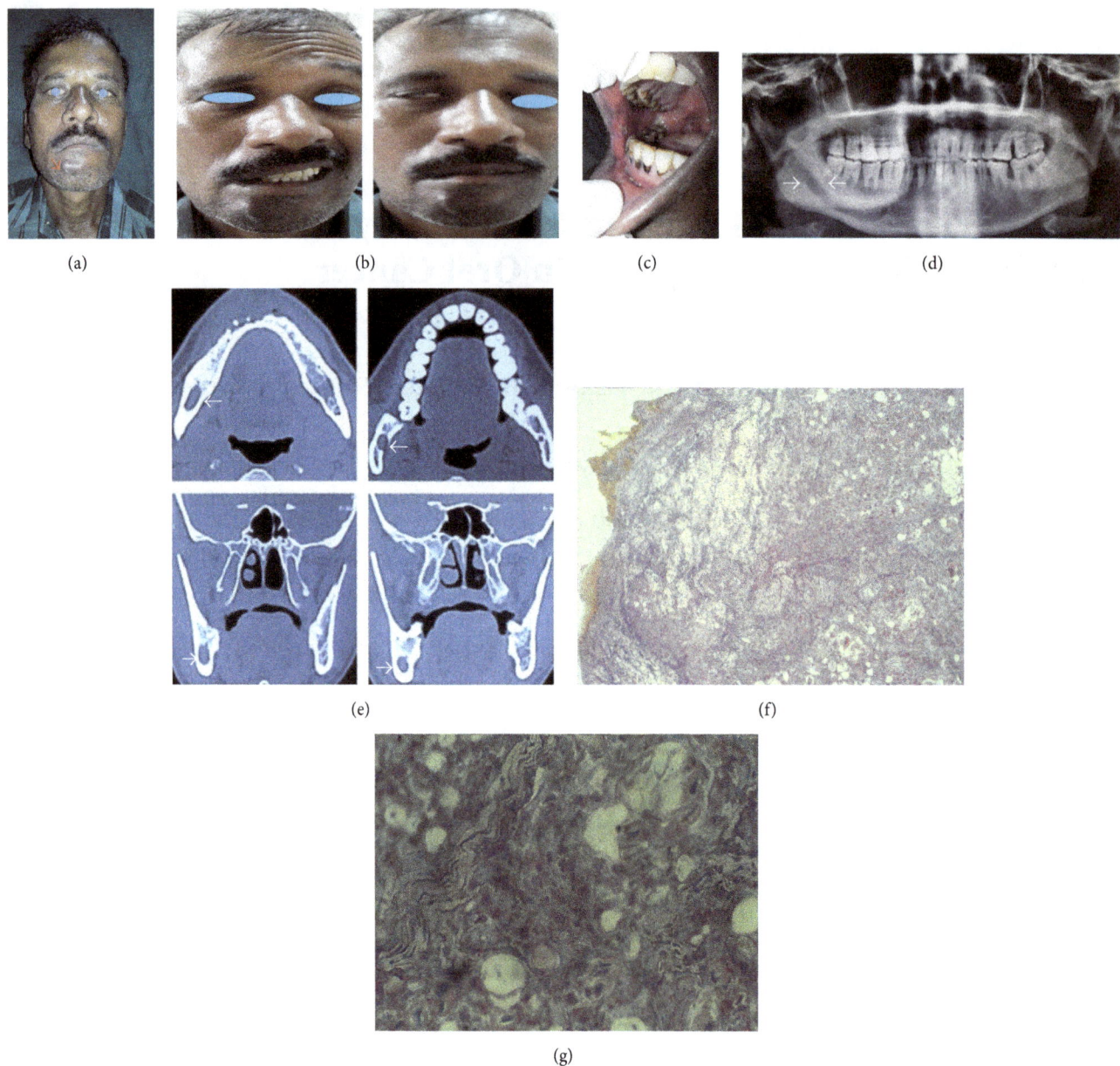

FIGURE 1: (a) Extraoral draining sinus. (b) Bells sign positive with absence of wrinkles on the affected side of the forehead. (c) Erosive ulcer extending from the corner of the mouth to retromolar trigone. (d) Diffuse widening of the mandibular canal extending from the mandibular foramen to the mental foramen. (e) Axial CT scan showing widening of the mandibular canal. (f) 10x view showing extensive PNI with the presence of tumour cells in the form of islands approximating the neural tissue. (g) 40x view showing intraneural tissue intermixed with tumour islands.

positive bells sign, flattening of the nasolabial fold [7], and deviation of the angle of the mouth on smile to the left side (Figure 1(b)). Paraesthesia of lower lip and chin suggested infiltration of the inferior alveolar nerve.

Intraoral examination revealed an erosive lesion approximately 6 × 2 cm in size, extending from the angle of the mouth on the right side anteriorly up to the retromolar trigone posteriorly. The floor was covered with a pseudomembranous slough, with rolled edges and erythematous margins. On palpation, there was induration, tenderness, and the presence of fibrous bands (Figure 1(c)). Soft, discrete, mobile submental lymph nodes and bilateral palpable soft submandibular lymph nodes were noted.

The panoramic radiograph revealed the presence of generalized bone loss with diffuse uniform enlargement of the mandibular canal, starting from the mandibular foramen to the mental foramen (Figure 1(d)). Spherical radiolucency and enlargement in the (R) mandibular canal were appreciated in multislice CT [8]. No breach in the cortical plates was seen (Figure 1(e)).

Incisional biopsy of the right buccal mucosa confirmed the clinical diagnosis of squamous cell carcinoma of right gingival-buccal sulcus. Histopathology sections revealed pleomorphic tumour cells with individual cell keratinization and dense peritumoural inflammatory response. Representative histological section demonstrating PNI (Modified Liebig Type A Classification) and infiltration of the epineurium was also seen [9, 10] (Figures 1(f) and 1(g))

The treatment plan included full-thickness, wide local excision of buccal mucosa, segmental mandibulectomy, and modified radical neck dissection preserving internal jugular vein, spinal accessory nerve, followed by reconstruction with the free fibula graft using reconstruction plate. The resected specimen showed well differentiated squamous cell carcinoma with margins and nodes free of tumour. Adjuvant radiotherapy was planned considering the PNI.

3. Discussion

Perineural invasion is well defined when at least 33% of the circumference of the nerve is surrounded by tumour cells. The biologic mechanism of PNI pathogenesis remains elusive with postulations that it relates to reciprocal signaling interactions and the intrinsic capacity of tumour cells to retort to signals within the peripheral nerve and promote invasion [11].

PNI is "a tropism of tumour cells for nerve bundles in the surrounding tissues" [4]. It is often linked with an aggressive behaviour, poor prognosis, recurrence, and higher likelihood of regional and distant occult micro and macro metastasis [12]. PNI has also been linked to stimulation of axogenesis that can lead to increased nerve density in and around neurotropic malignancies and further exacerbate tumour progression. PNI detection criteria include histopathological examination of the neural invasion, radiographic examination for osseous canal or foramen widening, and sensory complaints along the nerve distribution [13].

PNI is an important predictor for outcome of patients with SCC of the oral cavity and oropharynx. It is significantly associated with tumour differentiation, lymph node metastasis, depth of invasion, locoregional recurrence, and distant metastasis. Rahima et al. [14] concluded in their study that the 5-year disease-specific survival for patients with and without PNI was 56.6% and 94.6%, respectively ($P < .0001$).

The centrifugal and centripetal propagation of squamous cell carcinoma along the perineural space can demonstrate intracranial spread and jeopardise the available treatment options.

PNI in adenoid cystic carcinoma is well recognized; however, it should also be corroborated in oral squamous cell carcinoma specimens that have of late demonstrated PNI. The presence of PNI can connote a late stage disease and is a hallmark of subclinical invasion that can necessitate the need for aggressive resection, coincident management of neck lymph nodes, and the addition of adjuvant therapy. Targeted drug therapy for PNI in oral cancer is still at its infancy and can be a boon in the years to come. Patients with oral cancer often undergo adjuvant radiation for pathologically high risk features including positive nodal disease, extracapsular spread, and positive tumour margins. Excluding these high risk features, PNI is an independent risk factor necessitating the need for adjuvant radiation [15].

Widening of the mandibular canal is a classical sign of neurofibromatosis but it has been unusual so far in oral cancer. Intraosseous schwannomas may sometimes cause distension of the inferior alveolar canal; they typically produce well-defined unilocular radiolucency mimicking an odontogenic cyst or a tumour. The other causes of mandibular canal widening like perineuroma, multiple endocrine neoplasia syndrome type 2b, vascular leiomyoma, arteriovenous malformation, and traumatic neuroma have been reported in the literature [8].

The persistent paraesthesia of lower lip and chin region is a warning sign of a tumour or a malignancy compressing or invading the nerve.

Facial nerve and the trigeminal nerve are assumed to form a synapse at three strategic locations:

(1) Sphenopalatine ganglion

(2) Junction of the chorda tympani and the lingual nerve

(3) Parotid gland along the auriculotemporal branch of the mandibular nerve

Koivisto et al. (2016) [16] advocated that these synaptic points could provide a viable route for interneural spread of carcinoma from one nerve to another. The facial nerve palsy observed in our patient could be attributed to facial nerve involvement by the tumour cells that might have spread via the mandibular nerve.

The prognostic utility of PNI with respect to the diameter of the nerves is debated with conflicting results being reported from different series of cases. It has been postulated that the stroma of the perineural sheath promotes tumour growth, with the perineural space as a conduit for tumour growth. In view of this large diameter, nerves closer to the surgical margins may be associated with recurrence [17]. Contrary to this, Fagan et al. [18] in their study opined that PNI of small nerves is associated with an increased risk of local recurrence and cervical metastasis and is independent of extracapsular spread, a significant prognostic factor. A review by Woolgar cites OSCC demonstrating that PNI are all related to reduced survival rates and a significant risk of locoregional recurrence irrespective of the diameter of the nerves [19].

4. Conclusion

Oral squamous cell carcinoma often presents with a nonhealing exophytic/endophytic ulcer fixed to the underlying skin or the mucosa. This case differs from its usual presentation by its aggressive nature, multiple neural invasion, synchronization of submucous fibrosis and oral cancer, and diffuse widening of the mandibular canal. PNI is an independent risk factor for occult metastasis along with depth of invasion, size of primary tumour, differentiation, and immunosuppression. Further studies are warranted to elucidate its molecular biology of pathogenesis, histopathological pattern of PNI, and its significance in the prognosis. With a better understanding of the mechanisms involved, we can progress to develop therapeutic agents that can target this form of intriguing tumour spread.

Consent

Written consent was obtained by the authors for clinical photography and submission of patient photographs for publication.

Competing Interests

The authors declare that they have no competing interests.

References

[1] A. G. Farman and C. J. Nortje, "Panoramic radiographic appearance of the mandibular canal in health and in disease," in *Panoramic Radiology: Seminars on Maxillofacial Imaging and Interpretation*, pp. 107–118, Springer, Berlin, Germany, 2007.

[2] N. Raakesh, P. Sasikumar, V. Manojkumar, and G. K. Govind, "Progressively enlarging inferior alveolar nerve canal radiolucency-schwannoma?: a rare intraosseous lesion," *IJSS Case Reports & Reviews*, vol. 2, no. 2, pp. 10–12, 2015.

[3] K. Ikeda, K.-C. Ho, B. H. Nowicki, and V. M. Haughton, "Multiplanar MR and anatomic study of the mandibular canal," *American Journal of Neuroradiology*, vol. 17, no. 3, pp. 579–584, 1996.

[4] N. O. Binmadi and J. R. Basile, "Perineural invasion in oral squamous cell carcinoma: a discussion of significance and review of the literature," *Oral Oncology*, vol. 47, no. 11, pp. 1005–1010, 2011.

[5] J. Roh, T. Muelleman, O. Tawfik, and S. M. Thomas, "Perineural growth in head and neck squamous cell carcinoma: a review," *Oral Oncology*, vol. 51, no. 1, pp. 16–23, 2015.

[6] G. D. Parker and H. R. Harnsberger, "Clinical-radiologic issues in perineural tumor spread of malignant diseases of the extracranial head and neck," *Radiographics*, vol. 11, no. 3, pp. 383–399, 1991.

[7] D. H. Gilden, "Bell's palsy," *The New England Journal of Medicine*, vol. 351, no. 13, pp. 1323–1331, 2004.

[8] V. M. Vartiainen, M. Siponen, T. Salo, J. Rosberg, and M. Apaja-Sarkkinen, "Widening of the inferior alveolar canal: a case report with atypical lymphocytic infiltration of the nerve," *Oral Surgery, Oral Medicine, Oral Pathology, Oral Radiology, and Endodontology*, vol. 106, no. 4, pp. e35–e39, 2008.

[9] R. D. Laske, I. Scholz, K. Ikenberg et al., "Perineural invasion in squamous cell carcinoma of the oral cavity: histology, tumor stage, and outcome," *Laryngoscope Investigative Otolaryngology*, vol. 1, no. 1, pp. 13–18, 2016.

[10] R. P. Ekanayaka and W. M. Tilakaratne, "Oral submucous fibrosis: review on mechanisms of malignant transformation," *Oral Surgery, Oral Medicine, Oral Pathology and Oral Radiology*, vol. 122, no. 2, pp. 192–199, 2016.

[11] H. Liu, Q. Ma, Q. Xu et al., "Therapeutic potential of perineural invasion, hypoxia and desmoplasia in pancreatic cancer," *Current Pharmaceutical Design*, vol. 18, no. 17, pp. 2395–2403, 2012.

[12] J. Massano, F. S. Regateiro, G. Januário, and A. Ferreira, "Oral squamous cell carcinoma: review of prognostic and predictive factors," *Oral Surgery, Oral Medicine, Oral Pathology, Oral Radiology and Endodontology*, vol. 102, no. 1, pp. 67–76, 2006.

[13] M. Bagatin, Z. Orihovac, and A. M. Mohammed, "Perineural invasion by carcinoma of the lower lip," *Journal of Cranio-Maxillo-Facial Surgery*, vol. 23, no. 3, pp. 155–159, 1995.

[14] B. Rahima, S. Shingaki, M. Nagata, and C. Saito, "Prognostic significance of perineural invasion in oral and oropharyngeal carcinoma," *Oral Surgery, Oral Medicine, Oral Pathology, Oral Radiology, and Endodontology*, vol. 97, no. 4, pp. 423–431, 2004.

[15] B. K. Varsha, M. B. Radhika, S. Makarla, M. Kuriakose, G. V. V. Satya Kiran, and G. V. Padmalatha, "Perineural invasion in oral squamous cell carcinoma: case series and review of literature," *Journal of Oral and Maxillofacial Pathology*, vol. 19, no. 3, pp. 335–341, 2015.

[16] T. Koivisto, D. Chiona, L. L. Milroy, S. B. McClanahan, M. Ahmad, and W. R. Bowles, "Mandibular canal location: cone-beam computed tomography examination," *Journal of Endodontics*, vol. 42, no. 7, pp. 1018–1021, 2016.

[17] A. D. Merrilees, P. B. Bethwaite, G. L. Russell, R. G. Robinson, and B. Delahunt, "Parameters of perineural invasion in radical prostatectomy specimens lack prognostic significance," *Modern Pathology*, vol. 21, no. 9, pp. 1095–1100, 2008.

[18] J. J. Fagan, B. Collins, L. Barnes, F. D'Amico, E. N. Myers, and J. T. Johnson, "Perineural invasion in squamous cell carcinoma of the head and neck," *Archives of Otolaryngology—Head and Neck Surgery*, vol. 124, no. 6, pp. 637–640, 1998.

[19] J. A. Woolgar, "Histopathological prognosticators in oral and oropharyngeal squamous cell carcinoma," *Oral Oncology*, vol. 42, no. 3, pp. 229–239, 2006.

An Endocrine Jaw Lesion: Dentist Perspective in Diagnosis

Lavanya Kalapala,[1] Surapaneni Keerthi sai,[1] Suresh Babburi,[1] Aparna Venigalla,[1] Soujanya Pinisetti,[1] Ajay Benarji Kotti,[1] and Kiranmai Ganipineni[2]

[1]Department of Oral & Maxillofacial Pathology, Drs. Sudha & Nageswara Rao Siddhartha Institute of Dental Sciences, Chinoutpalli, Gannavaram, India
[2]Government Dental College, Vijayawada, India

Correspondence should be addressed to Surapaneni Keerthi sai; keethu.surapaneni@gmail.com

Academic Editor: Yuk-Kwan Chen

Brown tumor is a rare nonneoplastic focal giant cell lesion that occurs in hyperparathyroidism patients with a prevalence rate of 0.1% in jaws. We report an extremely rare case of brown tumor in mandible of a 40-year-old female patient that presented as the first clinical manifestation of hyperparathyroidism. Dentist played a pivotal role in the present case by the early diagnosis of lesion and its intervention.

1. Introduction

Hyperparathyroidism (HPT) is an endocrine disorder occurring due to increased secretion of paratharmone resulting in a complex of clinical, anatomical, and biochemical alterations [1]. HPT is categorized into 4 types: primary HPT is caused by parathyroid adenomas (85%), hyperplasias (10%), and carcinomas (5%). Secondary HPT occurs as a compensatory increase in paratharmone levels due to hypocalcemia or vitamin D deficiency. Tertiary HPT presents in patients with long-standing secondary HPT resulting in autonomous functioning of parathyroid gland. Fourth type is an ectopic variant seen in patients with other malignancies [2]. Many a times, hyperparathyroidism is discovered accidentally on routine biochemical and radiological investigations [3].

One of the skeletal lesions observed in HPT is brown tumor [4], also termed as Von Recklinghausen's disease of bone or osteitis cystica fibrosa. Due to the presence of excessive hemorrhage, vascularization, and hemosiderin deposits grossly, a characteristic brown color is attained and thus the name "BROWN TUMOR" is derived [5]. However, the term is a misnomer since it is not a true neoplasm [6].

Brown tumor is mostly asymptomatic, but occasionally it may present as a painful exophytic mass [1]. Radiographically it appears as a unilocular or multilocular lesion with an irregular periphery. Histologically it is a focal giant cell lesion which shows multinucleated giant cells within a fibrovascular stroma admixed with areas of hemorrhage and hemosiderin deposits [7].

We report a rare case of brown tumor occurring in mandible of a 40-year-old female patient that was the first clinical manifestation and presented as a multilocular radiolucency, which on further biochemical assessment confirmed the diagnosis of adenoma of parathyroid. Along with this case report other giant cell mimickers of oral cavity are also discussed.

2. Case Report

A 40-year-old female reported to the outpatient department with a chief complaint of pain in the lower left back tooth region since 6 months and associated swelling since 3 months. The swelling was initially small in size and gradually attained present size. Patient gave a history of weight loss since 1 year and traumatic incident 3 months before. Patient was hypertensive since 3 months and is under medication.

Extraorally, a swelling was observed on the left lower third of the face (Figures 1(a) and 1(b)) and on intraoral examination a swelling of 1×3 cm was observed extending from distal aspect of 34 to mesial aspect of 37 with no sulcus

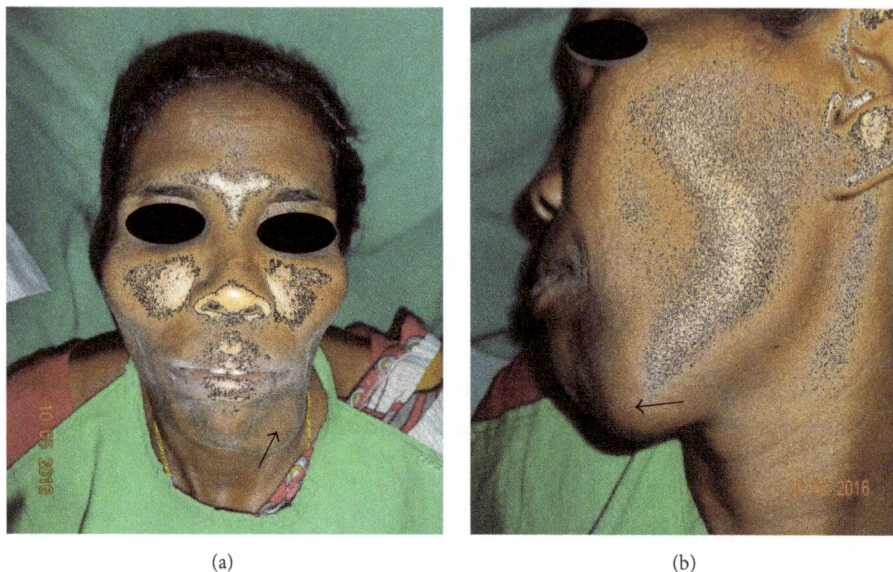

(a)   (b)

FIGURE 1: (a, b) Swelling in the left lower side of the mandible.

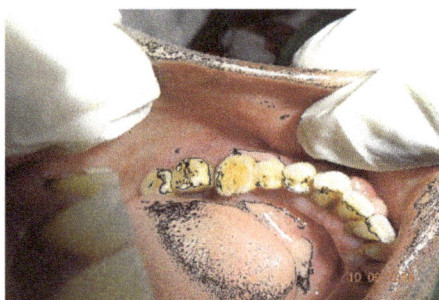

FIGURE 2: Intraoral swelling with no obliteration of sulcus.

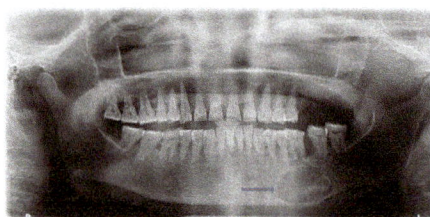

FIGURE 3: Radiolucent lesion extending from 34 to 37.

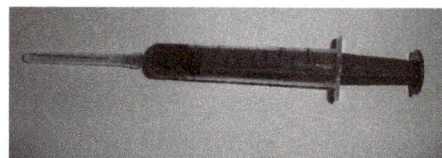

FIGURE 4: Aspirated fluid.

On microscopic examination, numerous osteoclast like multinucleated giant cells of varying sizes and shapes which were composed of 10–20 nuclei and dispersed in the background of mononuclear spindle shaped stromal cells were seen. Areas of osteoid, trabecular bone, hemorrhage, and inflammatory component were seen (Figures 5(a) and 5(b)). A giant cell lesion was diagnosed. But to rule out any metabolic disorders, the patient was advised a series of further investigations.

Hematological investigations demonstrated elevated serum calcium and phosphorus levels (13.1 mg% and 10 mg%, resp.) (normal: 8.8–11 mg%; 2.5–4.8 mg%, resp.) along with increased levels of paratharmone (711.3 pg/mL; normal: 12–72 pg/mL). Ultrasound of neck revealed a well-defined hypoechoic lesion of $2.2 \times 2 \times 3.1$ cm, located posteriorly and inferiorly to the right lobe of thyroid causing an indentation which was suggestive of a parathyroid adenoma. Skull radiographs revealed multiple well-defined osteolytic radiolucent lesions in the parietal and occipital areas (Figure 6).

Based on the clinical, radiographic, histological, and biochemical analyses, a final diagnosis of brown tumor associated with primary hyperparathyroidism was derived.

3. Discussion

Primary hyperparathyroidism is the 3rd most common endocrine disease [8], caused due to parathyroid adenomas,

obliteration and associated tooth mobility. Overlying mucosa was normal (Figure 2). On palpation the swelling was hard and tender.

OPG revealed a multilocular radiolucent lesion with well-defined margins was seen in relation to 35 and 36 with thinning out of inferior border of mandible. Loss of lamina dura in relation to 35 and 36 along with loss of continuity of mandibular canal was also observed (Figure 3).

FNAC revealed a reddish colored aspirate (Figure 4), composed of RBCs, lymphocytes, and neutrophils. Incisional biopsy was done and sent for histopathological evaluation.

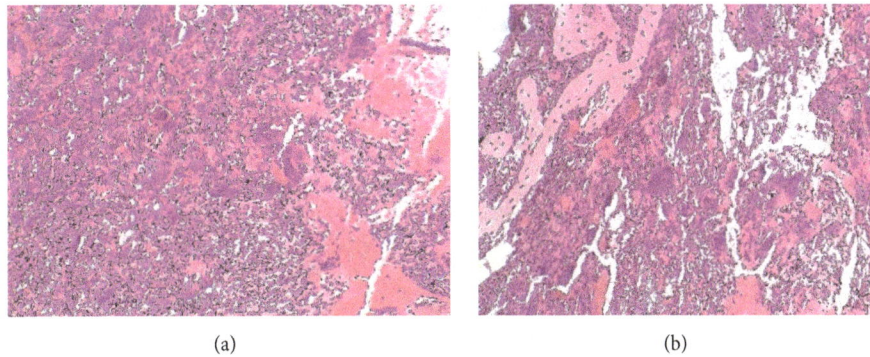

FIGURE 5: (a) Photomicrograph of 10x view shows numerous multinucleated giant cells and hemorrhagic areas. (b) Photomicrograph of 40x view shows multinucleated giant cells of varying size and shape and areas of osteoid.

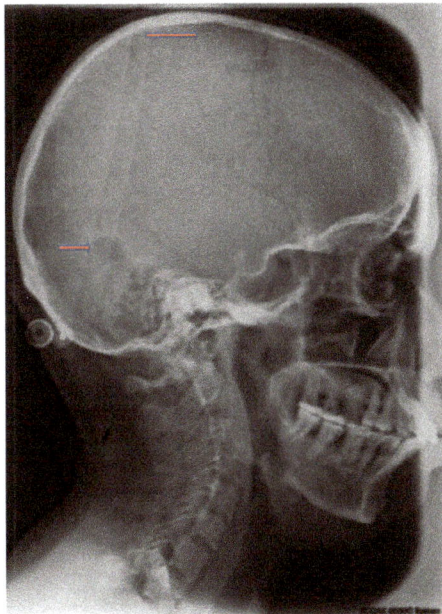

FIGURE 6: Skull radiograph showing osteolytic areas.

hyperplasias, or carcinomas [9]. Mostly it is a sporadic disease but may also occur in a familial pattern as autosomal dominant condition like hyperparathyroidism-jaw tumor syndrome (HPT-JT syndrome) and multiple endocrine neoplasia (MEN) syndrome [10].

HPT is commonly asymptomatic; however some patients may present with nonspecific symptoms like weight loss, GIT, and musculoskeletal disturbances [3] which was in concordance with our patient.

Classic skeletal lesions like bone resorption, bone cysts, brown tumors, and generalized osteopenia occur in less than 5% of all HPT cases [4]. The incidence of these skeletal lesions in HPT patients has fallen from 80% to 15% currently, which is attributed to better biochemical monitoring of calcium levels [5].

Brown tumor accounts for 10% of all skeletal lesions with a 0.1% incidence in jaws [5]. It is more common in females

older than 50 years. Gender predilection may be attributed to hormonal imbalances which are common in females more than males [7]. In the present case also the patient was a 40-year-old female.

Brown tumor may involve any part of skeleton but is commonly seen in ribs, clavicle, and pelvis. In head and neck region, mandible is commonly involved compared to maxilla especially the posterior region [11]. The present case was also reported in the posterior mandible.

Symptoms caused by the lesion depend on their size and location. Clinically, brown tumor may present as small asymptomatic swelling in jaws or as a painful exophytic mass which was observed in the present case.

Radiographically brown tumors appear as a well-defined unilocular or multilocular radiolucent lesion with expansion of affected bone. Additional features include subperiosteal resorption of phalanges of index and middle fingers, generalized osteopenia, and focal areas of skull demineralization-salt and pepper appearance [12]. Similar changes were noted in skull radiograph of the present patient. In the jaws, radiolucent lesions are observed with altered trabecular pattern, root resorption, root displacement, and loss of cortication around inferior alveolar canal. A characteristic feature in the jaws is loss of lamina dura surrounding the roots of involved teeth which is also seen in this case [3].

Histopathologically brown tumor exhibits dense fibroblastic stroma, areas of cystic degeneration, osteoid, hemorrhage, macrophages with hemosiderin, and multinucleated osteoclastic giant cells [7]. Cystic appearance is due to intraosseous bleeding and tissue degeneration [5]. Similar features were reported in the present case also.

Histologically brown tumor mimics many other giant cell lesions of head and neck region. Clinical, radiographic, and histological features of giant cell mimickers are discussed in Table 1.

On biochemical investigations, the present case showed hypercalcemia and hyperphosphatemia, along with increased parathyroid hormone level which aided in the confirmatory diagnosis. These alterations may be due to elevated parathyroid hormone which activates the osteolytic pump causing loss of calcium from bone to extracellular fluid resulting in elevated serum calcium levels. Ultrasound, CT scan, or

Table 1: Differential diagnosis of giant cell lesions.

S. number	Name of the lesion	Clinical features	Radiographic features	Histological features	Biochemical analysis		
					PTH	Ca	P
(1)	*Primary hyper-parathyroidism (present case)*	*Older aged women are commonly affected by predilection for mandible*	*Unilocular or multilocular radiolucency*	*Numerous multinucleated giant cells, areas of hemosiderin, and osteoid are seen*	√	√	√
(2)	Central giant cell granuloma	Common in younger individuals and occur in the anterior region of the jaw	Unilocular or multilocular radiolucency	Prominent but not numerous multinucleated giant cells, groups of collagen fibers, numerous foci of extravasated blood, and hemosiderin	—	—	—
(3)	Giant cell tumor or osteoclastoma	Common in third decade of life	Unilocular or multilocular radiolucency	Giant cells are scattered uniformly; areas of necrosis are seen	—	—	—
(4)	Aneurysmal bone cyst	Younger individuals	Multilocular with honeycomb or soap bubble appearance	Cavernous or sinusoidal blood filled spaces, multinucleated giant cells, hemosiderin pigment, and new osteoid formation are seen	—	—	—
(5)	Noonan-like multiple giant cell lesion syndrome	Autosomal dominant multiple congenital anomaly disorder, characterised by short stature, craniofacial dysmorphisms, and congenital heart defects (CHD)	Multilocular radiolucency	Numerous multinucleated giant cells, spindle shaped fibroblasts, and perivascular cuffing are seen	—	—	—
(6)	Cherubism	Painless, symmetric jaw lesions involving common maxilla	Multilocular radiolucencies with ground glass appearance	Numerous multinucleated giant cells, spindle shaped fibroblasts, and perivascular cuffing are seen	—	—	—

technetium scan techniques can also be used to detect the diseased parathyroid gland [10]. Ultrasound of our patient revealed a hypoechoic lesion lateral to thyroid gland suggesting a parathyroid adenoma.

Treatment of HPT is the first step in the management of brown tumor. After parathyroid excision, if the jaw lesions are smaller in size, they tend to regress spontaneously, either completely or partially. If the lesion is large and disfiguring or if the affected bone is weakened, surgical excision of the brown tumors is indicated. Some suggest systemic corticosteroids initially to decrease the size, followed by surgical excision of the residual lesion [11]. Recurrence is very rare once the hormonal levels revert back. Prognosis of the lesion mainly depends on the evaluation of biochemical parameters after extirpation of parathyroid tumor.

Even though the advancement of various diagnostic process and biochemical tests aids in early diagnosis of HPT, dentists should be aware of possible occurrence of brown tumor involving the jaws of undiagnosed patients as it may be presenting as the first manifestation. Hence it is essential that dentist should have the knowledge about oral manifestations associated with various systemic diseases leading to their early diagnosis.

4. Conclusion

Although the diagnosis of asymptomatic primary hyperparathyroidism is indicated by detection of elevated levels of calcium on routine biochemical analysis, still there is a possibility of patients presenting with advanced bony lesions.

Therefore all giant cell lesions occurring in the jaws have to be further evaluated biochemically to rule out primary hyperparathyroidism.

Competing Interests

There is no conflict of interests.

References

[1] A. D. Shetty, J. Namitha, L. James et al., "Brown tumor of mandible in association with primary hyperparathyroidism: a case report," *Journal of International Oral Health*, vol. 7, no. 2, pp. 50–52, 2015.

[2] A. L. S. Guimarães, L. Marques-Silva, C. C. Gomes, W. H. Castro, R. A. Mesquita, and R. S. Gomez, "Peripheral brown tumour of hyperparathyroidism in the oral cavity," *Oral Oncology Extra*, vol. 42, no. 3, pp. 91–93, 2006.

[3] S. Mittal, S. Sekhri, D. Gupta, and S. Goyal, "Oral manifestations of parathyroid disorders and its dental management," *Journal of Dental and Allied Sciences*, vol. 3, no. 1, pp. 34–38, 2014.

[4] G. Elbuken, O. Ozturk, B. Yazicioglu et al., "Primary hyperparathyroidism presented with peripheral brown tumor in the oral cavity: a case report," *Medicine Science*, vol. 3, no. 4, pp. 1751–1561, 2014.

[5] E. Proimos, T. S. Chimona, D. Tamiolakis, M. G. Tzanakakis, and C. E. Papadakis, "Brown tumor of the maxillary sinus in a patient with primary hyperparathyroidism: a case report," *Journal of Medical Case Reports*, vol. 3, article 7495, 2009.

[6] N. Soundarya, P. Sharada, N. Prakash, and G. L. Pradeep, "Bilateral maxillary brown tumors in a patient with primary hyperparathyroidism: report of a rare entity and review of literature," *Journal of Oral and Maxillofacial Pathology*, vol. 15, no. 1, pp. 56–59, 2011.

[7] M. M. Lessa, F. A. Sakae, R. K. Tsuji, B. C. Araújo Filho, R. L. Voegels, and O. Butugan, "Brown tumor of the facial bones: case report and literature review," *Ear, Nose and Throat Journal*, vol. 84, no. 7, pp. 432–434, 2005.

[8] S. Rai, S. K. Bhadada, V. Rattan, A. Bhansali, D. S. Rao, and V. Shah, "Oro-mandibular manifestations of primary hyperparathyroidism," *Indian Journal of Dental Research*, vol. 23, no. 3, pp. 384–387, 2012.

[9] K. T. Shanmugam, K. M. K. Masthan, A. Babu et al., "Hyperparathyroidism (Brown tumor)—a case report," *International Journal of Contemporary Dentistry*, vol. 2, no. 4, pp. 12–15, 2011.

[10] J. S. M. Daniels, "Primary hyperparathyroidism presenting as a palatal brown tumor," *Oral Surgery, Oral Medicine, Oral Pathology, Oral Radiology and Endodontology*, vol. 98, no. 4, pp. 409–413, 2004.

[11] M. M. Suarez-Cunqueiro, R. Schoen, A. Kersten, J. Klisch, and R. Schmelzeisen, "Brown tumor of the mandible as first manifestation of atypical parathyroid adenoma," *Journal of Oral and Maxillofacial Surgery*, vol. 62, no. 8, pp. 1024–1028, 2004.

[12] B. Chami, L. Benrachadi, N. El Omri et al., "Brown tumor of the palate as first manifestation of primary hyperparathyroidism: a case report," *Médecine Buccale Chirurgie Buccale*, vol. 17, pp. 287–291, 2011.

Geminated Maxillary Lateral Incisor with Two Root Canals

**Nayara Romano, Luis Eduardo Souza-Flamini, Isabela Lima Mendonça,
Ricardo Gariba Silva, and Antonio Miranda Cruz-Filho**

Department of Restorative Dentistry, School of Dentistry of Ribeirão Preto, University of São Paulo, Ribeirão Preto, SP, Brazil

Correspondence should be addressed to Antonio Miranda Cruz-Filho; cruz@forp.usp.br

Academic Editor: Daniel Torrés-Lagares

This paper reports a case of gemination in a maxillary lateral incisor with two root canals and crown-root dilaceration. A 16-year-old male patient was referred for endodontic treatment of the maxillary left lateral incisor and evaluation of esthetic and functional complaints in the anterior region. The patient reported trauma to the anterior primary teeth. There was no spontaneous pain, but the tooth responded positively to the vertical percussion test and negatively to the pulp vitality test. Clinical examination showed esthetic and functional alterations and normal periodontal tissues. CBCT imaging confirmed the suspicion of gemination and crown-root dilaceration and also revealed the presence of two root canals and periapical bone rarefaction. The root canals were instrumented with Reciproc R40 and 1% NaOCl irrigation and were filled by lateral condensation of gutta-percha and AH Plus sealer. The tooth was definitely restored with composite resin to recover esthetics. Continued follow-up over 6 months has shown absence of pain or clinical alterations as well as radiographic image suggestive of apical repair.

1. Introduction

Deep knowledge of the root canal system anatomy is critical to the success of endodontic therapy [1]. Anatomical complexities might interfere hindering the exploration, shaping, cleaning, and disinfection of root canals [2]. Maxillary lateral incisors normally have a single root and single canal [3]. However, morphological variations for these teeth include the presence of two [4, 5], three [6, 7], four [8], and even five canals [9], usually associated with the occurrence of traumatic stimuli during tooth development process [10]. Other morphological variations such as dens invagination [9, 11], radicular groove [12], and fusion [13] have also been reported.

Gemination is considered a rare developmental dental anomaly affecting the morphology of teeth. It is defined as a failed attempt at division of a single tooth germ by invagination, resulting in a tooth with a larger, incompletely separated crown having a single root and a single root canal [14]. There is no specific cause for the occurrence of this dental anomaly, which can be directly associated with genetic predisposition, racial characteristics, trauma to the primary dentition, and environmental factors, such as fetal exposure to alcohol, embryopathy by thalidomide, or hypervitaminosis A in pregnant women [15].

Although gemination can also occur in premolars and molars, it is more common in anterior teeth [16]. In most cases, the geminated tooth has a bifid crown with a single root and a single root canal and may cause aesthetic and functional impairments. Geminated and fused teeth have similar clinical appearance and clinical and radiographic examination is necessary for a differential diagnosis [17, 18].

In certain cases, two-dimensional imaging modalities, such as conventional and digital radiography, do not provide sufficient information for an accurate detection of anatomical variations and the use of more advanced auxiliary imagining resources is necessary. Imaging modalities that provide an undistorted three-dimensional vision of the tooth and surrounding structures should be used to improve the diagnostic potential. Cone-beam computed tomography (CBCT) provides three-dimensional images with high precision and sensitivity, offering a more detailed analysis of the case, a more adequate planning of root canal treatment, and guidance throughout the operative phase [19, 20].

This paper reports a case of gemination in a maxillary lateral incisor with two root canals and crown-root dilaceration.

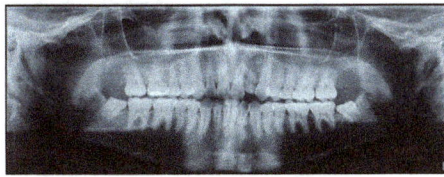

FIGURE 1: Panoramic radiograph.

2. Case Report

A 16-year-old male patient was referred to the clinic of our Department of Restorative Dentistry for evaluation and endodontic treatment of the maxillary left lateral incisor with main complaint of aesthetic and functional impairment.

Review of the patient's dental history revealed trauma to the anterior region of the maxilla around the age of 5 due to a fall. The traumatic injury caused intrusion of the primary maxillary left lateral incisor, which exfoliated after approximately 30 days. Orthodontic traction of the impacted permanent maxillary left lateral incisor was necessary at that time.

Clinical examination showed an amorphous, small, darkened crown and normal adjacent gingival tissues. There was no spontaneous pain, but the tooth responded positively to the vertical percussion test and negatively to the pulp vitality test.

Panoramic (Figure 1) and periapical (Figure 2(a)) radiographic examination suggested the existence of a developmental dental anomaly, with the presence of more than one root canal and apical rarefaction, as well as crown-root dilaceration. CBCT scanning was requested for a more detailed evaluation of the canal system and identification of dental structures (Figure 3) and confirmed gemination of the maxillary left lateral incisor and also revealed the presence of two root canals, one mesiobuccal and one distopalatal, and an apical hypodense lesion with destruction of the vestibular cortical bone (Figure 3, IMG 10 and 11).

Under local anesthesia and rubber dam isolation, access to the pulp chamber was achieved with round bur number 2 (KG Sorensen, São Paulo, SP, Brazil) and Endo-Z bur (Dentsply Maillefer, Ballaigues, Switzerland). Because of the difficulty in locating the canal openings, an ultrasonic insert (E3D; Helse Indústria e Comércio, Santa Rosa de Viterbo, SP, Brazil) was used to remove dentin tissue until finding the entrances of the mesiobuccal and distopalatal canals. The pulp chamber was flooded with 1% NaOCl solution and the canals were explored with a size 10 K file. In both canals, the working length was determined at 18 mm using an electronic apex locator (Root ZX mini, J Morita Mfg Corp., Japan). The canals were instrumented with R40 file of the Reciproc system (Reciproc, VDW, Germany) under irrigation with 1% NaOCl. Root canal treatment was carried out in two sessions. At the end of the first session, a calcium hydroxide paste was used as an intracanal medication and restorative glass-ionomer cement was used as temporary restoration. In the second session, after 15 days, the intracanal medication was removed and the canals were filled with 17% EDTA

for 3 minutes for smear layer removal, irrigated again with 1% NaOCl, dried with absorbent paper points, and filled by lateral condensation of gutta-percha and AH Plus sealer (Dentsply/De Trey, Konstanz, Germany) (Figure 2(b)). The patient returned after 30 days for evaluation. Clinically, the tooth presented no painful symptomatology or discomfort and the adjacent gingival tissue was normal. Radiographic examination showed no signs of failure in root canal filling or periapical lesions. The tooth crown was definitely restored with composite resin (Charisma A3, Heraeus Kulzer GmbH, Hanau, Germany) to recover esthetics and function.

Continued follow-up over 6 months has shown a successful outcome with absence of pain, no clinical alterations, and radiographic image suggestive of apical repair (Figure 2(c)).

3. Discussion

An accurate diagnosis and the precise determination of the number of root canals are mandatory for the success of endodontic treatment. Overlooking dental anomalies and anatomical variations can have a negative impact on treatment outcome, with persistence or exacerbation of preexisting apical periodontitis [21].

Radiographic examination is an important part in diagnosis and treatment planning [22]. Periapical radiographs with variations of angulation can be obtained to increase their accuracy in identifying anatomical anomalies [23]. However, conventional radiography offers limited information because it provides a two-dimensional image and there is a possibility of distortion and superimposition of structures. Computed tomography provides three-dimensional images, reproducing the structures more precisely and allowing a more accurate diagnosis [24]. In the present case, CBCT was essential to confirm the diagnosis of gemination as well as to determine the exact number and the precise location of the canals in order to have a safer access to the canal system during shaping, cleaning, and filling procedures. It should also be mentioned that the use of a surgical microscope is a widely employed clinical resource for the cases in which difficulty is experienced in the localization of root canals [25].

The maxillary lateral incisor usually has a single root and a single canal [3, 26]. However, cases of maxillary lateral incisors with more than one canal and separate roots have been reported [4, 8, 27]. Variations in the number of canals are associated with dental anomalies or intrusive trauma to the primary teeth during the development of the permanent successors [27, 28].

Gemination is less prevalent in the permanent dentition than in the primary dentition, affecting mainly maxillary incisors and canines [29]. The incidence of gemination in permanent teeth has been shown to range from 0.1% to 1% [30]. This dental anomaly has a direct impact on the development of the dentition, altering the mesiodistal dimension of the anomalous tooth and its alignment in the dental arch [31]. In the present case, the remainder of the crown showed a deviation relative to the long axis of the root, which was diagnosed as crown-root dilaceration. Dilaceration can affect any region of the tooth from the crown

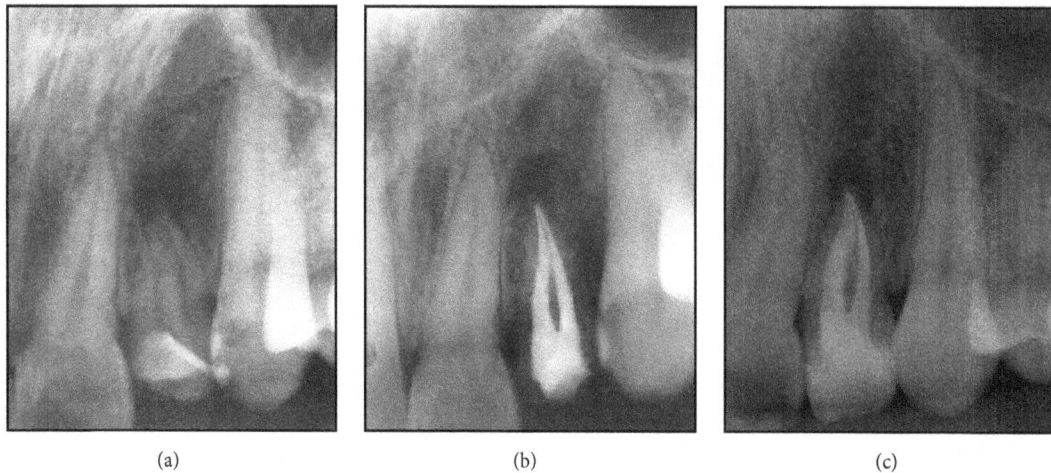

(a)   (b)   (c)

FIGURE 2: Operative imaging sequence. (a) Initial radiograph suggesting a geminated tooth; (b) final radiograph; (c) follow-up over 6 months' radiograph.

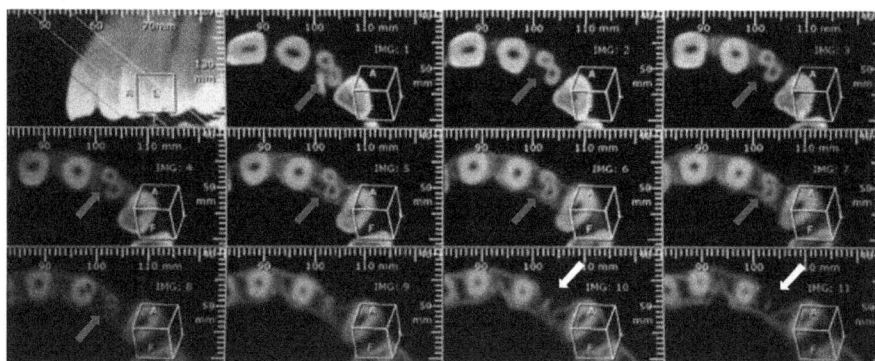

FIGURE 3: 3D reconstruction of CBCT images with 0.25 mm axial slice thickness and 0.25 mm slice interval. Images 1–8 indicate the presence of two root canals in the maxillary left lateral incisor. Images 10 and 11 show apical rarefaction with destruction of the vestibular cortical bone.

to the root apex. Crown dilaceration in permanent teeth is more frequent in cases with history of avulsion or intrusion of the primary predecessor. Traumatic dental injuries in the primary dentition occur more often in children between 1.5 and 3.5 years old [22, 32].

The etiology of gemination is not clear, but it is known to be associated with trauma to the primary dentition during the development of the permanent tooth germ. Some authors have also claimed that gemination could be the result of the interaction of hereditary genetic variations and environmental factors [33, 34]. In the present case, the diagnosis of gemination was established based on patient's dental history, CBCT imaging, and the concept of gemination reported in the literature.

Gemination can often be confused with fusion, which is a developmental dental anomaly characterized by the union of two adjacent tooth germs, resulting in a reduction in the number of teeth in affected arch. The differential diagnosis is usually made by counting the number of teeth in the arch, which is not altered in the cases of gemination [18, 35].

Developmental dental anomalies like gemination can cause functional, orthodontic, endodontic, and esthetic impairments and represent a challenge for dentists because, in most cases, a multidisciplinary approach is required to obtain the best treatment and a successful outcome [36].

4. Conclusion

Although it is considered a rare developmental dental anomaly with low prevalence, the occurrence of gemination deserves attention in clinical practice. Knowledge of the literature-based definition of this anomaly, review of dental history, and the use of accurate imaging resources, such as CBCT, are essential for a correct diagnosis and establishment of an adequate treatment plan in geminated teeth.

Consent

A written informed consent was obtained from the patient's parents for the publication of this case report and disclosure of images.

Disclosure

The study was conducted at School of Ribeirão Preto, University of São Paulo, Brazil.

Competing Interests

The authors declare that they have no competing interests regarding the publication of this manuscript.

References

[1] F. J. Vertucci, "Root canal morphology and its relationship to endodontic procedures," *Endodontic Topics*, vol. 10, no. 1, pp. 3–29, 2005.

[2] J. O. Andreasen, B. Sundström, and J. J. Ravn, "The effect of traumatic injuries to primary teeth on their permanent successors: I. A clinical and histologic study of 117 injured permanent teeth," *European Journal of Oral Sciences*, vol. 79, no. 3, pp. 219–283, 1971.

[3] F. J. Vertucci, "Root canal anatomy of the human permanent teeth," *Oral Surgery, Oral Medicine, Oral Pathology*, vol. 58, no. 5, pp. 589–599, 1984.

[4] M.-H. Lee, J.-H. Ha, M.-U. Jin, Y.-K. Kim, and S.-K. Kim, "Endodontic treatment of maxillary lateral incisors with anatomical variations," *Restorative Dentistry & Endodontics*, vol. 38, no. 4, pp. 253–257, 2013.

[5] A. Mohan, A. Rajesh Ebenezar, L. George, Sujathan, and S. Josy, "Maxillary lateral incisors with two canals and two separate curved roots," *Contemporary Clinical Dentistry*, vol. 3, no. 4, pp. 519–521, 2012.

[6] M. Jung, "Endodontic treatment of dens invaginatus type III with three root canals and open apical foramen," *International Endodontic Journal*, vol. 37, no. 3, pp. 205–213, 2004.

[7] M. Peix-Sánchez and R. Miñana-Laliga, "A case of unusual anatomy: a maxillary lateral incisor with three canals," *International Endodontic Journal*, vol. 32, no. 3, pp. 236–240, 1999.

[8] A. Nosrat and S. C. Schneider, "Endodontic management of a maxillary lateral incisor with 4 root canals and a dens invaginatus tract," *Journal of Endodontics*, vol. 41, no. 7, pp. 1167–1171, 2015.

[9] S. Jaikailash, M. Kavitha, M. S. Ranjani, and B. Saravanan, "Five root canals in peg lateral incisor with dens invaginatus: a case report with new nomenclature for the five canals," *Journal of Conservative Dentistry*, vol. 17, no. 4, pp. 379–381, 2014.

[10] M. Diab and H. E. El Badrawy, "Intrusion injuries of primary incisors. Part III: effects on the permanent successors," *Quintessence International*, vol. 31, no. 6, pp. 377–384, 2000.

[11] M. Bahmani, A. Adl, S. Javanmardi, and S. Naghizadeh, "Diagnosis and treatment of a type III dens invagination using cone-beam computed tomography," *Iranian Endodontic Journal*, vol. 11, no. 4, pp. 341–346, 2016.

[12] K. Kishan, V. Hegde, K. Ponnappa, T. Girish, and M. Ponappa, "Management of palato radicular groove in a maxillary lateral incisor," *Journal of Natural Science, Biology and Medicine*, vol. 5, no. 1, pp. 178–181, 2014.

[13] A. Yagci, K. Cantekin, S. K. Buyuk, and K. Pala, "The multidisciplinary management of fused maxillary lateral incisor with a supernumerary tooth in cleft lip adolescence," *Case Reports in Dentistry*, vol. 2014, Article ID 459416, 5 pages, 2014.

[14] A. J. Pereira, R. A. Fidel, and S. R. Fidel, "Maxillary lateral incisor with two root canals: fusion, gemination or dens invaginatus?" *Brazilian dental journal*, vol. 11, no. 2, pp. 141–146, 2000.

[15] T. Cetinbas, S. Halil, M. O. Akcam, S. Sari, and S. Cetiner, "Hemisection of a fused tooth," *Oral Surgery, Oral Medicine, Oral Pathology, Oral Radiology, and Endodontics*, vol. 104, no. 4, pp. 120–124, 2007.

[16] G. Shashirekha and A. Jena, "Prevalence and incidence of gemination and fusion in maxillary lateral incisors in odisha population and related case report," *Journal of Clinical and Diagnostic Research*, vol. 7, no. 10, pp. 2326–2329, 2013.

[17] J. M. Hernández-Guisado, D. Torres-Lagares, P. Infante-Cossío, and J. L. Gutiérrez-Pérez, "Dental gemination: report of case," *Medicina Oral*, vol. 7, no. 3, pp. 231–236, 2002.

[18] S. Sener, N. Unlu, F. A. Basciftci, and G. Bozdag, "Bilateral geminated teeth with talon cusps: a case report," *European Journal of Dentistry*, vol. 6, no. 4, pp. 440–444, 2012.

[19] S. Talwar, S. Utneja, R. R. Nawal, A. Kaushik, D. Srivastava, and S. S. Oberoy, "Role of cone-beam computed tomography in diagnosis of vertical root fractures: a systematic review and meta-analysis," *Journal of Endodontics*, vol. 42, no. 1, pp. 12–24, 2016.

[20] T. Venskutonis, G. Plotino, G. Juodzbalys, and L. Mickevičiene, "The importance of cone-beam computed tomography in the management of endodontic problems: a review of the literature," *Journal of Endodontics*, vol. 40, no. 12, pp. 1895–1901, 2014.

[21] P. N. R. Nair, "On the causes of persistent apical periodontitis: a review," *International Endodontic Journal*, vol. 39, no. 4, pp. 249–281, 2006.

[22] S. Sharma, S. Grover, V. Sharma, D. Srivastava, and M. Mittal, "Endodontic and esthetic management of a dilacerated maxillary central incisor having two root canals using cone beam computed tomography as a diagnostic aid," *Case Reports in Dentistry*, vol. 2014, Article ID 861942, 7 pages, 2014.

[23] R. Garlapati, B. S. Venigalla, R. Chintamani, and J. Thumu, "Re-treatment of a two-rooted maxillary central incisor—a case report," *Journal of Clinical and Diagnostic Research*, vol. 8, no. 2, pp. 253–255, 2014.

[24] N. Cohenca and H. Shemesh, "Clinical applications of cone beam computed tomography in endodontics: a comprehensive review," *Quintessence International*, vol. 46, no. 8, pp. 657–668, 2015.

[25] E. Shadmehr, S. Kiaani, and P. Mahdavian, "Nonsurgical endodontic treatment of a maxillary lateral incisor with dens invaginatus type II: a case report," *Dental Research Journal*, vol. 12, no. 2, pp. 187–191, 2015.

[26] S. Sert and G. S. Bayirli, "Evaluation of the root canal configurations of the mandibular and maxillary permanent teeth by gender in the Turkish population," *Journal of Endodontics*, vol. 30, no. 6, pp. 391–398, 2004.

[27] N. Shokouhinejad, M. S. Sheykhrezaee, and H. Assadian, "Endodontic treatment of two-canalled maxillary central and lateral incisors: a case report," *Iranian Endodontic Journal*, vol. 4, no. 2, pp. 79–80, 2009.

[28] T. S. Mellara, P. Nelson-Filho, A. M. Queiroz, M. Santamaria Júnior, R. A. Silva, and L. A. Silva, "Crown dilaceration in permanente teeth after trauma to the primary predecessor: report of three cases," *Brazilian Dental Journal*, vol. 23, no. 5, pp. 591–596, 2012.

[29] L. Mahendra, S. Govindarajan, M. Jayanandan, S. M. Shamsudeen, N. Kumar, and R. Madasamy, "Complete bilateral

gemination of maxillary incisors with separate root canals," *Case Reports in Dentistry*, vol. 2014, Article ID 425343, 4 pages, 2014.

[30] W. K. Duncan and M. L. Helpin, "Bilateral fusion and gemination: a literature analysis and case report," *Oral Surgery, Oral Medicine, Oral Pathology*, vol. 64, no. 1, pp. 82–87, 1987.

[31] R. L. Spuller and M. Harrington, "Gemination of a maxillary permanent central incisor treated by autogenous transplantation of a supernumerary incisor: case report," *Pediatric Dentistry*, vol. 8, no. 4, pp. 299–302, 1986.

[32] J. O. Andreasen, F. M. Andreasen, and L. Andersson, *Textbook and Color Atlas of Traumatic Injuries to the Teeth*, Blackwell, Oxford, UK, 4th edition, 2007.

[33] P. S. Grover and L. Lorton, "Gemination and twinning in the permanent dentition," *Oral Surgery, Oral Medicine, Oral Pathology*, vol. 59, no. 3, pp. 313–318, 1985.

[34] F. S. F. Tomazinho, F. Baratto-Filho, D. P. Leonardi, G. A. Haragushiku, and E. A. de Campos, "Occurrence of talon cusp on a geminated maxillary central incisor: a case report," *Journal of Oral Science*, vol. 51, no. 2, pp. 297–300, 2009.

[35] E. B. Tuna, M. Yildirim, F. Seymen, K. Gencay, and M. Ozgen, "Fused teeth: a review of the treatment options," *Journal of Dentistry for Children*, vol. 76, no. 2, pp. 109–116, 2009.

[36] G. Sammartino, V. Cerone, R. Gasparro, F. Riccitiello, and O. Trosino, "Multidisciplinary approach to fused maxillary central incisors: a case report," *Journal of Medical Case Reports*, vol. 8, article 398, 2014.

Apical Revascularization after Delayed Tooth Replantation: An Unusual Case

**Marília Pacífico Lucisano, Paulo Nelson-Filho,
Lea Assed Bezerra Silva, Raquel Assed Bezerra Silva, Fabricio Kitazono de Carvalho,
and Alexandra Mussolino de Queiroz**

Department of Pediatric Dentistry, School of Dentistry of Ribeirão Preto, University of São Paulo, Ribeirão Preto, SP, Brazil

Correspondence should be addressed to Marília Pacífico Lucisano; marilia.lucisano@forp.usp.br

Academic Editor: Muawia A. Qudeimat

The aim of this paper is to present the clinical and radiological outcome of the treatment involving a delayed tooth replantation after an avulsed immature permanent incisor, with a follow-up of 1 year and 6 months. An 8-year-old boy was referred after dental trauma that occurred on the previous day. The permanent maxillary right central incisor (tooth 11) had been avulsed. The tooth was hand-held during endodontic therapy and an intracanal medication application with calcium hydroxide-based paste was performed. An apical plug with mineral trioxide aggregate (MTA) was introduced into the apical portion of the canal. When the avulsed tooth was replanted with digital pressure, a blood clot had formed within the socket, which moved the MTA apical plug about 2 mm inside of the root canal. These procedures developed apical revascularization, which promoted a successful endodontic outcome, evidenced by apical closure, slight increase in root length, and absence of signs of external root resorption, during a follow-up of 1 year and 6 months.

1. Introduction

Tooth avulsion is one of the most severe types of trauma, which often affects young permanent dentition [1]. In this type of injury, a tooth is completely displaced from its alveolar socket, affecting the pulp tissue, periodontal ligament, dental hard tissues, and alveolar bone [2]. Although the best therapy for avulsed teeth is immediate replantation [3], it is not always possible in clinical conditions [4]. Consequently, delayed replantation is often required [5].

Replacement [6] and inflammatory external root resorption [7] commonly affect delayed reimplanted teeth. Both are progressive processes that damage the root structure, potentially leading to tooth loss [8].

Recently, revascularization therapy has been proposed as an alternative approach for immature necrotic teeth, with the advantage of inducing root-end development, thickening of radicular dentin, and reinforcement [9, 10].

The revascularization treatment protocol basically involves the following procedures: disinfection of the pulp space with an effective intracanal medication between sessions, commonly using a bi- or triantibiotic paste [11] or a calcium hydroxide-based paste [12, 13]; overinstrumentation to induce bleeding and production of a scaffold into the canal space; and placement of an MTA barrier on the blood clot followed by a tight sealing of the coronal access cavity [11]. It has been proposed that blood clot formation in the canal space is the source of stem cells from the apical papilla [14], which play a key role during wound healing [15].

This study aimed to describe an unusual case in which apical revascularization associated with delayed tooth replantation was performed.

2. Case Report

An 8-year-old boy was referred to the Pediatric Dentistry Clinic after dental trauma occurred on the previous day as a result of a bicycle accident. The patient arrived at the dental clinic about 17 hours after the trauma. During the clinical examination, the permanent maxillary right central incisor (tooth 11) had been avulsed, which was kept at an extraoral dry time of 13 hours. After this period, the avulsed tooth was transferred to a bottle with milk. The child was systemically healthy and there was no relevant medical history. A signed, written informed consent form was obtained from the patient's guardian.

Intraoral and radiographic examination revealed that, besides tooth avulsion, extrusion of the permanent maxillary left central incisor (tooth 21), slight intrusion of the permanent maxillary right lateral incisor (tooth 12), and lateral luxation of the permanent maxillary left lateral incisor (tooth 22) had occurred. Additionally, all of these teeth presented uncomplicated crown fractures (involving only enamel).

The chosen treatment sequence for this case is described below.

First, the avulsed tooth (tooth 11) was gently washed with saline solution and the nonvital periodontal fibers were removed from the root surface. Thereafter, the tooth was hand-held (by the coronal portion) during endodontic therapy, including access cavity preparation, pulpectomy, and root canal instrumentation with a K-file # 80 (Maillefer, Ballaigues, Switzerland) at 1 mm short of the root canal length, under irrigation with 1% sodium hypochlorite (NaOCl). After biomechanical preparation, the root canal was dried with sterile paper points and an intracanal medication with calcium hydroxide-based paste (Calen®, SS White Artigos Dentários Ltda., Rio de Janeiro, RJ, Brazil) was performed. The Calen paste is composed of 2.5 g calcium hydroxide, 0.5 g zinc oxide p.a., 0.05 g colophony, and 2 mL polyethylene glycol 400 (vehicle). Then, the coronal access was temporarily sealed with a sterile cotton pellet and glass-ionomer cement (Vidrion R®, SS White Artigos Dentários Ltda., Rio de Janeiro, RJ, Brazil). After that, mineral trioxide aggregate (ProRoot MTA, Dentsply Tulsa Dental, Tulsa, OK) was introduced into the apical portion of the canal, creating an apical plug, as recommended by the American Academy of Pediatric Dentistry (2014) [16]. No treatment was performed on the root surface after removal of nonviable periodontal ligament fibers [17]. After local anesthesia, the socket was gently curetted to remove any coagulum or granulation tissue and was washed with saline solution. When the avulsed tooth was replanted with digital pressure, a blood clot was formed within the socket, which moved the MTA apical plug about 2 mm to the inside of root canal. This unintentional procedure worked like apical revascularization, since the apical third of the canal was filled with a blood clot rich in stem cells, which were biostimulated by MTA (Figure 1(a)).

The teeth were then prepared for receiving splinting, involving acid etching, application of a bonding agent, and repositioning of the extruded tooth (tooth 21). The teeth were splinted from canine to canine, excluding the slightly intruded right lateral incisor (tooth 12), with composite resin and a 0.4 orthodontic wire. Systemic treatment included 7 days of 250 mg amoxicillin 3 times daily. The patient received instructions to have a soft diet and was informed on the importance of maintaining oral hygiene and the use of chlorhexidine mouthwash was recommended twice a day for 2 weeks. After 4 weeks, the splint was removed and the patient did not present any postoperative clinical or radiographic complications. The enamel fractures were restored with composite resin (Filtek Z250 XT, 3M ESPE, St. Paul, MN, USA).

After one month, it was necessary to endodontically treat the left central incisor (tooth 21) due to negative response to the cold sensitivity test. Endodontic treatment included access cavity preparation, root canal instrumentation up to a K-file # 80 under irrigation with 1% NaOCl, intracanal dressing with calcium hydroxide-based paste for 2 weeks, and obturation with gutta-percha points and a calcium hydroxide-based sealer (Sealapex; Kerr Corporation, Orange, CA, USA).

The patient was followed up regularly and, after 2 months, the radiographic examination revealed that the replanted tooth (tooth 11) showed apical closure and a slight increase in root length (Figure 1(b)).

The replanted tooth (tooth 11) was then obturated with gutta-percha points and a calcium hydroxide-based sealer, up to the limit of the apical plug.

The patient was followed up every month and after 1 year and 6 months. As shown in Figures 1(c) and 1(d), periapical radiographic examination showed apical closure and no sign of external root resorption of the replanted right central incisor (tooth 11). Clinically, the tooth remained with no symptomatology and mobility. Also, the left central incisor (tooth 21) remained with no radiographic signs of external root resorption and the lateral incisors (teeth 12 and 22) have shown continued root development.

3. Discussion

Currently, clinical management of delayed tooth replantation still represents a challenge for dentists. The literature has extensively demonstrated that 1 hour of extraoral dry time is critical, and after this period the periodontal ligament (PDL) cells remaining on the root surface of the avulsed tooth are less likely to be viable [7]. According to Guidelines from the International Association of Dental Traumatology, in conditions of dry time longer than 1 hour, like the present case, the PDL cells will be necrotic and are not expected to heal and thus need to be removed. In this situation, the delayed replanted tooth has a poor long-term prognosis and the expected outcome will be replacement due to external root resorption [17].

In the case described in this study, the treatment protocol was based on current guidelines for avulsed permanent teeth, which developed apical revascularization. It is highlighted that when the treatments were performed, pulp revascularization was not yet well established in the literature as a safe and effective treatment. Thus, it was decided to perform conventional treatment for both teeth. The procedure performed on the replanted tooth apparently promoted a successful endodontic outcome, as evidenced radiographically by apical closure and slight increase in root length. This response is consistent with previous reports on pulp revascularization in immature necrotic permanent teeth [12]. Recently, regenerative endodontic procedures have been applied to replanted permanent teeth after a brief [18] or >8 hours' extra-alveolar period [19] with promising results.

(a)

(b)

(c)

(d)

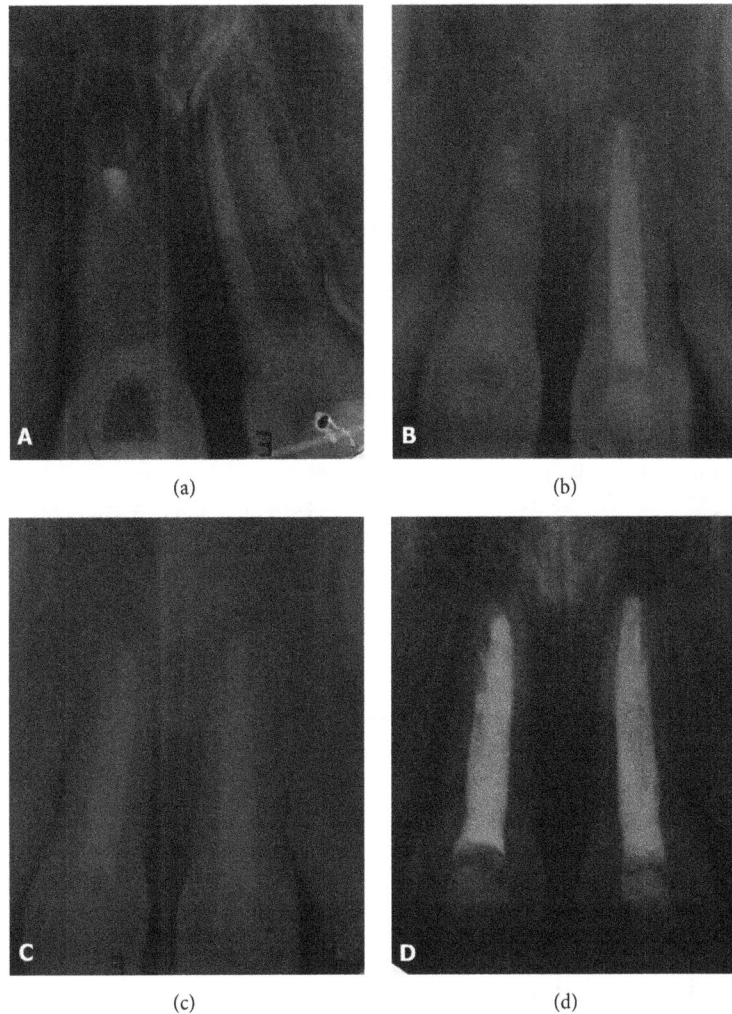

FIGURE 1: (a) Initial radiograph after tooth replantation (tooth 11), evidencing the incomplete root formation, the MTA apical plug about 2 mm inside of root canal, and the intracanal medication with calcium hydroxide-based paste. (b) Radiographic examination after 2 months, revealing apical closure and slight increase in root length of the replanted tooth (tooth 11). Endodontic treatment was performed on the left central incisor (tooth 21). (c) Radiographic examination 6 months after treatment of tooth 11, revealing apical closure. (d) Final radiographic examination, after a follow-up of 1 year and 6 months, revealing apical closure and no sign of external root resorption of the replanted right central incisor (tooth 11).

It is noteworthy that the revascularization of pulp space and methods to promote it are among the future areas of research on promising treatment procedures for avulsed teeth recommended by Guidelines for the Management of Traumatic Dental Injuries [17].

Revascularization has emerged as a promising alternative treatment to conventional apexification, presenting advantages such as root-end development and radicular reinforcement [10, 20]. The nature of tissues formed in the canal after revascularization therapy was first described by Thibodeau et al. [21] after performing a study in immature dog teeth. It was observed that cementum-, bone-, and periodontal ligament-like tissues were formed, which was subsequently confirmed by other *in vivo* studies [22–24]. According to Simon and Smith [25], the origin of the formed tissue may not be so important from a clinical perspective, since the objective is to induce apical closure and healing of the periapical tissues

and to keep the patient free from signs and symptoms, like in this current case report.

Recruitment of stem cells to the injured site and their differentiation into specific tissue-committed cells are required for wound healing [26]. It was suggested that stem cells of apical papilla (SCAP) can be considered an endogenous cell source for pulp revascularization [23, 27]. However, in cases of loss of apical papilla, which probably occurs with avulsed teeth, stem cells can be migrated from the periapical tissues or from a distance source into the canal space [28]. According to Ostby [29], bleeding induced into the root canal space is a source of viable cells, which are derived from circulating cells, cementum, periodontal ligament, or alveolar bone. In the present case, the clinical procedure allowed the blood clot to fill the apical portion of the root canal, which was most likely the source of stem cells for healing and mineralized tissue formation.

Additionally, the procedure performed in the present case enabled direct contact of the blood clot with MTA. As extensively reported in the literature, MTA is a biomaterial with excellent tissue compatibility, good sealing capacity, and a mineralized tissue inducing effect [30, 31], which may have played a key role in the apical closure reached in this case.

It is known that infection control is essential for apical repair of immature teeth [20]. In cases of delayed tooth replantation, endodontic treatment and systemic antibiotic therapy must be performed in order to control the contamination [32], as was carried out in the present case report. The use of an intracanal medication in pulp revascularization is a critical aspect since the disinfection of the root canal should be achieved with minimum mechanical instrumentation [13, 18]. Due to its ideal properties for removal of endodontic infections, induction of a mineralizing effect, and control of root resorptive processes [32], calcium hydroxide-based paste was used as intracanal medication during the root canal treatment performed prior to replantation, as is still currently recommended [13].

Therefore, all efforts and cautions to manage this case were conducted with the aim to improve the prognosis. After 1 year and 6 months, radiographic examination showed apical closure and no sign of external root resorption of the replanted tooth. However, it should be emphasized that in the long term ankylosis and replacement resorption can take place because of the loss of the PDL cells, as is common after performing a delayed replantation [17].

In conclusion, the clinical procedures performed in the present case of delayed replantation of an avulsed immature tooth, which worked like apical revascularization, promoted a successful endodontic outcome after a follow-up of 1 year and 6 months. However, studies with this protocol and a longer period of follow-up are needed to scientifically demonstrate the efficacy and safety of this therapy.

Competing Interests

The authors deny any competing interests.

References

[1] N. Moradi Majd, H. Zohrehei, A. Darvish, H. Homayouni, and M. Adel, "Continued root formation after delayed replantation of an avulsed immature permanent tooth," *Case Reports in Dentistry*, vol. 2014, Article ID 832637, 5 pages, 2014.

[2] A. R. Casaroto, M. M. Hidalgo, A. M. Sell et al., "Study of the effectiveness of propolis extract as a storage medium for avulsed teeth," *Dental Traumatology*, vol. 26, no. 4, pp. 323–331, 2010.

[3] E. B. Tuna, D. Yaman, and S. Yamamato, "What is the best root surface treatment for avulsed teeth?" *Open Dentistry Journal*, vol. 8, no. 1, pp. 175–179, 2014.

[4] F. Chen, S. Qi, L. Lu, and Y. Xu, "Effect of storage temperature on the viability of human periodontal ligament fibroblasts," *Dental Traumatology*, vol. 31, no. 1, pp. 24–28, 2015.

[5] L. Andersson and I. Bodin, "Avulsed human teeth replanted within 15 minutes—a long-term clinical follow-up study," *Endodontics & Dental Traumatology*, vol. 6, no. 1, pp. 37–42, 1990.

[6] J. V. B. Barbizam, R. Massarwa, L. A. B. da Silva et al., "Histopathological evaluation of the effects of variable extraoral dry times and enamel matrix proteins (enamel matrix derivatives) application on replanted dogs' teeth," *Dental Traumatology*, vol. 31, no. 1, pp. 29–34, 2015.

[7] J. V. Bastos, M. I. S. Côrtes, J. F. C. Silva et al., "A study of the interleukin-1 gene cluster polymorphisms and inflammatory external root resorption in replanted permanent teeth," *International Endodontic Journal*, vol. 48, no. 9, pp. 878–887, 2015.

[8] M. Cvek, "Prognosis of luxated non-vital maxillary incisors treated with calcium hydroxide and filled with gutta-percha. A retrospective clinical study," *Endodontics & Dental Traumatology*, vol. 8, no. 2, pp. 45–55, 1992.

[9] R. Bansal and R. Bansal, "Regenerative endodontics: a state of the art," *Indian Journal of Dental Research*, vol. 22, no. 1, pp. 122–131, 2011.

[10] L. S. Antunes, A. G. Salles, C. C. Gomes, T. B. Andrade, M. P. Delmindo, and L. A. Antunes, "The effectiveness of pulp revascularization in root formation of necrotic immature permanent teeth: a systematic review," *Acta Odontologica Scandinavica*, vol. 74, no. 3, pp. 161–169, 2015.

[11] P. McCabe, "Revascularization of an immature tooth with apical periodontitis using a single visit protocol: a case report," *International Endodontic Journal*, vol. 48, no. 5, pp. 484–497, 2015.

[12] M. Y.-H. Chen, K.-L. Chen, C.-A. Chen, F. Tayebaty, P. A. Rosenberg, and L. M. Lin, "Responses of immature permanent teeth with infected necrotic pulp tissue and apical periodontitis/abscess to revascularization procedures," *International Endodontic Journal*, vol. 45, no. 3, pp. 294–305, 2012.

[13] M. H. C. Silva, C. N. Campos, and M. S. Coelho, "Revascularization of an immature tooth with apical periodontitis using calcium hydroxide: a 3-year follow-up," *Open Dentistry Journal*, vol. 9, pp. 482–485, 2015.

[14] S. R. J. Simon, P. L. Tomson, and A. Berdal, "Regenerative endodontics: regeneration or repair?" *Journal of Endodontics*, vol. 40, no. 4, pp. S70–S75, 2014.

[15] L. M. Lin, D. Ricucci, and G. T.-J. Huang, "Regeneration of the dentine-pulp complex with revitalization/revascularization therapy: challenges and hopes," *International Endodontic Journal*, vol. 47, no. 8, pp. 713–724, 2014.

[16] American Academy of Pediatric Dentistry (AAPD), "Guideline on pulp therapy for primary and immature permanent teeth," *Journal of Pediatric Dentistry*, vol. 36, pp. 242–250, 2014.

[17] L. Andersson, J. O. Andreasen, P. Day et al., "International association of dental traumatology guidelines for the management of traumatic dental injuries: 2. Avulsion of permanent teeth," *Dental Traumatology*, vol. 28, no. 2, pp. 88–96, 2012.

[18] J. Y. Nagata, T. F. Rocha-Lima, B. P. Gomes et al., "Pulp revascularization for immature replanted teeth: a case report," *Australian Dental Journal*, vol. 60, no. 3, pp. 416–420, 2015.

[19] H. Priya M, P. B. Tambakad, and J. Naidu, "Pulp and periodontal regeneration of an avulsed permanent mature incisor using platelet-rich plasma after delayed replantation: a 12-month Clinical Case Study," *Journal of Endodontics*, vol. 42, no. 1, pp. 66–71, 2016.

[20] J. Y. Nagata, B. P. Figueiredo De Almeida Gomes, T. F. Rocha Lima et al., "Traumatized immature teeth treated with 2 protocols of pulp revascularization," *Journal of Endodontics*, vol. 40, no. 5, pp. 606–612, 2014.

[21] B. Thibodeau, F. Teixeira, M. Yamauchi, D. J. Caplan, and M. Trope, "Pulp revascularization of immature dog teeth with

apical periodontitis," *Journal of Endodontics*, vol. 33, no. 6, pp. 680–689, 2007.

[22] L. A. B. da Silva, P. Nelson-Filho, R. A. B. da Silva et al., "Revascularization and periapical repair after endodontic treatment using apical negative pressure irrigation versus conventional irrigation plus triantibiotic intracanal dressing in dogs' teeth with apical periodontitis," *Oral Surgery, Oral Medicine, Oral Pathology, Oral Radiology and Endodontology*, vol. 109, no. 5, pp. 779–787, 2010.

[23] C. M. Pagliarin, C. d. Londero, M. C. Felippe, W. T. Felippe, C. C. Danesi, and F. B. Barletta, "Tissue characterization following revascularization of immature dog teeth using different disinfection pastes," *Brazilian Oral Research*, vol. 30, no. 1, 2016.

[24] C. Stambolsky, S. Rodríguez-Benítez, J. L. Gutiérrez-Pérez, D. Torres-Lagares, J. Martín-González, and J. J. Segura-Egea, "Histologic characterization of regenerated tissues after pulp revascularization of immature dog teeth with apical periodontitis using tri-antibiotic paste and platelet-rich plasma," *Archives of Oral Biology*, vol. 71, pp. 122–128, 2016.

[25] S. Simon and A. J. Smith, "Regenerative endodontics," *British Dental Journal*, vol. 216, no. 6, article E13, 2014.

[26] S. Maxson, E. A. Lopez, D. Yoo, A. Danilkovitch-Miagkova, and M. A. LeRoux, "Concise review: role of mesenchymal stem cells in wound repair," *Stem Cells Translational Medicine*, vol. 1, no. 2, pp. 142–149, 2012.

[27] W. Sonoyama, Y. Liu, T. Yamaza et al., "Characterization of the apical papilla and its residing stem cells from human immature permanent teeth: A Pilot Study," *Journal of Endodontics*, vol. 34, no. 2, pp. 166–171, 2008.

[28] G. T.-J. Huang and F. Garcia-Godoy, "Missing concepts in de novo pulp regeneration," *Journal of Dental Research*, vol. 93, no. 8, pp. 717–724, 2014.

[29] B. N. Ostby, "The role of the blood clot in endodontic therapy. An experimental histologic study," *Acta Odontologica Scandinavica*, vol. 19, no. 3-4, pp. 323–353, 2009.

[30] R. K. Subay, B. Ilhan, and H. Ulukapi, "Mineral trioxide aggregate as a pulpotomy agent in immature teeth: long-term case report," *European Journal of Dentistry*, vol. 7, no. 1, pp. 133–138, 2013.

[31] L. K. Bakland and J. O. Andreasen, "Will mineral trioxide aggregate replace calcium hydroxide in treating pulpal and periodontal healing complications subsequent to dental trauma? A review," *Dental Traumatology*, vol. 28, no. 1, pp. 25–32, 2012.

[32] S. R. Panzarini, C. L. Trevisan, D. A. Brandini et al., "Intracanal dressing and root canal filling materials in tooth replantation: a literature review," *Dental Traumatology*, vol. 28, no. 1, pp. 42–48, 2012.

17

Regional Odontodysplasia with Generalised Enamel Defect

A. M. Al-Mullahi[1] and K. J. Toumba[2]

[1]*Oral Health Department, Sultan Qaboos University Hospital, Sultan Qaboos University, Muscat, Oman*
[2]*Paediatric Dentistry, Leeds Dental Institute, University of Leeds, Leeds, UK*

Correspondence should be addressed to A. M. Al-Mullahi; mullahi.ama@gmail.com

Academic Editor: Alberto C. B. Delbem

Regional odontodysplasia (ROD) is uncommon developmental anomaly, which tends to be localised and involves the ectodermal and mesodermal tooth components. A five-year-old female was referred to Department of Child Dental Health at the Leeds Dental Institute regarding malformed primary teeth. On examination 64, 74, and 72 had localised hypomineralized enamel defect. The crown of 55 was broken down with only the root remaining below the gingival level. 54 has a yellowish brown discolouration with rough irregular surface. The upper anterior teeth show mild enamel opacity. Radiographically, 55 and 54 had thin radioopaque contour, showing poor distinction between the enamel and dentine and the classic feature of a wide pulp chamber. 15, 16, and 17 were developmentally delayed and were displaying the characteristic "ghost appearance." Comprehensive dental care was done under local anaesthesia and it included extraction of the primary molars affected by ROD, stainless steel crown on 64, and caries prevention program. Fifteen months following the initial assessment the patient's oral condition remains stable and she is under regular follow-up at the department. Paediatric dentists should be aware of this anomaly as it involves both dentitions and usually requires multidisciplinary care.

1. Introduction

Regional odontodysplasia (ROD) is uncommon developmental anomaly, which tends to be localised and involves the ectodermal and mesodermal tooth components [1]. This anomaly has no reported association with any specific racial group; however female is slightly more affected than male at ratio of 1.4:1 [1]. Although this anomaly usually affects dental tissues, case reports have documented the presence of regional odontodysplasia with epidermal nevus syndrome [2, 3], hypoplasia of the affected side of the face [4], hypophosphatasia [5], hydrocephalus and mental retardation [6], and ipsilateral vascular nevi [4, 7]. The etiology remains uncertain of many possible causes that have been proposed in the literature. This included somatic mutation of the dental lamina [8], viral infection [9], medication taken during pregnancy [10], local circulating disorder like vascular nevi on the skin of the affected side of the face [11, 12], failure of migration, and differentiation of neural crest cells [2].

Regional odontodysplasia typically affects one quadrant of the jaw, although it does occasionally cross the midline [7, 13–15]; however there are few cases where this anomaly has affected either the maxillary and mandibular quadrants of the same side [16, 17] or both quadrants of the same jaw [16, 18] and it is extremely rare for the anomaly to affect all four quadrants [13, 19]. Affected teeth are usually in a continuous series, although it may skip a tooth or a group of teeth [12]. Primary teeth affected by this anomaly are usually followed by affected permanent successors; however it is very rare to find normal permanent teeth to follow affected primary ones [20]. Patients with regional odontodysplasia usually present with pain and dental abscess formation [21–23] which can be seen even in the absence of dental caries [24]. Other presenting complaints include delay or failure of eruption [14, 25], gingival swelling [26, 27], and abnormal clinical appearance of the teeth [1]. Clinically, affected teeth are usually smaller than normal with a rough surface texture and extensive pits and grooves. The enamel is hypocalcified and/or hypoplastic with a yellow or brown discolouration and can be soft on exploration with a dental probe [27]. Affected teeth are more susceptible to dental caries due to defective mineralisation [28, 29]. Radiographically, teeth with ROD have shortened roots

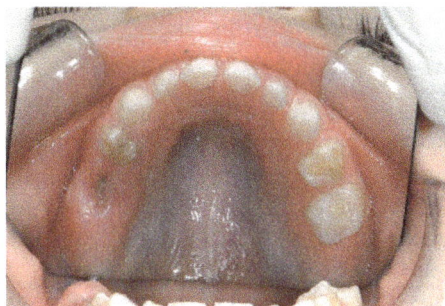

FIGURE 1: Broken down 55 to subgingival level and hypomineralization and hypoplasia of 54 and 64.

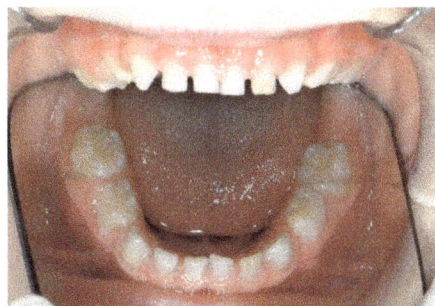

FIGURE 2: The lower arch.

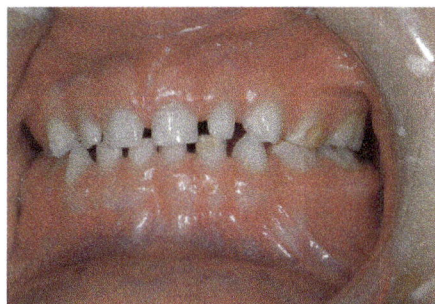

FIGURE 3: Photograph showing the enamel hypomineralization affecting the labial surface of the upper anterior teeth, hypoplasia in 72, and hypomineralization in 64 and 74.

with open apices [30]. The distinctive "ghost appearance" of these teeth is due to the wide pulp chamber [1, 22, 24] and the reduced thickness of enamel and dentine with loss of demarcation between these tissues.

In this report, we describe a case of regional odontodysplasia with generalised enamel defects in the primary dentition.

2. Case Report

A 5-year-old Caucasian female attended the consultant clinic at Paediatric Dental Department of Leeds Dental Institute, following a referral by her general dental practitioner regarding malformed deciduous teeth. The child's chief complaint on presentation was pain from the teeth in upper right quadrant. The pain started one week ago; it was associated with eating and it lasted for a short period. She did not suffer from any dental infection or associated facial swelling. The patient's perinatal and medical history was noncontributory and the mother reported no previous family history of dental anomalies.

2.1. Clinical Examination. Extraoral examination revealed no pathological features. Intraorally the mucosa had normal colour and texture. In the maxillary arch, the first primary molars had hypomineralized and hypoplastic enamel defects with 54 more severely affected with rough and irregular surface, which had a yellow brown discolouration (Figure 1). The crown of 55 was broken down with only the root remaining below the gingival level. The upper incisors had mild enamel opacity on the labial surfaces and 53 showed enamel pitting (Figure 2). The mandibular arch had a normal number of teeth and the primary molars appear more yellowish in colour (Figure 3). The mesial marginal ridge of 74 had localised enamel opacity and the incisal half of the 72's labial surface had a hypoplastic defect.

2.2. Radiographic Examination. The patient's general dental practitioner sent an orthopantomogram (OPG) radiograph (Figure 4) and we have taken bitewing radiographs for caries assessment and diagnosis. The radiographic image showed 55 and 54 with classical radiographic features of "ghost teeth," with a thin radioopaque contour, showing poor distinction

between the enamel and dentine and wide pulp chamber. 55 had very thin retained roots with complete loss of the crown. 15, 16, and 17 are developmentally delayed in relation to the corresponding teeth on the contralateral side of the arch and displaying the characteristic features seen in teeth with regional odontodysplasia. Although 54 is affected by ROD, the permanent successor appears to be in the same developing stage as the other first premolars. Based on the clinical and radiographic findings, our diagnosis was regional odontodysplasia and generalised enamel defects.

2.3. Treatment. The initial treatment plan included extraction of 55, stainless steel restoration of 54 and 64 under local anaesthesia, and caries preventative program that included regular fluoride varnish, casein phosphopeptides and amorphous calcium phosphate applications, and fissure sealant of the primary molars. However, on a subsequent visit, 54 become infected and a draining sinus developed buccal to that tooth. Hence, the treatment plan has changed to include extraction of 54 and removal of the remaining roots of 55 under local anaesthesia. The planned treatment was done under local anaesthesia over several visits (Figures 5 and 6). The removal of the remaining roots of 55 was not possible without raising a flab and bone removal because of the thin roots. Hence, the clinical decision was to remove the superficial part and leave the remaining part of the root as it is not infected. Extracted 54 and remaining roots of 55 were sent for histopathological examination. Following the eruption of the upper left first permanent molar there was deep fissure

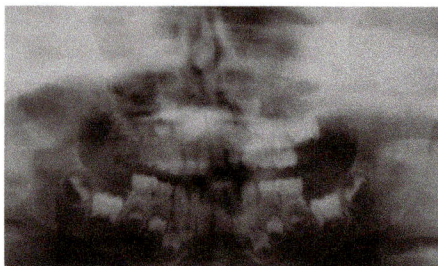

FIGURE 4: OPG radiograph.

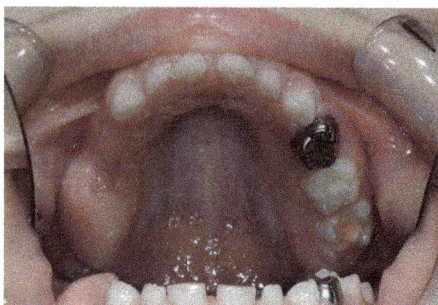

FIGURE 5: Upper arch, posttreatment.

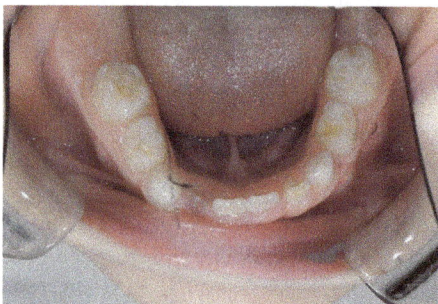

FIGURE 6: Lower arch, posttreatment.

with area of enamel opacity on the mesial aspect of the palatal wall. Hence, the tooth was fissure sealed using Fuji Triage™ to prevent plaque accumulation.

2.4. Histology Report. The histopathology report for the sent specimen (54 and remaining roots of 55) described malformed enamel with underlying irregular, poorly mineralised dysplastic dentine. The pulp shows nonfusion of one pulp horn. The center of the pulp shows necrotic material with inflammatory cells associated with mineralisation. The report confirmed the clinical and radiographic diagnosis of regional odontodysplasia.

2.5. Follow-Up. Fifteen months following the initial assessment the patient's oral condition remains stable with no evidence of dental disease. The patient was placed on a regular follow-up schedule at the department to monitor the eruption of the teeth affected by this anomaly and the presence of mineralisation defects in the remaining permanent teeth and

assessing its severity to consider the treatment options and future dental care.

3. Discussion

The presented case shares many features abundantly described in patients with regional odontodysplasia; these include slight gender tendency toward female [1] and unilateral involvement of maxilla which is twice as common to mandibular involvement [1]. However, there are few features which are rarely reported like radiographic evidence of a normally developing permanent successor (upper right first premolar) to follow affected primary predecessor (upper right first primary molar) [20] or the generalised enamel hypomineralization and hypoplasia affecting the other primary teeth which have not been reported in any case of regional odontodysplasia. The enamel defects seen in teeth with ROD are usually severe [13, 27]; however the remaining teeth usually have normal enamel and dentine [1]. In this case, the severity and pattern of mineralisation defects seen in the unaffected teeth by ROD, mineralization of the permanent successors, size of the pulp, and radiographic features do not conform with the diagnosis of ROD. These defects are likely to be developmental defect of enamel (DDE) in the primary dentition. The DDE in primary teeth are relatively common with prevalence ranging from 8.4% to 48.0% [31, 32] and in primary teeth of healthy children in developed countries ranging from 24% to 49% [33, 34]. Many risk factors have been associated with the development of DDE and it includes medical conditions [35, 36], social factors [37], medical problems during pregnancy [38], absence of breast feeding [38], nutritional problems [37], and mutation in the amino acid sequence of amelogenin gene [39]. The high prevalence of developmental defect of enamel in the primary dentition, the diversity of the risk factors, and clinical presentation favour the diagnosis of DDE.

Treatment of ROD remains a clinical dilemma as it is controversial with lack of consensuses in managing this anomaly. Early extraction of the affected teeth has been proposed by many authors [13, 16, 22, 27] as these teeth might develop dental pathology even in the absence of dental caries due to the thin enamel layer and the presence of enamel and dentinal cleft which allow ingress of microorganism to the dental pulp [1]. In addition, the defective mineralisation of the involved teeth results in undesirable appearance and poor dental aesthetics. The extraction was followed in some cases by prosthetic replacement [40, 41]. Some authors have argued for maintaining the noninfected affected teeth to allow normal jaw development and reduce the risk of psychological trauma associated with premature tooth loss [24, 27]. Other treatment approaches in ROD include coverage restorations [25] and autotransplantation of teeth in the permanent dentition [20]. The management of ROD involves interventional dental care in both dentitions and it requires multidisciplinary care. The present case was managed by extraction of the affected teeth which is in agreement with previous reports in the literature [16] and stabilising the remaining primary teeth. The patient is under regular follow-up in the department to assess the developing permanent dentition affected by ROD and to determine the extent of involvement and severity of the generalised enamel hypomineralization and plan future dental care accordingly.

4. Conclusion

ROD in the primary dentition can be easily mistaken for grossly carious teeth. However early diagnosis of this condition is important as it involves both dentitions and usually requires multidisciplinary care.

Competing Interests

The authors declare that they have no conflict of interests in producing this paper.

References

[1] P. J. M. Crawford and M. J. Aldred, "Regional odontodysplasia: a bibliography," *Journal of Oral Pathology and Medicine*, vol. 18, no. 5, pp. 251–263, 1989.

[2] P. J. Slootweg and P. R. M. Meuwissen, "Regional odontodysplasia in epidermal nevus syndrome," *Journal of Oral Pathology*, vol. 14, no. 3, pp. 256–262, 1985.

[3] S. M. R. Prakash, S. Gupta, N. Kamarthi, and S. Goel, "Inflammatory linear verrucous epidermal nevus and regional odontodysplasia: a rare sorority," *Indian Journal of Dentistry*, vol. 6, no. 4, pp. 203–206, 2015.

[4] E. Schmid-Meier, "Unilateral odontodysplasia with ipsilateral hypoplasia of the mid-face," *Journal of Maxillofacial Surgery*, vol. 10, pp. 119–122, 1982.

[5] K. Russell and R. Yacobi, "Generalized odontodysplasia concomitant with mild hypophosphatasia—a case report," *Journal (Canadian Dental Association)*, vol. 59, no. 2, pp. 187–190, 1993.

[6] G. Dahllöf, S. Lindskog, K. Theorell, and R. Ussisoo, "Concomitant regional odontodysplasia and hydrocephalus," *Oral Surgery, Oral Medicine, Oral Pathology*, vol. 63, no. 3, pp. 354–357, 1987.

[7] J. Lustmann, H. Klein, and M. Ulmansky, "Odontodysplasia. Report of two cases and review of the literature," *Oral Surgery, Oral Medicine, Oral Pathology*, vol. 39, no. 5, pp. 781–793, 1975.

[8] M. A. Rushton, "Odontodysplasia: "ghost teeth"," *British Dental Journal*, vol. 119, pp. 109–113, 1965.

[9] P. C. Reade, B. G. Radden, and J. J. Barke, "Regional odontodysplasia. A review and a report of two cases," *Australian Dental Journal*, vol. 19, no. 3, pp. 152–161, 1974.

[10] J. Lustmann and M. Ulmansky, "Structural changes in odontodysplasia," *Oral Surgery, Oral Medicine, Oral Pathology*, vol. 41, no. 2, pp. 193–202, 1976.

[11] W. N. Alexander, G. E. Lilly, and W. B. Irby, "Odontodysplasia," *Oral Surgery, Oral Medicine, Oral Pathology*, vol. 22, no. 6, pp. 814–820, 1966.

[12] S.-H. Yuan, P. R. Liu, and N. K. Childers, "An alternative restorative method for regional odontodysplasia: case report," *Pediatric Dentistry*, vol. 19, no. 6, pp. 421–424, 1997.

[13] M. A. Hamdan, F. A. Sawair, L. D. Rajab, A. M. Hamdan, and I. K. Al-Omari, "Regional odontodysplasia: a review of the literature and report of a case," *International Journal of Paediatric Dentistry*, vol. 14, no. 5, pp. 363–370, 2004.

[14] A. Al-Tuwirqi, D. Lambie, and W. K. Seow, "Regional odontodysplasia: literature review and report of an unusual case located in the mandible," *Pediatric Dentistry*, vol. 36, no. 1, pp. 62–67, 2014.

[15] E. Barbería, A. Sanz Coarasa, A. Hernández, and C. Cardoso-Silva, "Regional odontodysplasia. A literature review and three case reports," *European Journal of Paediatric Dentistry*, vol. 13, no. 2, pp. 161–166, 2012.

[16] M. P. Gomes, A. Modesto, A. S. Cardoso, and W. Hespanhol, "Regional odontodysplasia: report of a case involving two separate affected areas," *Journal of Dentistry for Children*, vol. 66, no. 3, pp. 203–207, 1999.

[17] J. Fearne, D. M. Williams, and A. H. Brook, "Regional odontodysplasia: a clinical and histological evaluation," *Journal of the International Association of Dentistry for Children*, vol. 17, no. 1, pp. 21–25, 1986.

[18] H. R. Steiman, C. L. Cullen, and J. R. Geist, "Bilateral mandibular regional odontodysplasia with vascular nevus," *Pediatric Dentistry*, vol. 13, no. 5, pp. 303–306, 1991.

[19] G. T. Hankey and R. Duckworth, "Odontodysplasia in the deciduous dentition," *The Dental practitioner and dental record*, vol. 19, no. 3, pp. 93–95, 1968.

[20] M. Ibrahim Mostafa, N. Samir Taha, and M. A. Ismail Mehrez, "Generalised versus regional odontodysplasia: diagnosis, transitional management, and long-term followup—a report of 2 Cases," *Case Reports in Dentistry*, vol. 2013, Article ID 519704, 5 pages, 2013.

[21] M. J. Kinirons, F. V. O'Brien, and T. A. Gregg, "Regional odontodysplasia: an evaluation of three cases based on clinical, microradiographic and histopathological findings," *British Dental Journal*, vol. 165, no. 4, pp. 136–139, 1988.

[22] L. Lowry, R. R. Welbury, and J. V. Soames, "An unusual case of regional odontodysplasia," *International Journal of Paediatric Dentistry*, vol. 2, no. 3, pp. 171–176, 1992.

[23] Y. Melamed, J. Harnik, A. Becker, and J. Shapira, "Conservative multidisciplinary treatment approach in an unusual odontodysplasia," *ASDC Journal of Dentistry for Children*, vol. 61, no. 2, pp. 119–124, 1994.

[24] A. Cahuana, Y. González, and C. Palma, "Clinical management of regional odontodysplasia," *Pediatric Dentistry*, vol. 27, no. 1, pp. 34–39, 2005.

[25] E. M. Sadeghi and M. H. Ashrafi, "Regional odontodysplasia: clinical, pathologic, and therapeutic considerations," *The Journal of the American Dental Association*, vol. 102, no. 3, pp. 336–339, 1981.

[26] K. B. Fanibunda and J. V. Soames, "Odontodysplasia, gingival manifestations, and accompanying abnormalities," *Oral Surgery, Oral Medicine, Oral Pathology, Oral Radiology, and Endodontics*, vol. 81, no. 1, pp. 84–88, 1996.

[27] A. C. Marques, W. H. Castro, and M. A. do Carmo, "Regional odontodysplasia: an unusual case with a conservative approach," *British Dental Journal*, vol. 186, no. 10, pp. 522–524, 1999.

[28] J. R. Pinkham and E. J. Burkes Jr., "Odontodysplasia," *Oral Surgery, Oral Medicine, Oral Pathology*, vol. 36, no. 6, pp. 841–850, 1973.

[29] R. J. Pruhs, C. R. Simonsen, P. S. Sharma, and B. Fodor, "Odontodysplasia," *The Journal of the American Dental Association*, vol. 91, no. 5, pp. 1057–1066, 1975.

[30] S.-Y. Cho, "Conservative management of regional odontodysplasia: case report," *Journal of the Canadian Dental Association*, vol. 72, no. 8, pp. 735–738, 2006.

[31] S. Kar, S. Sarkar, and A. Mukherjee, "Prevalence and distribution of developmental defects of enamel in the primary dentition of IVF children of West Bengal," *Journal of Clinical and Diagnostic Research*, vol. 8, no. 7, pp. ZC73–ZC76, 2014.

[32] J. C. Carvalho, E. F. Silva, R. R. Gomes, J. A. C. Fonseca, and H. D. Mestrinho, "Impact of enamel defects on early caries development in preschool children," *Caries Research*, vol. 45, no. 4, pp. 353–360, 2011.

[33] R. L. Slayton, J. J. Warren, M. J. Kanellis, S. M. Levy, and M. Islam, "Prevalence of enamel hypoplasia and isolated opacities in the primary dentition," *Pediatric Dentistry*, vol. 23, no. 1, pp. 32–36, 2001.

[34] M.-J. Robles, M. Ruiz, M. Bravo-Perez, E. González, and M.-A. Peñalver, "Prevalence of enamel defects in primary and permanent teeth in a group of schoolchildren from Granada (Spain)," *Medicina Oral, Patologia Oral y Cirugia Bucal*, vol. 18, no. 2, pp. e187–e193, 2013.

[35] C. Massignan, M. Ximenes, C. da Silva Pereira, L. Dias, M. Bolan, and M. Cardoso, "Prevalence of enamel defects and association with dental caries in preschool children," *European Archives of Paediatric Dentistry*, vol. 17, no. 6, pp. 461–466, 2016.

[36] E. Farmakis, J. W. Puntis, and K. J. Toumba, "Enamel defects in children with coeliac disease," *European Journal of Paediatric Dentistry*, vol. 6, no. 3, pp. 129–132, 2005.

[37] A. M. B. Chaves, A. Rosenblatt, and O. F. B. Oliveira, "Enamel defects and its relation to life course events in primary dentition of Brazilian children: a longitudinal study," *Community Dental Health*, vol. 24, no. 1, pp. 31–36, 2007.

[38] S. E. Lunardelli and M. A. Peres, "Breast-feeding and other mother-child factors associated with developmental enamel defects in the primary teeth of Brazilian children," *Journal of Dentistry for Children*, vol. 73, no. 2, pp. 70–78, 2006.

[39] R. Saha, P. B. Sood, M. Sandhu, A. Diwaker, and S. Upadhyaye, "Association of amelogenin with high caries experience in indian children," *The Journal of clinical pediatric dentistry*, vol. 39, no. 5, pp. 458–461, 2015.

[40] R. F. Gerlach, J. Jorge Jr., O. P. De Almeida, R. Della Coletta, and A. A. Zaia, "Regional odontodysplasia: report of two cases," *Oral Surgery, Oral Medicine, Oral Pathology, Oral Radiology, and Endodontics*, vol. 85, no. 3, pp. 308–313, 1998.

[41] R. Guzman, M. A. Elliott, and K. M. Rossie, "Odontodysplasia in a pediatric patient: literature review and case report," *Pediatric Dentistry*, vol. 12, no. 1, pp. 45–48, 1990.

18

A Conservative Approach to a Peripheral Ameloblastoma

Rocco Borrello,[1] **Elia Bettio,**[1] **Christian Bacci,**[1] **Marialuisa Valente,**[2] **Stefano Sivolella,**[1] **Sergio Mazzoleni,**[1] **and Mario Berengo**[1]

[1]*Section of Dentistry, Department of Neurosciences, University of Padova, Padova, Italy*
[2]*Department of Cardiac Thoracic and Vascular Sciences, University of Padova, Padova, Italy*

Correspondence should be addressed to Rocco Borrello; rocco.borrello@unipd.it

Academic Editor: Tommaso Lombardi

Peripheral Ameloblastoma (PA) is the rarest variant of ameloblastoma. It differs from the other subtypes of ameloblastoma in its localization: it arises in the soft tissues of the oral cavity coating the tooth bearing bones. Generally, it manifests nonaggressive behavior and it can be treated with complete removal by local conservative excision. In this study we report a case of PA of the maxilla in a 78-year-old female patient and we describe the four different histopathological patterns revealed by histological examination. After local excision and diagnosis, we planned a long term follow-up: in one year no recurrence had been reported. The choice of treatment is illustrated in Discussion.

1. Introduction

Ameloblastoma is a benign odontogenic tumour which originates from ameloblasts. It commonly arises between the third and the fourth decade of life [1–3] and it can occur either in the jawbones or in the gingival soft tissue. There are three subtypes of ameloblastoma: solid and multicystic ameloblastoma, unicystic ameloblastoma, and Peripheral Ameloblastoma (PA) [4, 5]. The first two subtypes are localized in the bone tissue of maxilla and mandible; both are locally aggressive tumours with recurrence potential. PA, also known as extraosseous ameloblastoma, is an extremely rare variant, representing 1-2% of all ameloblastomas [6]. It develops in the gingiva [3, 7, 8], usually in the area of mandibular canine/premolar [7], and can be clinically observed as an exophytic sessile nodule with firm consistency [4, 8]. It is generally painless and nonradiolucent and it is thought to derive from the gingival epithelium or from remnants of the dental lamina [8, 9].

2. Case Report

A 78-year-old female patient was referred to the Dental Clinic of the University of Padua in order to evaluate a painless swelling on the palatal mucosa located near the superior left canine. The lesion, as described by the patient, was first noticed 10 years before. The patient was a nonsmoker and was under treatment for hypertension (with ACE inhibitor, beta blocker, and low-dose aspirin). Oral examination revealed two adjacent lesions, covered with normal coloured mucosa, measuring $7 \times 5 \times 5$ mm and $4 \times 3 \times 3$ mm (Figure 1). The main lesion appeared as a hard painless gingival swelling with smooth surface; the smaller one was a pedunculated outgrowth of the palatal mucosa with soft consistency. No associated lymphadenopathy was detected. X-ray examinations (intraoral radiograph and computed tomography) showed slight bone resorption in correspondence of the lesion (Figures 2 and 3).

Excisional biopsy of the two lesions was performed under local anaesthesia, and the tissues were submitted to histopathological examination. Microscopic examination of the main lesion showed a mucosal mass covered by stratified squamous epithelium (Figure 4). The lamina propria contained multiple cords and small islands of epithelial tumour cells with ameloblastic features. The peripheral tumour cells often exhibited hyperchromatic, columnar nuclei with a palisaded arrangement and areas of reverse nuclear polarity. In some areas, the cells of the tumour islands showed an acanthomatous pattern with central squamous differentiation (Figure 5, left side). Other parts of the lesion consisted of

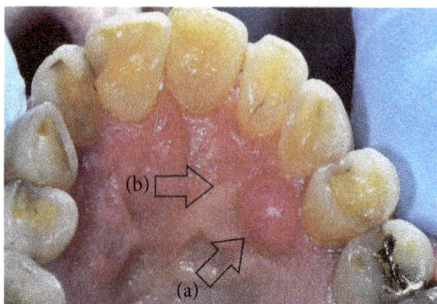

FIGURE 1: Clinical aspect of the PA. (a) The main lesion. (b) The smaller lesion.

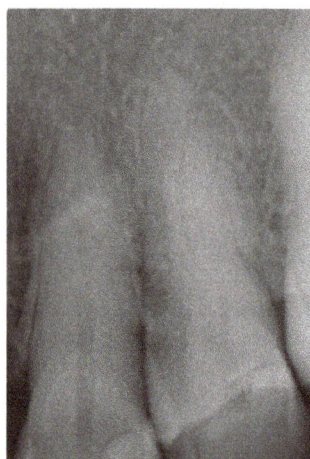

FIGURE 2: Intraoral radiograph of the PA.

narrow ribbon-like cords that were suggestive of an early plexiform pattern (Figure 6). The minor lesion also revealed the presence of tumour cells with a desmoplastic pattern, consisting of thin cords (only a few cells in width) of odontogenic epithelium dispersed in a dense collagenous stroma (Figure 7).

According to the clinical, radiographic, and histopathological exams, a PA was diagnosed. Four months after the excisional biopsy the surgical wound appeared healed by secondary intention. Further surgical approach (a radical resection) was deemed unnecessary and a two-month follow-up was planned. After two months the lesion area was clinically unchanged. A second CT performed 10 months later did not show the superficial bone resorption, confirming the tumour was not infiltrating the bone (Figure 8). After one year no relevant clinical alteration could be observed (Figure 9).

3. Discussion

Treatment of the subtypes of ameloblastoma is still controversial and it is based on recurrence potential and aggressivity of each subtype. In addition, the choice of treatment depends not only on the apparent microscopic pattern on biopsy, but also on the tumour location, size of the lesion, age of the patient, and reliance of the patient for good long term follow-up.

Whereas radiotherapy and chemotherapy are not recommended techniques, surgical intervention, radical or conservative resection, is the preferred management for ameloblastomas [2].

Radical resection can be marginal or segmental and it is associated with a recurrence rate ranging from 0% to 10% [2, 4]. Such a treatment can be beneficial in maxillary ameloblastoma (which acts clinically more aggressively for the lack of the thick cortical bone found in mandible that can slow down the tumour growth) [2].

Solid and multicystic ameloblastoma can be treated with a surgical approach extended up to 1–1.5 cm around radiographic or histologic margins of the lesion since, because of its capacity of infiltrating the bone, it is regarded as a locally aggressive tumour [2, 4]; conservative resection, such as curettage and enucleation, is associated with a high recurrence rate (solid and multicystic 60–80%, unicystic 30–60%) [2–5, 10–19]; for this reason it can be paired with cryotherapy, electrocautery, or tissue fixatives like Carnoy's solution [2].

Unicystic ameloblastoma, which is thought to be less aggressive than solid or multicystic ameloblastoma, often can be treated with enucleation and peripheral ostectomy sometimes supplemented by physicochemical treatment (cryotherapy, electrocautery, or tissue fixatives) [4]. However, some cases may require more aggressive surgical resection to be performed [4, 20].

PA, per contra, manifests a benign behaviour with an average growth rate lower than other subtypes of ameloblastoma (0.17 versus $0.81 \, cm^3$/month, resp.) [2, 21]. Moreover, bone involvement of PA is absent or irrelevant, appearing as a small depression of the bone surface in correspondence of the tumour (named "cupping" or "saucerization") (Figure 3) [3–5, 8, 9]. The surgical treatment of choice for PA consists in conservative local excision without removing bone or teeth [2, 4, 8, 9, 13].

In the reported case the tumour appeared as an exophytic sessile lesion and the patient had no symptoms. Intraoral

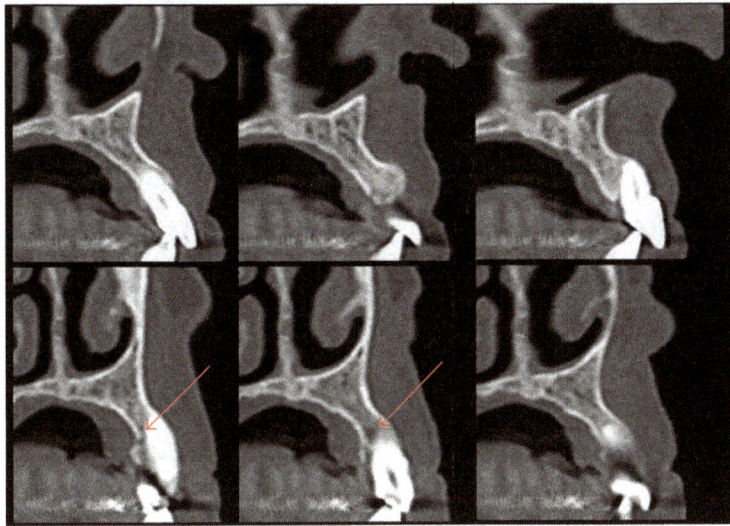

FIGURE 3: Preoperative CT. The red arrows point to the small depression of the bone surface in correspondence of the tumour ("cupping" or "saucerization").

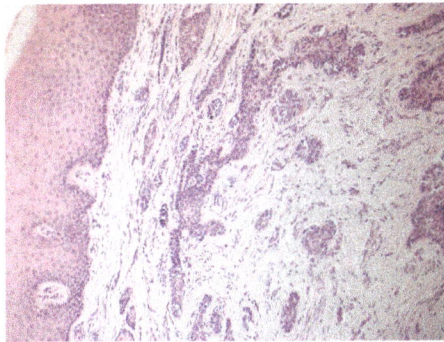

FIGURE 4: Histological aspect of the PA.

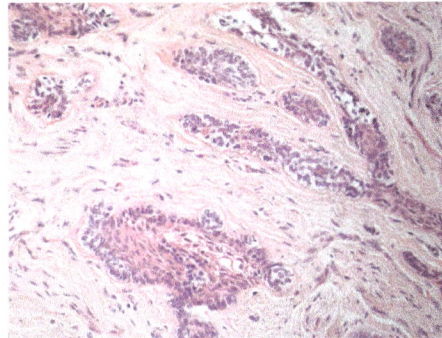

FIGURE 6: Plexiform pattern.

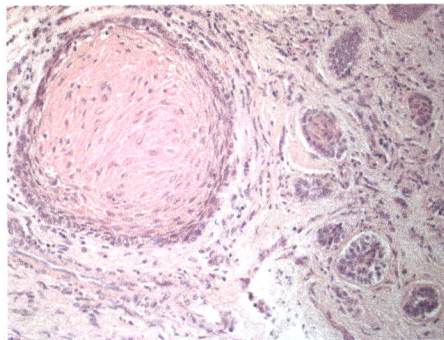

FIGURE 5: Follicular and acanthomatous cell patterns.

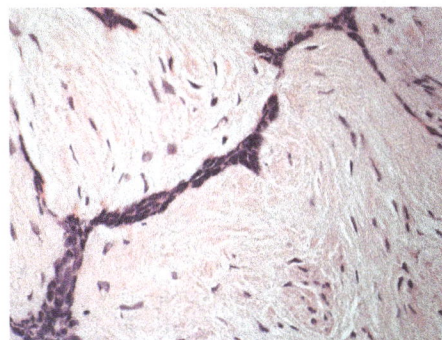

FIGURE 7: Desmoplastic pattern.

examination as well as the radiographs gave no useful indication in order to formulate the correct diagnosis. The lesion was treated with local excision and, after the response of the histopathologic laboratory, further surgical approaches were judged as unnecessary overtreatments. Nevertheless, considering the recurrence rate of the PA (from 16% to 19%) [8, 22, 23] a long term follow-up was planned with the

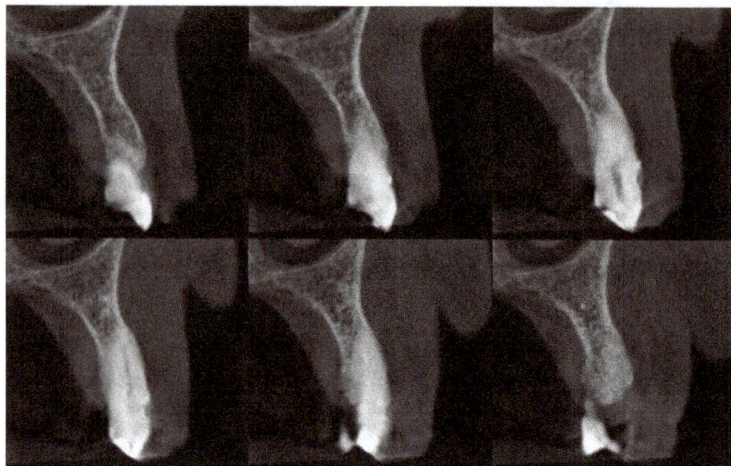

FIGURE 8: CT 10 months after biopsy.

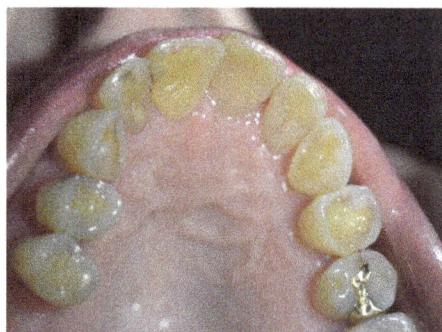

FIGURE 9: Palate clinical view 1 year after biopsy.

purpose of detecting any recurrence which could possibly develop in the future.

Competing Interests

The authors declare that there is no conflict of interest regarding the publication of this paper.

References

[1] P. A. Reichart, H. P. Philipsen, and S. Sonner, "Ameloblastoma: biological profile of 3677 cases," *European Journal of Cancer Part B: Oral Oncology*, vol. 31, no. 2, pp. 86–99, 1995.

[2] M. P. Chae, N. R. Smoll, D. J. Hunter-Smith, and W. M. Rozen, "Establishing the natural history and growth rate of ameloblastoma with implications for management: systematic review and meta-analysis," *PLoS ONE*, vol. 10, no. 2, Article ID e0117241, 2015.

[3] W. M. Mendenhall, J. W. Werning, R. Fernandes, R. S. Malyapa, and N. P. Mendenhall, "Ameloblastoma," *American Journal of Clinical Oncology: Cancer Clinical Trials*, vol. 30, no. 6, pp. 645–648, 2007.

[4] M. A. Pogrel and D. M. Montes, "Is there a role for enucleation in the management of ameloblastoma?" *International Journal of Oral and Maxillofacial Surgery*, vol. 38, no. 8, pp. 807–812, 2009.

[5] D. G. Gardner, "Some current concepts on the pathology of ameloblastomas," *Oral Surgery, Oral Medicine, Oral Pathology, Oral Radiology, and Endodontics*, vol. 82, no. 6, pp. 660–669, 1996.

[6] H. Goda, K. Nakashiro, I. Ogawa, T. Takata, and H. Hamakawa, "Peripheral ameloblastoma with histologically low-grade malignant features of the buccal mucosa: a case report with immunohistochemical study and genetic analysis," *International Journal of Clinical and Experimental Pathology*, vol. 8, no. 2, pp. 2085–2089, 2015.

[7] A. Buchner, P. W. Merrell, and W. M. Carpenter, "Relative frequency of peripheral odontogenic tumors: a study of 45 new cases and comparison with studies from the literature," *Journal of Oral Pathology and Medicine*, vol. 35, no. 7, pp. 385–391, 2006.

[8] H. P. Philipsen, P. A. Reichart, H. Nikai, T. Takata, and Y. Kudo, "Peripheral ameloblastoma: biological profile based on 160 cases from the literature," *Oral Oncology*, vol. 37, no. 1, pp. 17–27, 2001.

[9] D. G. Gardner, "Peripheral ameloblastoma. A study of 21 cases, including 5 reported as basal cell carcinoma of the gingiva," *Cancer*, vol. 39, no. 4, pp. 1625–1633, 1977.

[10] D. Ghandhi, A. F. Ayoub, M. A. Pogrel, G. MacDonald, L. M. Brocklebank, and K. F. Moos, "Ameloblastoma: a Surgeon's dilemma," *Journal of Oral and Maxillofacial Surgery*, vol. 64, no. 7, pp. 1010–1014, 2006.

[11] L. Robinson and M. G. Martinez, "Unicystic ameloblastoma: a prognostically distinct entity," *Cancer*, vol. 40, no. 5, pp. 2278–2285, 1977.

[12] S. L. Lau and N. Samman, "Recurrence related to treatment modalities of unicystic ameloblastoma: a systematic review," *International Journal of Oral and Maxillofacial Surgery*, vol. 35, no. 8, pp. 681–690, 2006.

[13] D. G. Gardner and A. M. J. Pecak, "The treatment of ameloblastoma based on pathologic and anatomic principles," *Cancer*, vol. 46, no. 11, pp. 2514–2519, 1980.

[14] N. Nakamura, Y. Higuchi, T. Mitsuyasu, F. Sandra, and M. Ohishi, "Comparison of long-term results between different approaches to ameloblastoma," *Oral Surgery, Oral Medicine, Oral Pathology, Oral Radiology, and Endodontics*, vol. 93, no. 1, pp. 13–20, 2002.

[15] M. K. Sehdev, A. G. Huvos, E. W. Strong, F. P. Gerold, and G. W. Willis, "Ameloblastoma of maxilla and mandible," *Cancer*, vol. 33, no. 2, pp. 324–333, 1974.

[16] H. Müller and P. J. Slootweg, "The ameloblastoma, the controversial approach to therapy," *Journal of Maxillofacial Surgery*, vol. 13, no. 2, pp. 79–84, 1985.

[17] D.-Y. Luo, C.-J. Feng, and J.-B. Guo, "Pulmonary metastases from an Ameloblastoma: case report and review of the literature," *Journal of Cranio-Maxillofacial Surgery*, vol. 40, no. 8, pp. e470–e474, 2012.

[18] R. Dandriyal, A. Gupta, S. Pant, and H. Baweja, "Surgical management of ameloblastoma: conservative or radical approach," *National Journal of Maxillofacial Surgery*, vol. 2, no. 1, pp. 22–27, 2011.

[19] D. Hertog, E. A. J. M. Schulten, C. R. Leemans, H. A. H. Winters, and I. Van der Waal, "Management of recurrent ameloblastoma of the jaws; a 40-year single institution experience," *Oral Oncology*, vol. 47, no. 2, pp. 145–146, 2011.

[20] A. C. McClary, R. B. West, A. C. McClary et al., "Ameloblastoma: a clinical review and trends in management," *European Archives of Oto-Rhino-Laryngology*, vol. 273, pp. 1649–1661, 2016.

[21] O. Odukoya and O. A. Effiom, "Clinicopathological study of 100 Nigerian cases of ameloblastoma," *Nigerian Postgraduate Medical Journal*, vol. 15, no. 1, pp. 1–5, 2008.

[22] J. M. Nauta, A. K. Panders, C. J. F. Schoots, A. Vermey, and J. L. N. Roodenburg, "Peripheral ameloblastoma. A case report and review of the literature," *International Journal of Oral and Maxillofacial Surgery*, vol. 21, no. 1, pp. 40–44, 1992.

[23] A. Buchner and J. J. Sciubba, "Peripheral epithelial odontogenic tumors: a review," *Oral Surgery, Oral Medicine, Oral Pathology*, vol. 63, no. 6, pp. 688–697, 1987.

19

Effectiveness of Long Term Supervised and Assisted Physiotherapy in Postsurgery Oral Submucous Fibrosis Patients

S. Kale, N. Srivastava, V. Bagga, and A. Shetty

Department of Oral and Maxillofacial Surgery, Sri Rajiv Gandhi College of Dental Sciences and Hospital, Bangalore, India

Correspondence should be addressed to S. Kale; saurabh.dent@gmail.com

Academic Editor: Giuseppe Colella

Oral submucous fibrosis is one of the leading potentially malignant disorders prevailing in India. A number of conservative and surgical treatment options have been suggested for this potentially malignant disorder (Arakeri and Brennan, 2013). While the role of physiotherapy has been highlighted in the conservative management, its importance in postsurgical cases to avoid scar contracture and subsequent relapse has not been given due importance in the literature. The following is a case report of a male patient surgically treated for OSMF (oral submucous fibrosis) and meticulously followed up for recalls and physiotherapy. The constant supervision and motivation for physiotherapy along with the constant assistance helped achieve satisfying results.

1. Introduction

Oral submucous fibrosis (OSMF) is one of the leading potentially malignant disorders prevailing in India. T. Karemore and V. Karemore in their article estimate the number of patients suffering from OSMF in India to be approximately 5 million [1]. The risk of malignant transformation for these is also suggested to be ranging from 7% to 30% [2]. Of the many treatment modalities available for this condition, surgical release of the fibrous bands is one of these. However, treatment outcome relies heavily on patient compliance and cooperation and undeterred dedication towards active physiotherapy postoperatively. Relapses in many of the cases of OSMF treated by surgery have been attributed to insufficient physiotherapy on the part of the patient. This case report attempts to highlight a case of OSMF treated by surgery, followed up postoperatively twice a day for a period of 2 months to oversee and encourage sufficient physiotherapy.

2. Case Report

A patient, aged 30 years and a painter by profession, presented to a private clinic with a chief complaint of burning sensation over the cheek on both sides and a noticeable decline in the amount of mouth opening starting 7 years ago. He was advised on mouth opening exercises by the dental practitioner. However, due to the severe pain experienced by the patient during the mouth opening exercises, the patient discontinued the physiotherapy. The patient reported back to the practitioner and was prescribed intralesional injections of hyaluronidase and dexamethasone with strict instructions to abstain from areca nut consumption completely in all forms.

Despite completing the course of intralesional injections bilaterally, the patients complaints did not subside.

On reporting to our department, a thorough clinical examination was performed. The habit history revealed the following habits:

(1) A chronic cigarette smoker, smoking 5 cigarettes a day for the past 10 years

(2) A chronic gutka chewer, consuming 10 packets of gutka per day, for the past 6 years

(3) An occasional alcohol consumer for the past 10 years

(4) An occasional pan chewer for the past 6 years

Clinical findings revealed the following:

(1) A mouth opening of 22 mm (Figure 1)

(2) Blanching of the buccal mucosa bilaterally and over the soft palate

(3) Erythematous patches over the buccal mucosa

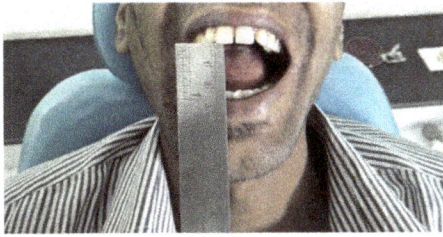

FIGURE 1: Preoperative MO—22 mm.

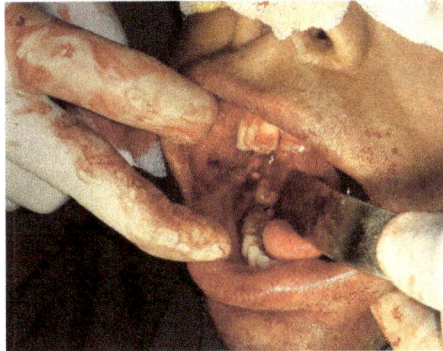

FIGURE 2: Surgical resection of fibrous bands.

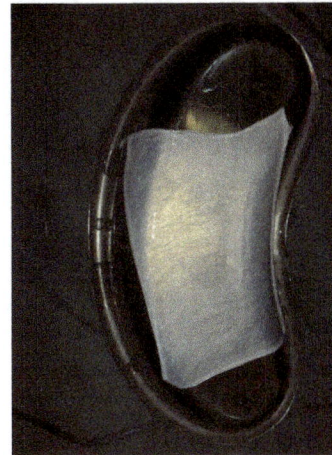

FIGURE 3: Collagen membrane impregnated with placental extract and hyaluronidase.

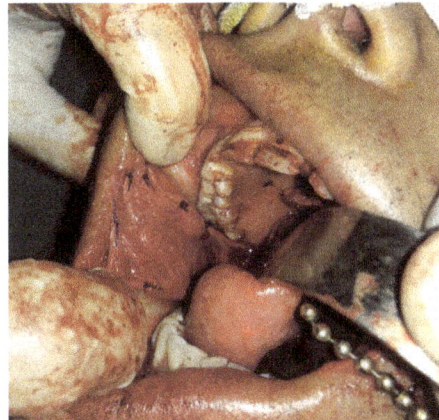

FIGURE 4: Collagen membrane sutured on the defect over the buccal mucosa.

(4) Hockey stick shaped uvula

(5) Restricted mobility of the tongue, with the tongue on protrusion, slightly overlapping the lower incisors

(6) Stains and calculus

(7) Palpation that confirmed the inspectory findings and exhibited presence of vertical fibrous bands over the buccal mucosa and horizontal bands circumorally

The previous history of intralesional injections and the minimal benefit from them drove the treatment plan in favour of surgical resection of the fibrous bands bilaterally in the region of the buccal mucosa.

The preoperative investigations were done and found to be within normal limits. Informed consent for surgery was obtained from the patient. Surgical resection of the fibrous bands was carried out under general anaesthesia (Figure 2). Postresection mouth opening achieved was 32 mm. To further enhance the mouth opening, a plan for bilateral coronoidectomy was decided on the operating table which further improved the mouth opening to 48 mm. The resultant defect over the buccal mucosa was covered with a collagen membrane impregnated with placental extract and hyaluronidase (Figure 3) [3]. The collagen membrane was sutured over the defect (Figure 4) and a bolster gauze was placed over it to stabilize the membrane. A Ryles tube was inserted postoperatively to aid in feeding.

Active physiotherapy was started from the 1st postoperative day under the cover of strong analgesics (intramuscular diclofenac sodium 3 mL BD). A Hester's jaw opener was used actively to open the mouth. The patient was discharged on the second postoperative day after a session of assisted physiotherapy. From the third postoperative day onwards, the patient was advised to report to our department every morning for a period of 2 months. Active physiotherapy using Hester's jaw opener was performed in the department. The patient was again attended to everyday in the evenings for a session of active physiotherapy and was also simultaneously encouraged. Targets were set for the patient to attain specific mouth openings till certain days to encourage him. In cases where a complaint of pain incapacitated the patient from doing physiotherapy, the attending surgeons personally helped the patient use the Hester's gradually. The patient was advised to perform physiotherapy himself using the jaw opener between these 2 assisted sessions of physiotherapy. Mouth opening was gradually increased and the wound was evaluated regularly. Wound was evaluated on the 10th postoperative day and certain loose sutures were removed. Betadine irrigation was also done. The characteristic hockey stick shaped uvula and the blanching of the palate associated with OSMF could also be observed clearly after surgery (Figure 5).

The improvement in mouth opening observed was as follows:

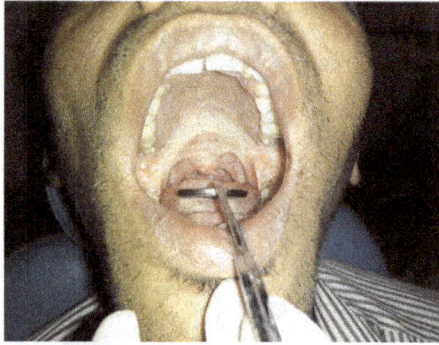

FIGURE 5: Hockey stick shaped uvula and the blanching of the palate.

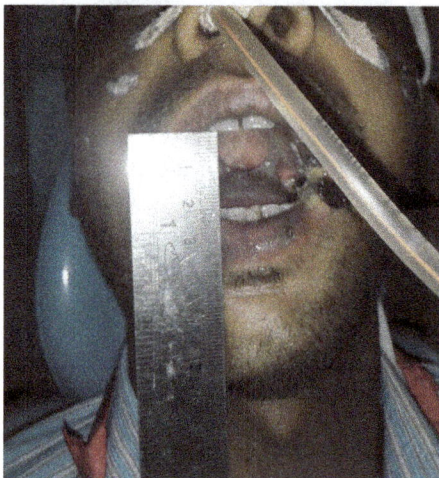

FIGURE 6: 3rd postoperative day *immediately after* assisted mouth opening—21 mm.

(1) 3rd postoperative day assisted mouth opening— 21 mm (Figure 6)

(2) 7th postoperative day assisted mouth opening— 33 mm (Figure 7)

(3) 1-month postoperative assisted mouth opening— 40 mm (Figure 8)

(4) 35-day postoperative passive mouth opening—35 mm (Figure 9)

(5) 6-month postoperative passive mouth opening— 43 mm (Figure 10)

3. Discussion

The association of OSMF with India dates back to the times of Sushruta, who recognized OSMF as a mouth and throat malady and termed it "Vidhari" in around 3000 BC [4]. Schwartz in 1952 first found the existence of this condition in five Indian women from Kenya [5]. Named initially as "atrophia idiopathica (tropica) mucosae oris" by him, it was later renamed "submucous fibrosis" by Joshi in 1953 [5]. Of the many reasons cited for the recurrence of OSMF after surgery or after other treatment modalities, insufficient

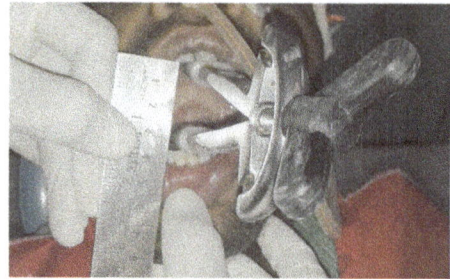

FIGURE 7: 7th postoperative day assisted mouth opening—33 mm.

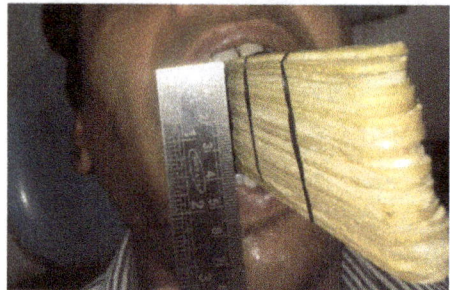

FIGURE 8: 30th postoperative day ice cream sticks assisted mouth opening—40 mm.

physiotherapy is one of the major causes. While nonstoppage of the habit can be attributed to the addictive nature of areca nut, insufficient physiotherapy mainly results from the following causes:

(1) Negligence and underestimation on part of the patient towards the importance of performing physiotherapy in the right way and for the right number of times

(2) Pain during the physiotherapy incapacitating the patient from doing active physiotherapy on his own

A number of studies have been performed to assess the effectiveness of physiotherapy as a conservative treatment modality for mild to moderate cases of OSMF. Thakur et al. [6] in their study on 64 patients observed physiotherapy to be a helpful adjunct to micronutrients for conservative management of patients with mild to moderate OSMF. The results were statistically significant when physiotherapy and micronutrient therapy were used in combination compared to physiotherapy being used alone.

Vijayakumar and Priya [7] in their study on 64 patients with grade 2 and 3 OSMF evaluated the role of physiotherapy and ultrasound therapy in conservative management of such patients. The mean improvement in mouth opening obtained was 6 mm suggesting that heating a muscle and subsequent physiotherapy can help achieve improved mouth opening.

Alam et al. [8] through their study on patients with OSMF advocated physiotherapy postsubmucosal injections of chemicals for treating OSMF. The main objective of the physiotherapy according to the author was to counteract the tendency of fibrosis, trismus, and dysphagia occurring after

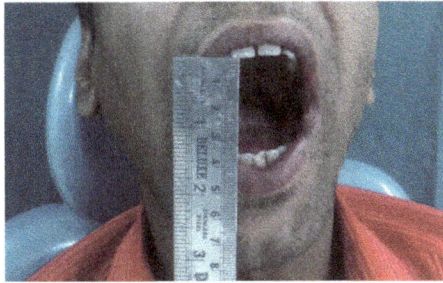

FIGURE 9: 35th postoperative day passive mouth opening—35 mm.

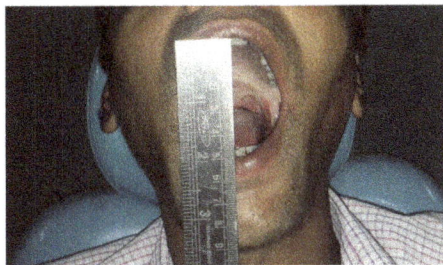

FIGURE 10: 6-month postoperative passive mouth opening—43 mm.

the trauma due to the injections and the irritative nature of the chemicals injected.

The literature however is scarce on the importance of physiotherapy after surgery to reduce chances of scar contracture and relapse. A study done by Cox and Zoellner on 54 OSMF patients highlighted the importance of physiotherapy in improving mouth opening [9]. Physiotherapy was employed as the sole modality of conservative treatment as compared to the use of local injections of hyaluronidase. The results of the study pointed towards a significant improvement in mouth opening in the physiotherapy group. Many studies invariably mention the need for physiotherapy after surgery to improve outcomes and prevent scar contracture and recurrence [10–12]. However, the initiation of physiotherapy, its importance, and the desirable duration to continue physiotherapy after surgery have not been discussed much. A common observation is the patients aversion towards immediate postoperative physiotherapy due to the associated severe pain. However, we promote starting active physiotherapy immediately 2 days postoperatively to minimize chances of scar contracture setting in. To overcome the pain, we advocate keeping the patient under a strong analgesic cover. Also, another reason for the disappointment noted with postsurgery outcomes is the poor compliance on part of the patient to perform physiotherapy to the desired extent, for the desired frequency and in the correct way. Home programmes of physiotherapy can be successful only if the patient is motivated and made to do the exercises once every day under supervision. Motivating the patient and a constant supervision and assistance towards physiotherapy were hence our main objectives. Without supervision and motivation, patients tend to fall short of the desired goal of mouth opening. Repeated over days, this results in a gradual decline

in the potential increase in mouth opening which could have been achieved.

The success towards achieving a satisfactory mouth opening in this patient can be attributed to the active supervised physiotherapy. The patient visited the hospital regularly for a period of 2 months for assisted physiotherapy and was in turn attended to for the same duration by an attending surgeon. This is not feasible for every patient as the routine and compliance will vary for every individual.

The following case report is an attempt to highlight the need for our intervention into the patients' home programmes of physiotherapy to maximize the benefits obtained from these. The results can be more definitively seen in controlled trials as are going on in our institution.

Competing Interests

The authors declare that they have no competing interests.

References

[1] T. Karemore and V. Karemore, "Etiopathogenesis and treatment strategies of oral submucous fibrosis," *Journal of Indian Academy of Oral Medicine and Radiology*, vol. 23, no. 4, pp. 598–602, 2011.

[2] G. Arakeri and P. A. Brennan, "Oral submucous fibrosis: an overview of the aetiology, pathogenesis, classification, and principles of management," *British Journal of Oral and Maxillofacial Surgery*, vol. 51, no. 7, pp. 587–593, 2013.

[3] Y. Raghavendra Reddy, N. Srinath, H. Nandakumar, and M. Rajini Kanth, "Role of collagen impregnated with dexamethasone and placentrix in patients with oral submucous fibrosis," *Journal of Maxillofacial and Oral Surgery*, vol. 11, no. 2, pp. 166–170, 2012.

[4] S. Samdariya, D. Kumar, A. Kumar, P. Porwal, and P. Pareek, "Oral submucous fibrosis—a short review," *International Journal of Medical Science and Public Health*, vol. 3, no. 11, pp. 1308–1312, 2014.

[5] C. B. More, S. Das, H. Patel, C. Adalja, V. Kamatchi, and R. Venkatesh, "Proposed clinical classification for oral submucous fibrosis," *Oral Oncology*, vol. 48, no. 3, pp. 200–202, 2012.

[6] N. Thakur, V. Keluskar, A. Bagewadi, and A. Shetti, "Effectiveness of micronutrients and physiotherapy in the management of oral submucous fibrosis," *International Journal of Contemporary Dentistry*, vol. 2, no. 1, pp. 101–105, 2011.

[7] M. Vijayakumar and D. Priya, "Physiotherapy for improving mouth opening & tongue protrution in patients with Oral Submucous Fibrosis (OSMF)—case series," *International Journal of Pharmaceutical Science and Health Care*, vol. 3, no. 2, pp. 52–58, 2013.

[8] S. Alam, I. Ali, K. Y. Giri et al., "Efficacy of aloe vera gel as an adjuvant treatment of oral submucous fibrosis," *Oral Surgery, Oral Medicine, Oral Pathology and Oral Radiology*, vol. 116, no. 6, pp. 717–724, 2013.

[9] S. Cox and H. Zoellner, "Physiotherapeutic treatment improves oral opening in oral submucous fibrosis," *Journal of Oral Pathology and Medicine*, vol. 38, no. 2, pp. 220–226, 2009.

[10] C. R. Bande, A. Datarkar, and N. Khare, "Extended nasolabial flap compared with the platysma myocutaneous muscle flap for reconstruction of intraoral defects after release of oral

submucous fibrosis: a comparative study," *British Journal of Oral and Maxillofacial Surgery*, vol. 51, no. 1, pp. 37–40, 2013.

[11] R. M. Borle, P. V. Nimonkar, and R. Rajan, "Extended nasolabial flaps in the management of oral submucous fibrosis," *British Journal of Oral and Maxillofacial Surgery*, vol. 47, no. 5, pp. 382–385, 2009.

[12] U. Lokesh, G. Veena, Anubhav Jann,, G. K. Vivek, and M. R. Shilpa, "Application of lasers for oral submucus fibrosis—an experimental study," *Archives of CraniOrofacial Sciences (ACOFS)*, vol. 1, no. 6, pp. 81–86, 2014.

20

Tardive Dyskinesia, Oral Parafunction, and Implant-Supported Rehabilitation

S. Lumetti,[1] G. Ghiacci,[1] G. M. Macaluso,[1] M. Amore,[2] C. Galli,[1] E. Calciolari,[3] and E. Manfredi[1]

[1]*Centro Universitario di Odontoiatria, SBiBiT, Università degli Studi di Parma, Parma, Italy*
[2]*Sezione di Psichiatria, Dipartimento di Neuroscienze, Riabilitazione, Oftalmologia, Genetica e Scienze Materno-Infantili, Università degli Studi di Genova, Genova, Italy*
[3]*Centre for Oral Clinical Research, Queen Mary University of London, London, UK*

Correspondence should be addressed to G. Ghiacci; giulia.ghiacci@gmail.com

Academic Editor: Miguel de Araújo Nobre

Oral movement disorders may lead to prosthesis and implant failure due to excessive loading. We report on an edentulous patient suffering from drug-induced tardive dyskinesia (TD) and oral parafunction (OP) rehabilitated with implant-supported screw-retained prostheses. The frequency and intensity of the movements were high, and no pharmacological intervention was possible. Moreover, the patient refused night-time splint therapy. A series of implant and prosthetic failures were experienced. Implant failures were all in the maxilla and stopped when a rigid titanium structure was placed to connect implants. Ad hoc designed studies are desirable to elucidate the mutual influence between oral movement disorders and implant-supported rehabilitation.

1. Introduction

Tardive dyskinesia (TD) is characterised by involuntary, repetitive, and purposeless movements, which may involve chewing motions, cheek puffing, tongue protrusion, and lip pursing. Movements of other body segments may also occur, and symptoms may appear during sleep and/or wakefulness [1, 2]. Most often TD represents a side effect of antipsychotic medications [3, 4]. Typical and, at a lower rate, atypical antipsychotics may induce TD probably by increasing dopamine sensitivity in the nigrostriatal pathway, especially for D2 dopamine receptor [5–9]. Other drugs, as antiemetic metoclopramide and antidepressants, have been linked to TD, although with much lower frequency [10–13]. It is important to underline the fact that these drugs are capable of inducing diverse movement disorders, as dystonia [14], myoclonus [15], "rabbit syndrome" [16], and sleep bruxism [17]. The latter has been linked particularly to selective serotonin reuptake inhibitors (SSRIs) [18, 19].

The term "tardive" was originally used to indicate the most frequent timing of dyskinesia onset, after at least 3 months of therapy. However, the appearance of dyskinetic symptoms is not dose-related and may occur either after a short or a long time of drug use, and it is generally accepted that most patients will eventually fall ill with the disorder if they remain on neuroleptics long enough.

Oral parafunctions (OP) include many activities occurring during the awake state, the commonest being prolonged steady mandibular postures and jaw clenching [20]. They can be classified in primary, or idiopathic, and secondary, when they originate from a neurological or psychiatric disease or represent a side effect of a medication or a recreational drug. Alcohol intake and cigarette smoking may also contribute [21]. They have been associated with psychiatric disorders as well as psychosocial factors like stress and anxiety [22–24].

TD may have dental implications, as it causes attritions and abfractions on natural teeth [25, 26]. It also represents a risk factor for the prosthetic management of the patient, worsening the stability of complete dentures and increasing the risk of prostheses breaks. Additionally, TD-provoking drugs can induce changes of salivary flow, which worsen patient's adaptation to removable prostheses [27–30]. Implant-supported fixed rehabilitation may appear as a valuable

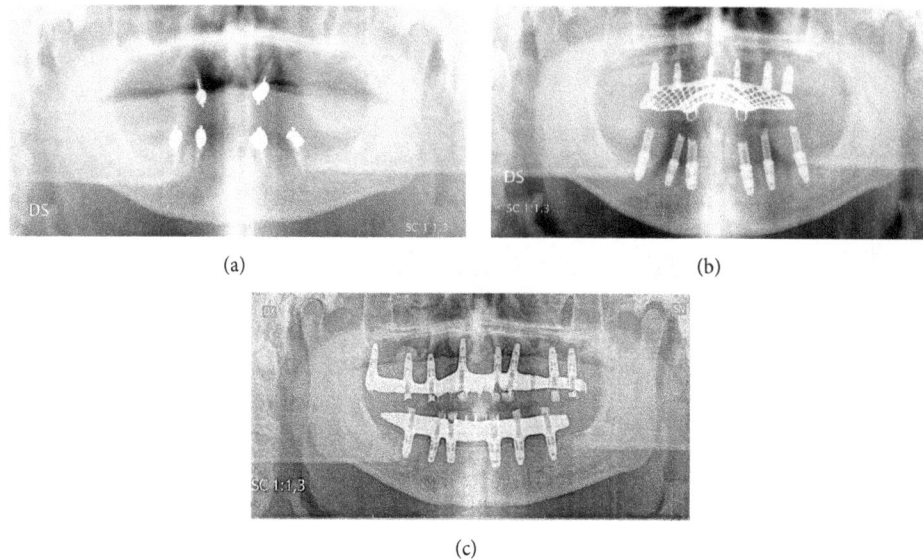

FIGURE 1: Orthopantomography of the patient at first visit (a), 18 weeks (b), and 96 weeks (c).

therapeutic option, as it improves prostheses stability and has positive psychosocial effects [31, 32]. However, oral movement disorders may cause excessive load of the prostheses, which in turn may affect implant outcome [33, 34], and jeopardise simple or complex rehabilitative procedures and tardive dyskinesia represents a particularly critical situation for implant rehabilitation [35, 36].

We here report a case of implant-supported fixed rehabilitation in an edentulous patient with extreme loading conditions due to TD and OP.

2. Case Presentation

A 58-year-old Caucasian man complaining of unsatisfactory removable prostheses was admitted to the dental clinic. Remote anamnesis revealed history of alcohol abuse associated with impulsive behaviour, with the start of medical therapies dating back to 2004. The patient was at that time suffering from major depression and narcissistic personality disorder and was administered a multiple pharmacotherapy. He was treated with Citalopram 40 mg/day, aimed at controlling depression, from 2004 to 2007; an occasional treatment with Paroxetine 30 mg/day was performed in 2004 for 90 days. During the same year, the patient took Promethazine 25 mg/day. Valproic acid 1 g/day and Oxcarbazepine 1.2 g/day were prescribed up to now as anticonvulsants. The patient was also administered benzodiazepines: Lorazepam 2.5 mg/day from 2004 to 2006, Triazolam 0.25 mg/day, and Diazepam 2 mg/day from 2005 to 2006. A temporary treatment with the second-generation antipsychotic Olanzapine 5 mg/day was carried out for 90 days in 2005. The patient also assumed Trazodone 75 mg/day. In 2007, the antidepressant Venlafaxine substituted Citalopram, with doses increasing to the current posology of 150 mg/day. Clonazepam 5 mg/day was administered since 2007, substituting previously used benzodiazepines. In 2008, the patient received Hydroxyzine

25 mg/day. During 2011, Zolpidem 4 mg/day was prescribed to the patient. Olanzapine 5 mg/day was permanently reintroduced into the therapy in April 2012.

The patient has been suffering from TD as a side effect of drugs since 2009. The involuntary movements he presented were repetitive stereotyped chewing motions and lip protruding. The movements were probably present also during sleep, but the patient did not accept further ambulatory sleep study.

OP was also evident, as prolonged steady mandibular postures and habit of teeth clenching: these activities, differently from the repetitive movements of TD, could be voluntarily stopped and were exacerbated in state of psychological anxiety.

The patient had been smoking 20 cigarettes/day since many years.

Clinical examination of the oral cavity revealed the presence of 2 residual teeth in the maxilla (canines) and 4 residual teeth in the mandible (2 canines and 2 premolars), restored with post and ball attachment to, respectively, stabilise maxillary and mandibular overdentures. All teeth were affected by severe reduction of periodontal support and showed class III mobility. Marked gingival inflammation was also evident. Orthopantomography attested horizontal bone loss around the remaining teeth and generalised vertical atrophy of the alveolar processes (Figure 1(a)).

Treatment consisted of extraction of the remaining hopeless teeth (time: T0) and subsequent full mouth rehabilitation with implant-supported fixed prostheses. After thorough discussion, the patient approved this therapeutic option.

Twelve weeks following T0, a CT scan (Siemens Somatom Emotion 6; Siemens, Erlangen, Germany) was performed to plan implant insertion (NobelGuide planning software; Nobel Biocare, Göteborg, Sweden). Two weeks later, the patient underwent bilateral sinus lift with lateral window approach. Autologous bone chips plus deproteinised bovine bone granules (Bio-Oss; Geistlich Pharma AG, Wolhusen,

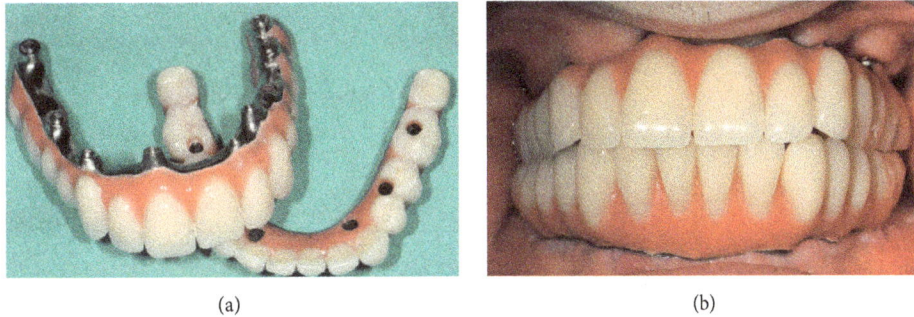

(a)   (b)

FIGURE 2: Final prostheses delivered to the patient at 96 weeks.

Switzerland) were used as grafting materials. In the course of the same surgical intervention, six dental implants (NobelReplace, Nobel Biocare, Göteborg, Sweden, as all the remaining implants employed) were placed in the maxilla with an insertion torque > 30 N/cm. The patient was provided with a provisional complete denture to wear during the planned 24-week healing period.

The mandible was rehabilitated 18 weeks after T0 by means of 6 dental implants inserted with a torque > 40 N/cm and immediately restored with a provisional screw-retained acrylic bridge. The implants were all 10 mm long and 4.3 diameter, except the 4.6 implant, which had a 5 mm diameter (Figure 1(b)). A group function occlusal scheme was created, with accurate control of contacts in intercuspal position and lateral and protrusive movements. This occlusal scheme was maintained in both provisional and final prostheses.

At 32 weeks, a complete mandibular implant-supported screw-retained prosthesis was finalised with composite teeth and milled titanium framework.

At 36 weeks, the implant in 1.1 position failed. At a routine control visit, the implant was exposed and mobile, with no symptoms. It was therefore removed and substituted with a larger implant. At the same time point, the remaining maxillary implants were loaded with a provisional implant-supported screw-retained acrylic prosthesis.

Four weeks later (at 40-week time point), the implants in 2.2 and 2.6 positions failed, with no apparent sign of infection. The implant in 2.2 site was replaced with a larger one. This was not possible for the 2.6 implant; thus an implant was inserted more distally, in 2.7 position. An additional implant was placed in 1.7. A provisional acrylic bridge was then placed, using all the maxillary implants.

At 44 weeks, the implant in 2.4 site showed severe marginal bone loss on the vestibular side, which was managed by means of a deproteinised bovine bone granular graft (Bio-Oss; Geistlich Pharma AG, Wolhusen, Switzerland). Despite this intervention, the implant failed at 48 weeks and was replaced with a longer implant, inserted apically. Another implant was positioned in the adjacent 2.3 area.

At the following monthly follow-up visits, the provisional maxillary bridge frequently showed cracks, which underwent mostly unnoticed by the patient. All cracks could be repaired.

At 60 weeks, the maxillary acrylic bridge broke into two pieces, and implants 2.4 and 2.7 were removed, due to their loss of osseointegration in the absence of infection signs. Implants were placed in 2.6 and 2.7 sites. A new acrylic full arch bridge was screwed to all the maxillary implants.

At 72 weeks, the patient was provided with a maxillary screw-retained prosthesis with composite teeth and milled titanium framework (Figures 2(a) and 2(b)). From this moment to the 96-week follow-up visit, no further maxillary implant was lost and the prosthesis performed satisfactorily. A time course of maxillary implant insertions and failures is described in Figure 3.

At 96 weeks, all mandibular implants were successful (Figure 1(c)), as they had good stability and showed no marginal bone loss, no inflammation, nor any symptoms. The mandibular full arch bridge performed adequately during the whole examination period, showing some sign of attrition.

TD appeared as a permanent condition during the observation period. It was not possible to prescribe a pharmacological therapy specifically aimed at controlling TD due to the underlying psychiatric disease of the patient. The patient refused night splint therapy.

Massive efforts to teach self-control of OP were undertaken, but the effect was highly variable in time and, overall, poor.

3. Discussion

Oral parafunctions may alter occlusal loads of natural teeth, prostheses, and dental implants, both in terms of force direction and intensity. Dental attrition, abraction, and occlusal pits on natural teeth have been documented in patients with self-reported parafunctions. Many authors suggested that oral parafunctions represent a risk factor for marginal bone loss around implants and implant failure [37–40].

TD and other oral movement disorders can similarly generate increased tooth or implant loads. A case of traumatic granulomatous tissue at the implant site of a patient with TD has been reported [41]. Other studies showed successful results of implant-retained overdentures in patients with neurological movement disorders involving oral and perioral areas [35, 36, 42–46].

As a matter of fact, the influence of increased load on implants still represents a matter of debate and no clear-cut conclusion can be drawn from the published literature [47–54]. This is in part due to the inherent difficulty in quantifying

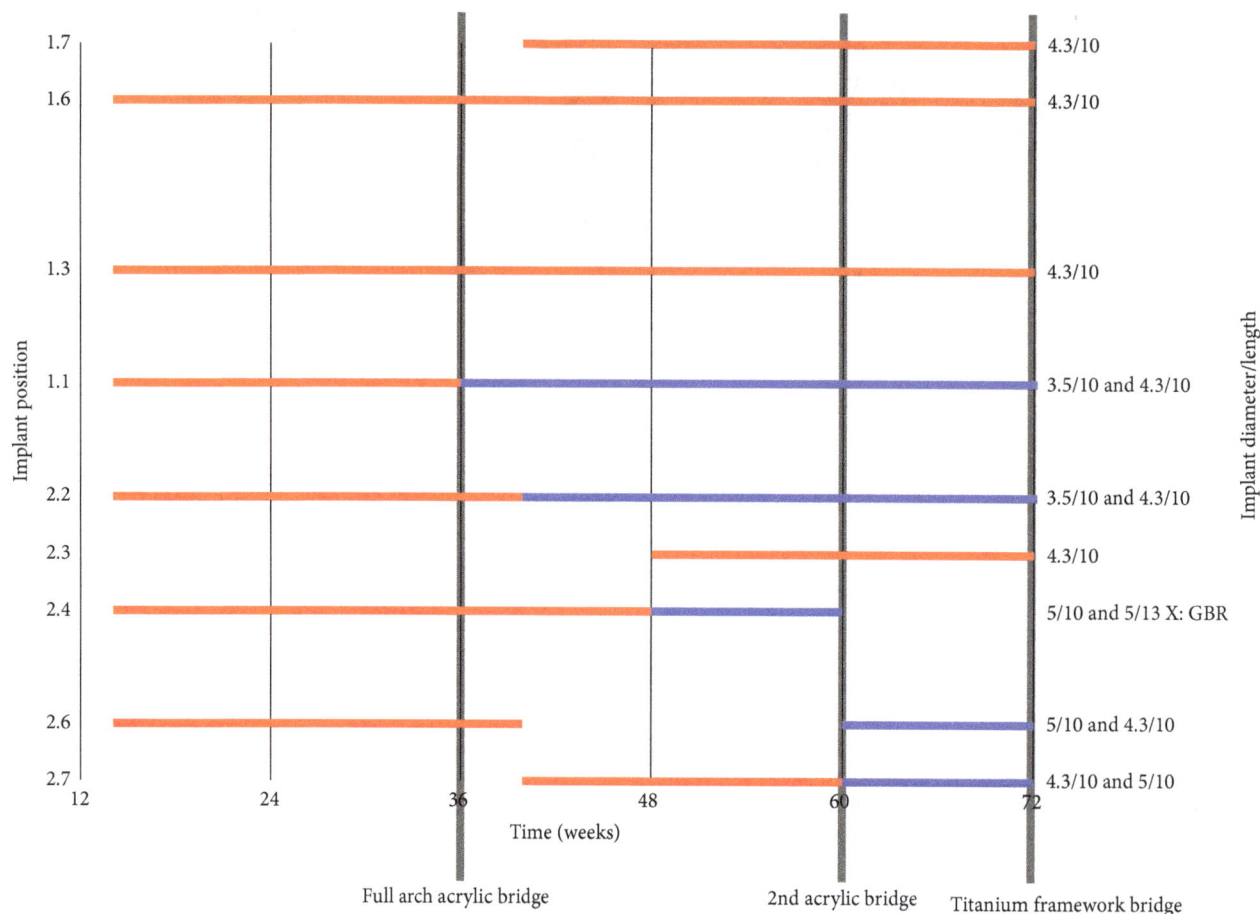

FIGURE 3: Time course of maxillary implant insertions and failures, ordered by position. In red a given implant first positioning and in blue the substituting implant. The initial planning included 6 implants with delayed loading. Five implants failed. The maxilla was finally rehabilitated at 72 weeks with a screwed titanium milled framework with acrylic composite teeth supported by 8 implants. No additional implant failures occurred.

the load transferred to implants in a clinical setting. In the present case, all implant failures occurred in absence of infection. They were likely due to the extreme mechanical loads caused by coexisting severe TD and OP.

The different survival rate of maxillary versus mandibular implants (57% versus 100%) may be related to different factors. The anatomical characteristics of the jaws arguably play a role, the mandible being mainly composed of cortical compact bone. The literature has consistently reported high implant success rates in the mandible, also employing immediate loading protocols. Maxillary bone is generally less favourable, due to its lower density and higher amount of trabecular bone [55, 56], which may hinder the rehabilitation techniques that are applied [57, 58]. Moreover, sinus lift interventions and grafted materials used may play an influence on implant outcome [59, 60]. In our case, implants placed in areas of sinus lifts were successful in 1.6 and 1.7 positions, while they failed on the opposite side in 2.6 and 2.7 positions.

Prosthetic aspects are of the utmost importance in determining the load transfer to implants. Unfortunately, as of today, there is no clear evidence-based concept of "ideal

occlusal scheme" to apply in implant-supported prosthodontics [61, 62]. A review assessed the importance of decreasing cuspal interferences, centralising forces along implant axes and avoiding cantilevers [63]. Klineberg recommended an occlusal design with narrow occlusal table, with central fossa loading in intercuspal contact and low cusp inclination [64, 65]. Occlusal canine guidance instead of group function in patients with OP has also been proposed [66].

Prosthetic breaks represent one of the commonest complications in the rehabilitation of patients suffering from oral parafunctions: it has been reported that ceramic crowns have high risk of fracture, especially when they articulate one with the other [67, 68]. Skalak first hypothesised that resilient prosthetic materials help reducing overloads and so recommended the use of acrylic resin teeth in implant-supported prostheses [69]. Others proposed to use a metal occlusal surface, which combine resiliency and resistance properties [70].

In this case, the patient frequently broke the unreinforced acrylic resin maxillary full arch prosthesis. Such loss of integrity may have represented a further cause of mechanical stress build-up at certain implant areas, together with the inherent flexibility of this type of prosthesis. We believe that the latter characteristic was of the utmost importance, since implant failure stopped after installing a prostheses with rigid titanium milled framework. This was probably due to a better load distribution among implants. It is also possible that specific implant surfaces may prove better suitability to withstand abnormal mechanical loads [71], and this aspect should be further explored. This could be consistent with a previous report by Amornvit et al. showing a successful implant rehabilitation with a balanced occlusal scheme, which may have compensated the excessive occlusal loading [36]. The patient's personal history as a heavy smoker should also be considered, as smoke has been shown to be related to risk for and severity of bruxism [72, 73] and may have affected the severity of the symptoms, but may also have impacted on implant survival as smoke has been associated with increased implant failure and complications [74–77].

We conclude that abnormal occlusal loads related to TD and OP played a key role in determining repeated prosthetic breaks and implant failures in the present case. The use of a bridge with a rigid framework stopped implants failures. Longitudinal controlled studies to investigate implant-supported rehabilitation in TD and other extreme load-generating movement disorders are needed.

Competing Interests

The authors have no conflict of interests to disclose.

References

[1] P. J. Blanchet, P. H. Rompré, G. J. Lavigne, and C. Lamarche, "Oral dyskinesia: a clinical overview," *International Journal of Prosthodontics*, vol. 18, no. 1, pp. 10–19, 2005.

[2] P. G. Aia, G. J. Revuelta, L. J. Cloud, and S. A. Factor, "Tardive dyskinesia," *Current Treatment Options in Neurology*, vol. 13, no. 3, pp. 231–241, 2011.

[3] J. Muench and A. M. Hamer, "Adverse effects of antipsychotic medications," *American Family Physician*, vol. 81, no. 5, pp. 617–622, 2010.

[4] D. Tarsy, C. Lungu, and R. J. Baldessarini, "Epidemiology of tardive dyskinesia before and during the era of modern antipsychotic drugs," *Handbook of Clinical Neurology*, vol. 100, pp. 601–616, 2011.

[5] W. M. Glazer, "Review of incidence studies of tardive dyskinesia associated with typical antipsychotics," *Journal of Clinical Psychiatry*, vol. 61, no. 4, pp. 15–20, 2000.

[6] W. M. Glazer, "Expected incidence of tardive dyskinesia associated with atypical antipsychotics," *Journal of Clinical Psychiatry*, vol. 61, supplement 4, pp. 21–26, 2000.

[7] P. Turrone, G. Remington, and J. N. Nobrega, "The vacuous chewing movement (VCM) model of tardive dyskinesia revisited: is there a relationship to dopamine D_2 receptor occupancy?" *Neuroscience and Biobehavioral Reviews*, vol. 26, no. 3, pp. 361–380, 2002.

[8] H. Tuppurainen, J. T. Kuikka, H. Viinamki, M. Husso, and J. Tiihonen, "Extrapyramidal side-effects and dopamine $D_{2/3}$ receptor binding in substantia nigra," *Nordic Journal of Psychiatry*, vol. 64, no. 4, pp. 233–238, 2010.

[9] R. J. Baldessarini and D. M. Gardner, "Incidence of extrapyramidal syndromes and tardive dyskinesia," *Journal of Clinical Psychopharmacology*, vol. 31, no. 3, pp. 382–384, 2011.

[10] S. D. Botsaris and J. M. Sypek, "Paroxetine and tardive dyskinesia," *Journal of Clinical Psychopharmacology*, vol. 16, no. 3, pp. 258–259, 1996.

[11] C. U. Correll and E. M. Schenk, "Tardive dyskinesia and new antipsychotics," *Current Opinion in Psychiatry*, vol. 21, no. 2, pp. 151–156, 2008.

[12] P.-Y. Chen, P.-Y. Lin, S.-C. Tien, Y.-Y. Chang, and Y. Lee, "Duloxetine-related tardive dystonia and tardive dyskinesia: a case report," *General Hospital Psychiatry*, vol. 32, no. 6, pp. 646.e9–646.e11, 2010.

[13] A. S. Rao and M. Camilleri, "Review article: metoclopramide and tardive dyskinesia," *Alimentary Pharmacology and Therapeutics*, vol. 31, no. 1, pp. 11–19, 2010.

[14] M. B. Detweiler and G. J. Harpold, "Bupropion-induced acute dystonia," *Annals of Pharmacotherapy*, vol. 36, no. 2, pp. 251–254, 2002.

[15] D. Kasantikul and B. Kanchanatawan, "Antipsychotic-induced tardive movement disorders: a series of twelve cases," *Journal of the Medical Association of Thailand*, vol. 90, no. 1, pp. 188–194, 2007.

[16] K. Sansare, D. Singh, V. Khanna, and F. R. Karjodkar, "Risperidone-induced rabbit syndrome: an unusual movement disorder," *The New York State Dental Journal*, vol. 78, no. 5, pp. 44–46, 2012.

[17] J. M. Ellison and P. Stanziani, "SSRI-associated nocturnal bruxism in four patients," *Journal of Clinical Psychiatry*, vol. 54, no. 11, pp. 432–434, 1993.

[18] G. J. Lavigne, T. Kato, A. Kolta, and B. J. Sessle, "Neurobiological mechanisms involved in sleep bruxism," *Critical Reviews in Oral Biology and Medicine*, vol. 14, no. 1, pp. 30–46, 2003.

[19] O. Sabuncuoglu, O. Ekinci, and M. Berkem, "Fluoxetine-induced sleep bruxism in an adolescent treated with buspirone: a case report," *Special Care in Dentistry*, vol. 29, no. 5, pp. 215–217, 2009.

[20] G. J. Lavigne, S. Khoury, S. Abe, T. Yamaguchi, and K. Raphael, "Bruxism physiology and pathology: an overview for clinicians," *Journal of Oral Rehabilitation*, vol. 35, no. 7, pp. 476–494, 2008.

[21] G. J. Lavigne, F. Lobbezoo, P. H. Rompré, T. A. Nielsen, and J. Montplaisir, "Cigarette smoking as a risk factor or an exacerbating factor for restless legs syndrome and sleep bruxism," *Sleep*, vol. 20, no. 4, pp. 290–293, 1997.

[22] J. Ahlberg, M. Rantala, A. Savolainen et al., "Reported bruxism and stress experience," *Community Dentistry and Oral Epidemiology*, vol. 30, no. 6, pp. 405–408, 2002.

[23] M. K. A. Van Selms, F. Lobbezoo, D. J. Wicks, H. L. Hamburger, and M. Naeije, "Craniomandibular pain, oral parafunctions, and psychological stress in a longitudinal case study," *Journal of Oral Rehabilitation*, vol. 31, no. 8, pp. 738–745, 2004.

[24] D. Manfredini and F. Lobbezoo, "Role of psychosocial factors in the etiology of bruxism," *Journal of Orofacial Pain*, vol. 23, no. 2, pp. 153–166, 2009.

[25] F. Lobbezoo and M. Naeije, "Dental implications of some common movement disorders: a concise review," *Archives of Oral Biology*, vol. 52, no. 4, pp. 395–398, 2007.

[26] N. Tsiggos, D. Tortopidis, A. Hatzikyriakos, and G. Menexes, "Association between self-reported bruxism activity and occurrence of dental attrition, abfraction, and occlusal pits on natural teeth," *Journal of Prosthetic Dentistry*, vol. 100, no. 1, pp. 41–46, 2008.

[27] U. Brägger, S. Aeschlimann, W. Bürgin, C. H. F. Hämmerle, and N. P. Lang, "Biological and technical complications and failures with fixed partial dentures (FPD) on implants and teeth after four to five years of function," *Clinical Oral Implants Research*, vol. 12, no. 1, pp. 26–34, 2001.

[28] S. K. Praharaj, A. K. Jana, K. Goswami, P. R. Das, N. Goyal, and V. K. Sinha, "Salivary flow rate in patients with schizophrenia on clozapine," *Clinical Neuropharmacology*, vol. 33, no. 4, pp. 176–178, 2010.

[29] J. Katsoulis, S. G. Nikitovic, S. Spreng, K. Neuhaus, and R. Mericske-Stern, "Prosthetic rehabilitation and treatment outcome of partially edentulous patients with severe tooth wear: 3-years results," *Journal of Dentistry*, vol. 39, no. 10, pp. 662–671, 2011.

[30] P. Zoidis and G. Polyzois, "Removable dental prosthesis splint: an occlusal device for nocturnal bruxing partial denture users," *Journal of Prosthodontics*, vol. 22, no. 8, pp. 652–656, 2013.

[31] M. Packer, V. Nikitin, T. Coward, D. M. Davis, and J. Fiske, "The potential benefits of dental implants on the oral health quality of life of people with Parkinson's disease," *Gerodontology*, vol. 26, no. 1, pp. 11–18, 2009.

[32] T. D. F. Borges, F. A. Mendes, T. R. de Oliveira, V. L. Gomes, C. J. do Prado, and F. D. das Neves, "Mandibular overdentures with immediate loading: satisfaction and quality of life," *The International Journal of Prosthodontics*, vol. 24, no. 6, pp. 534–539, 2011.

[33] F. Lobbezoo, J. E. I. G. Brouwers, M. S. Cune, and M. Naeije, "Dental implants in patients with bruxing habits," *Journal of Oral Rehabilitation*, vol. 33, no. 2, pp. 152–159, 2006.

[34] D. Manfredini, C. E. Poggio, and F. Lobbezoo, "Is bruxism a risk factor for dental implants? A systematic review of the literature," *Clinical Implant Dentistry and Related Research*, vol. 16, no. 3, pp. 460–469, 2014.

[35] A. G. Payne and L. Carr, "Can edentulous patients with orofacial dyskinesia be treated successfully with implants? A case report," *The Journal of the Dental Association of South Africa*, vol. 51, no. 2, pp. 67–70, 1996.

[36] P. Amornvit, D. Rokaya, and S. Bajracharya, "Prosthetic management of complete edentulous patient with oromandibular dyskinesia: a case report," *Academic Journal of Oral and Dental Medicine*, vol. 1, pp. 1–4, 2014.

[37] F. Lobbezoo, J. Van Der Zaag, and M. Naeije, "Bruxism: its multiple causes and its effects on dental implants—an updated review," *Journal of Oral Rehabilitation*, vol. 33, no. 4, pp. 293–300, 2006.

[38] D. Manfredini, M. B. Bucci, V. B. Sabattini, and F. Lobbezoo, "Bruxism: overview of current knowledge and suggestions for dental implants planning," *Cranio—Journal of Craniomandibular Practice*, vol. 29, no. 4, pp. 304–312, 2011.

[39] B. R. Chrcanovic, J. Kisch, T. Albrektsson, and A. Wennerberg, "Bruxism and dental implant failures: a multilevel mixed effects parametric survival analysis approach," *Journal of Oral Rehabilitation*, vol. 43, no. 11, pp. 813–823, 2016.

[40] K. Yadav, A. Nagpal, S. K. Agarwal, and A. Kochhar, "Intricate assessment and evaluation of effect of bruxism on long-term survival and failure of dental implants: a comparative study," *The Journal of Contemporary Dental Practice*, vol. 17, no. 8, pp. 670–674, 2016.

[41] M. G. Kelleher, B. J. Scott, and S. Djemal, "Case report: complications of rehabilitation using osseointegrated implants—tardive dyskinesia," *The European Journal of Prosthodontics and Restorative Dentistry*, vol. 6, no. 4, pp. 133–136, 1998.

[42] S. M. Heckmann, J. G. Heckmann, and H.-P. Weber, "Clinical outcomes of three Parkinson's disease patients treated with mandibular implant overdentures," *Clinical Oral Implants Research*, vol. 11, no. 6, pp. 566–571, 2000.

[43] J. Jackowski, J. Andrich, H. Kappeler, A. Zollner, P. Johren, and T. Muller, "Implant-supported denture in a patient with Huntington's disease: interdisciplinary aspects," *Special Care in Dentistry*, vol. 21, no. 1, pp. 15–20, 2001.

[44] M. Peñarrocha, J. M. Sanchis, J. Rambla, and M. A. Sánchez, "Oral rehabilitation with osseointegrated implants in a patient with oromandibular dystonia with blepharospasm (brueghel's syndrome): a patient history," *International Journal of Oral and Maxillofacial Implants*, vol. 16, no. 1, pp. 115–117, 2001.

[45] H. Sutcher, "Prosthetic dentistry in the treatment of movement disorders: dyskinesias and other neurological abnormalities," *Medical Hypotheses*, vol. 56, no. 3, pp. 318–320, 2001.

[46] E. Deniz, A. M. Kokat, and A. Noyan, "Implant-supported overdenture in an elderly patient with Huntington's disease," *Gerodontology*, vol. 28, no. 2, pp. 157–160, 2011.

[47] E. Engel, G. Gomez-Roman, and D. Axmann-Krcmar, "Effect of occlusal wear on bone loss and periotest value of dental implants," *International Journal of Prosthodontics*, vol. 14, no. 5, pp. 444–450, 2001.

[48] M. Davarpanah, M. Caraman, B. Jakubowicz-Kohen, M. Kebir-Quelin, and S. Szmukler-Moncler, "Prosthetic success with a maxillary immediate-loading protocol in the multiple-risk patient," *International Journal of Periodontics and Restorative Dentistry*, vol. 27, no. 2, pp. 161–169, 2007.

[49] S. Nagasawa, K. Hayano, T. Niino et al., "Nonlinear stress analysis of titanium implants by finite element method," *Dental Materials Journal*, vol. 27, no. 4, pp. 633–639, 2008.

[50] G. E. Salvi and U. Brägger, "Mechanical and technical risks in implant therapy," *International Journal of Oral & Maxillofacial Implants*, vol. 24, supplement, pp. 69–85, 2009.

[51] N. Alsabeeha, M. Atieh, and A. G. T. Payne, "Loading protocols for mandibular implant overdentures: a systematic review with meta-analysis," *Clinical Implant Dentistry and Related Research*, vol. 12, supplement 1, pp. e28–e38, 2010.

[52] T. Grandi, P. Garuti, P. Guazzi, L. Tarabini, and A. Forabosco, "Survival and success rates of immediately and early loaded implants: 12-month results from a multicentric randomized clinical study," *Journal of Oral Implantology*, vol. 38, no. 3, pp. 239–249, 2012.

[53] Y.-T. Hsu, J.-H. Fu, K. Al-Hezaimi, and H.-L. Wang, "Biomechanical implant treatment complications: a systematic review of clinical studies of implants with at least 1 year of functional loading," *The International Journal of Oral & Maxillofacial Implants*, vol. 27, no. 4, pp. 894–904, 2012.

[54] T.-J. Ji, J. Y. K. Kan, K. Rungcharassaeng, P. Roe, and J. L. Lozada, "Immediate loading of maxillary and mandibular implant-supported fixed complete dentures: A 1- to 10-year retrospective study," *Journal of Oral Implantology*, vol. 38, no. 1, pp. 469–476, 2012.

[55] R. Glauser, A. Rée, A. Lundgren, J. Gottlow, C. H. Hämmerle, and P. Schärer, "Immediate occlusal loading of Brånemark implants applied in various jawbone regions: a prospective, 1-year clinical study," *Clinical implant dentistry and related research*, vol. 3, no. 4, pp. 204–213, 2001.

[56] G. M. Raghoebar, B. Friberg, I. Grunert, J. A. Hobkirk, G. Tepper, and I. Wendelhag, "3-Year prospective multicenter study on one-stage implant surgery and early loading in the edentulous

mandible," *Clinical Implant Dentistry and Related Research*, vol. 5, no. 1, pp. 39–46, 2003.

[57] S. Lumetti, U. Consolo, C. Galli et al., "Fresh-frozen bone blocks for horizontal ridge augmentation in the upper maxilla: 6-month outcomes of a randomized controlled trial," *Clinical Implant Dentistry and Related Research*, vol. 16, no. 1, pp. 116–123, 2014.

[58] S. Lumetti, C. Galli, E. Manfredi et al., "Correlation between density and resorption of fresh-frozen and autogenous bone grafts," *BioMed Research International*, vol. 2014, Article ID 508328, 6 pages, 2014.

[59] W. Att, J. Bernhart, and J. R. Strub, "Fixed rehabilitation of the edentulous maxilla: possibilities and clinical outcome," *Journal of Oral and Maxillofacial Surgery*, vol. 67, no. 11, pp. 60–73, 2009.

[60] A. Barone, B. Orlando, P. Tonelli, and U. Covani, "Survival rate for implants placed in the posterior maxilla with and without sinus augmentation: a comparative cohort study," *Journal of Periodontology*, vol. 82, no. 2, pp. 219–226, 2011.

[61] B. J. Jackson, "Occlusal principles and clinical applications for endosseous implants," *Journal of Oral Implantology*, vol. 29, no. 5, pp. 230–234, 2003.

[62] Y. Kim, T.-J. Oh, C. E. Misch, and H.-L. Wang, "Occlusal considerations in implant therapy: clinical guidelines with biomechanical rationale," *Clinical Oral Implants Research*, vol. 16, no. 1, pp. 26–35, 2005.

[63] M. R. Wood and S. G. Vermilyea, "A review of selected dental literature on evidence-based treatment planning for dental implants: report of the Committee on Research in Fixed Prosthodontics of the Academy of Fixed Prosthodontics," *Journal of Prosthetic Dentistry*, vol. 92, no. 5, pp. 447–462, 2004.

[64] I. Klineberg, D. Kingston, and G. Murray, "The bases for using a particular occlusal design in tooth and implant-borne reconstructions and complete dentures," *Clinical Oral Implants Research*, vol. 18, no. S3, pp. 151–167, 2007.

[65] I. J. Klineberg, M. Trulsson, and G. M. Murray, "Occlusion on implants—is there a problem?" *Journal of Oral Rehabilitation*, vol. 39, no. 7, pp. 522–537, 2012.

[66] E. Göre and G. Evlioğlu, "Assessment of the effect of two occlusal concepts for implant-supported fixed prostheses by finite element analysis in patients with bruxism," *The Journal of Oral Implantology*, vol. 40, no. 1, pp. 68–75, 2014.

[67] R. P. Kinsel and D. Lin, "Retrospective analysis of porcelain failures of metal ceramic crowns and fixed partial dentures supported by 729 implants in 152 patients: patient-specific and implant-specific predictors of ceramic failure," *Journal of Prosthetic Dentistry*, vol. 101, no. 6, pp. 388–394, 2009.

[68] O. Komiyama, F. Lobbezoo, A. De Laat et al., "Clinical management of implant prostheses in patients with bruxism," *International Journal of Biomaterials*, vol. 2012, Article ID 369063, 6 pages, 2012.

[69] R. Skalak, "Biomechanical considerations in osseointegrated prostheses," *The Journal of Prosthetic Dentistry*, vol. 49, no. 6, pp. 843–848, 1983.

[70] W.-S. Lin, C. Ercoli, R. Lowenguth, L. M. Yerke, and D. Morton, "Oral rehabilitation of a patient with bruxism and cluster implant failures in the edentulous maxilla: a clinical report," *Journal of Prosthetic Dentistry*, vol. 108, no. 1, pp. 1–8, 2012.

[71] S. Lumetti, E. Manfredi, S. Ferraris et al., "The response of osteoblastic MC3T3-E1 cells to micro- and nano-textured, hydrophilic and bioactive titanium surfaces," *Journal of Materials Science: Materials in Medicine*, vol. 27, no. 4, article no. 68, 2016.

[72] D. Feu, F. Catharino, C. C. A. Quintão, and M. A. De Oliveira Almeida, "A systematic review of etiological and risk factors associated with bruxism," *Journal of Orthodontics*, vol. 40, no. 2, pp. 163–171, 2013.

[73] E. Bertazzo-Silveira, C. M. Kruger, I. Porto De Toledo et al., "Association between sleep bruxism and alcohol, caffeine, tobacco, and drug abuse," *The Journal of the American Dental Association*, vol. 147, no. 11, pp. 859.e4–866.e4, 2016.

[74] D. Nitzan, A. Mamlider, L. Levin, and D. Schwartz-Arad, "Impact of smoking on marginal bone loss," *International Journal of Oral and Maxillofacial Implants*, vol. 20, no. 4, pp. 605–609, 2005.

[75] S. DeLuca and G. Zarb, "The effect of smoking on osseointegrated dental implants. Part II: peri-implant bone loss," *International Journal of Prosthodontics*, vol. 19, no. 6, pp. 560–566, 2006.

[76] L. Levin, R. Hertzberg, S. Har-Nes, and D. Schwartz-Arad, "Long-term marginal bone loss around single dental implants affected by current and past smoking habits," *Implant Dentistry*, vol. 17, no. 4, pp. 422–429, 2008.

[77] S. Vervaeke, B. Collaert, S. Vandeweghe, J. Cosyn, E. Deschepper, and H. De Bruyn, "The effect of smoking on survival and bone loss of implants with a fluoride-modified surface: a 2-year retrospective analysis of 1106 implants placed in daily practice," *Clinical Oral Implants Research*, vol. 23, no. 6, pp. 758–766, 2012.

A Case of Primary Combined Squamous Cell Carcinoma with Neuroendocrine (Atypical Carcinoid) Tumor in the Floor of the Mouth

Kenji Yamagata, Kazuhiro Terada, Fumihiko Uchida, Naomi Kanno, Shogo Hasegawa, Toru Yanagawa, and Hiroki Bukawa

Department of Oral and Maxillofacial Surgery, Institute of Clinical Medicine, Faculty of Medicine, University of Tsukuba, Tsukuba, Japan

Correspondence should be addressed to Kenji Yamagata; y-kenji@md.tsukuba.ac.jp

Academic Editor: Giuseppe Colella

The combined squamous cell carcinoma (SCC) with neuroendocrine (atypical carcinoid (AC)) tumor is extremely rare in the head and neck. We present here the first case of SCC with AC arising in the floor of the mouth of 65-year-old man. The tumor is comprised of two components of SCC and AC in the biopsy specimen. Neuroendocrine tumor component was classified as AC from the punctate necrosis and 2–10>/10 HPF. Immunohistochemical staining was HMW-CK/34B (+) and P63 (+) in SCC and synaptophysin (+) and CD56 (+) in AC. The pathological diagnosis of SCC with AC was made from both the morphological and immunological exam. Concurrent chemoradiotherapy was performed with radiotherapy 70.2 Gy and chemotherapy of CDDP and VP-16. Although the treatment effect was complete response both of primary tumor and of neck metastases, the recurrence of the primary tumor was after 6 months. Bilateral modified radical neck dissection and tumor resection of the floor of the mouth with reconstructive surgery of anterior lateral thigh free flap were performed. Although the primary and neck tumor did not recur, the multiple lung metastases and mediastinum lymph node metastases occurred at 6 months after surgery.

1. Introduction

Neuroendocrine neoplasms are a heterogeneous group of tumors that vary from benign to highly malignant. WHO (2005) classified neuroendocrine tumor (NET) of the larynx into 4 types: (1) typical carcinoid, (2) atypical carcinoid (AC), (3) small cell carcinoma, neuroendocrine type, and (4) combined small cell carcinoma, neuroendocrine type, with nonsmall cell carcinoma [1]. The AC (synonyms of malignant carcinoid, moderately differentiated neuroendocrine carcinoma, and large cell neuroendocrine carcinoma) is the most frequent, constituting 54% of all NET in this site, followed by the small cell carcinoma, neuroendocrine type (34%), paraganglioma (9%), and the typical carcinoid (3%) [1]. Although the NET is a tumor that occurs particularly in the lung and larynx, oral cavity is a rare site for a primary NET [2]. Recently, neuroendocrine differentiation has also been found in some tumors not considered to be of neuroendocrine origin, including squamous cell carcinoma (SCC) of the lung and esophagus [3, 4]. The occurrence and possible role of NET in the head and neck SCC have not yet been analyzed. Combined-type SCC and AC instances in the head and neck area were reported only in 3 cases and very rare [5–7]. We report here the fast case of the combined SCC with AC of the floor of the mouth.

2. Case Report

A 65-year-old Japanese man referred to the Department of Oral and Maxillofacial Surgery, University of Tsukuba Hospital, complaining of pain in the floor of the mouth for one month. His medical history revealed diabetes mellitus, hypertension, chronic pancreatitis, reflux esophagitis, and iron deficiency anemia. His face was symmetrical and there was no trismus. The regional lymph nodes were swollen multiply in both sides from level I to level II. Intraoral examination

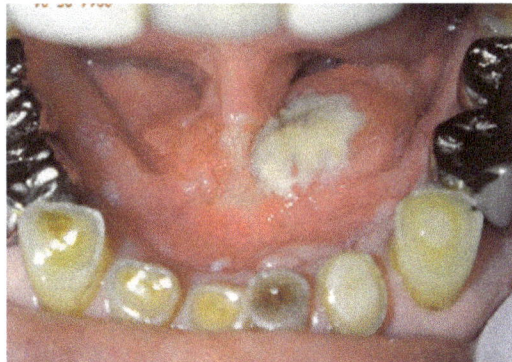

FIGURE 1: Intraoral examination shows relatively well defined elastic hard mass with ulcer in the left floor of the mouth, which measures approximately 36 × 33 mm.

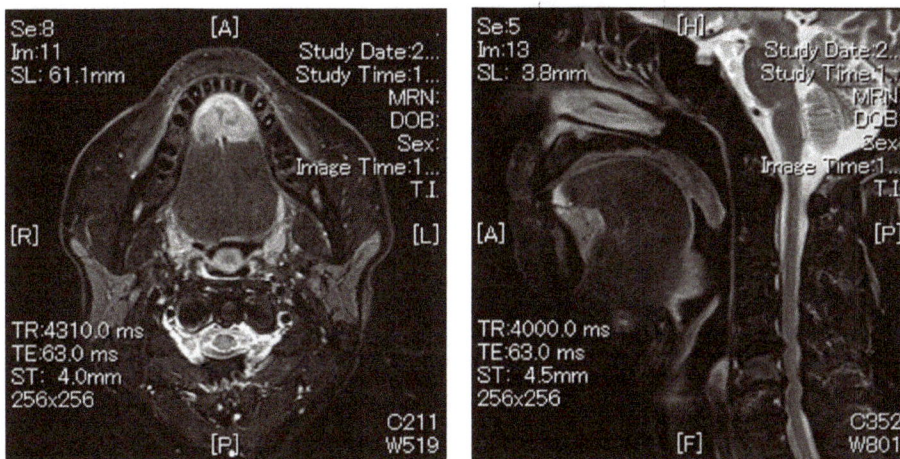

FIGURE 2: T2 weighted MRI sequence shows a 29 × 23 × 22 mm heterogeneous high signal mass in the floor of mouth.

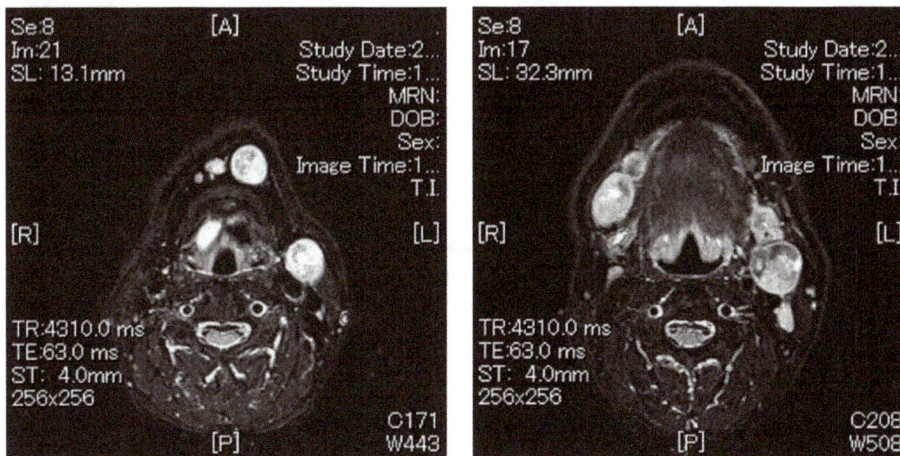

FIGURE 3: Bilateral multiple neck lymph node metastases are shown. The level Ia LNs are swollen in 16 mm and 7 mm, right level Ib LNs are swollen in 23 mm and 13 mm, left level Ib LN is swollen in 5 mm, and left level IIa LN is swollen in 37 mm.

shows relatively well defined elastic hard mass with necrotic ulcer in the right to left floor of the mouth, which measures approximately 36 × 33 mm (Figure 1).

T2 weighted MRI showed a sequence that shows a 29 × 23 × 22 mm heterogeneous high signal mass in the floor of mouth (Figure 2). Bilateral multiple neck lymph node metastases are depicted in MRI. The level Ia LNs are swollen in 16 mm and 7 mm, right level Ib LNs are swollen in 23 mm and 13 mm, left level Ib LN is swollen in 5 mm, and left level IIa LN is swollen in 37 mm (Figure 3). The 18F-fluorodeoxy-glucose positron-emission tomography combined with computed tomography (18F-FDG PET/CT) revealed FDG uptake

(a)

(HE ×100)   (HE ×400)

(b)

(HE ×100)   (HE ×400)

(c)

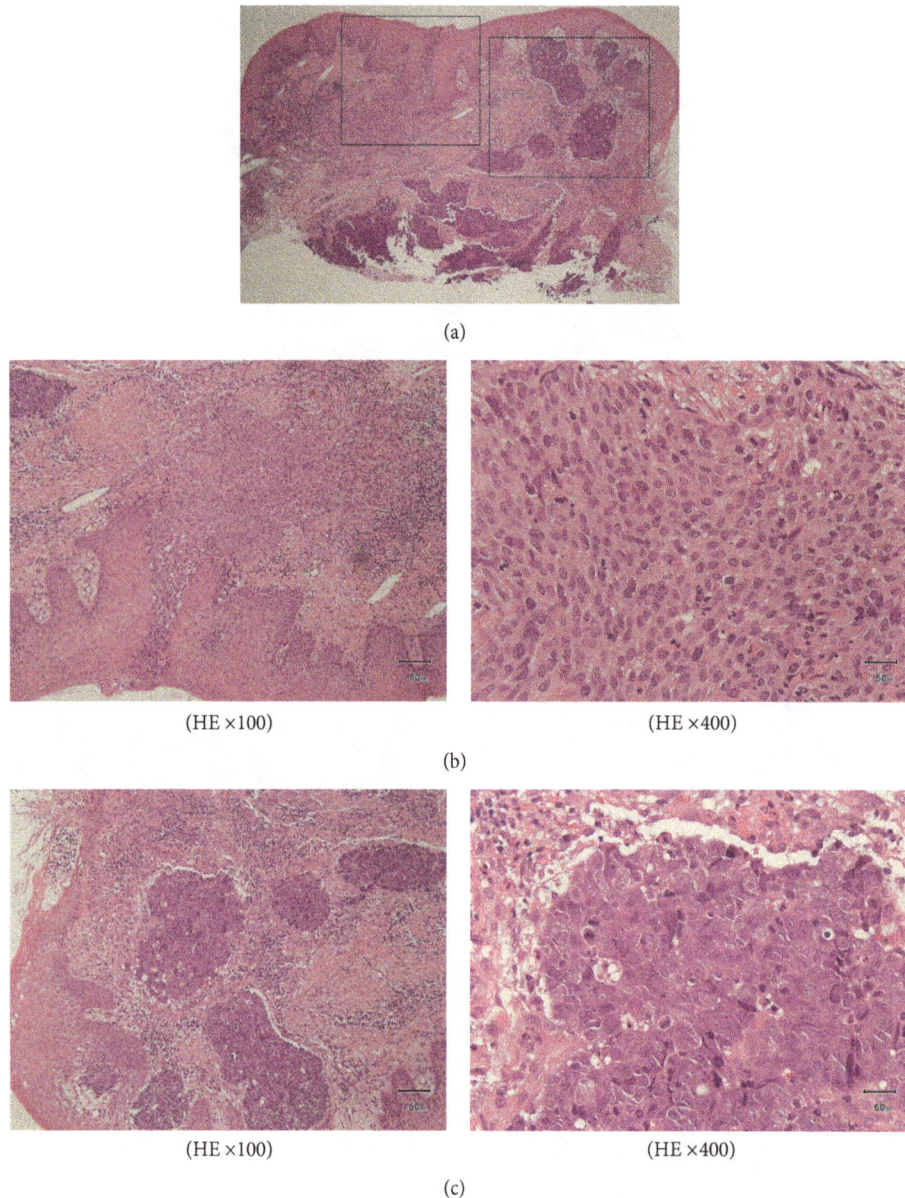

FIGURE 4: (a) The histopathology of biopsy specimen (HE ×40). The square of straight line was comprised of SCC, and dotted line was comprised of AC. Microscopically, the tumor consists of two components of SCC and AC. (b) The component of SCC. Nonkeratic dysplastic squamous cells proliferated with apoptosis and mitosis. (c) The component of AC. The cells change in a larger way and have high N/C rate and chromatin, a lot of mitosis and karyolysises are seen. A punctate necrosis is observed in the tumor nest, and the rosette structures are observed.

in the floor of the mouth mass measuring 28 × 13 mm with the SUV max 10.4 and bilateral multiple LNs.

The incisional biopsy was performed from floor of the mouth under local anesthesia. Microscopically, the tumor consisted of two components of SCC and AC. SCC consisted of nonkeratic dysplastic squamous cells proliferated with apoptosis and mitosis. The cells change larger and have high N/C rate and chromatin, a lot of mitosis and karyolysises are seen in component of NET. The punctate necrosis was observed and 2–10>/10 HPF. The NET component was classified as AC (Figures 4(a)–4(c)). Immunohistochemical staining was synaptophysin (+), CD56 (+), and chromogranin A

(−) in AC and HMW-CK/34B (+) and P63 (+) in SCC. There was no transitional part between SCC and AC (Figures 5(a) and 5(b)). From these findings pathological diagnosis of SCC with AC in the floor of the mouth was made.

Concurrent chemoradiotherapy was performed with radiotherapy 70.2 Gy and chemotherapy of CDDP and VP-16 for 4 times under the consideration of unresectable neck metastases. Chemotherapy regimen was day 1: CDDP 70 mg/m^2 + VP-16 100 mg/m^2, day 2: VP-16 100 mg/m^2, and day 3: VP-16 100 mg/m^2. The highest side effects according to CTCAE ver. 4.0 were leukocytopenia (G4), anemia (G3), and thrombocytopenia (G3). The aspiration pneumonia occurred

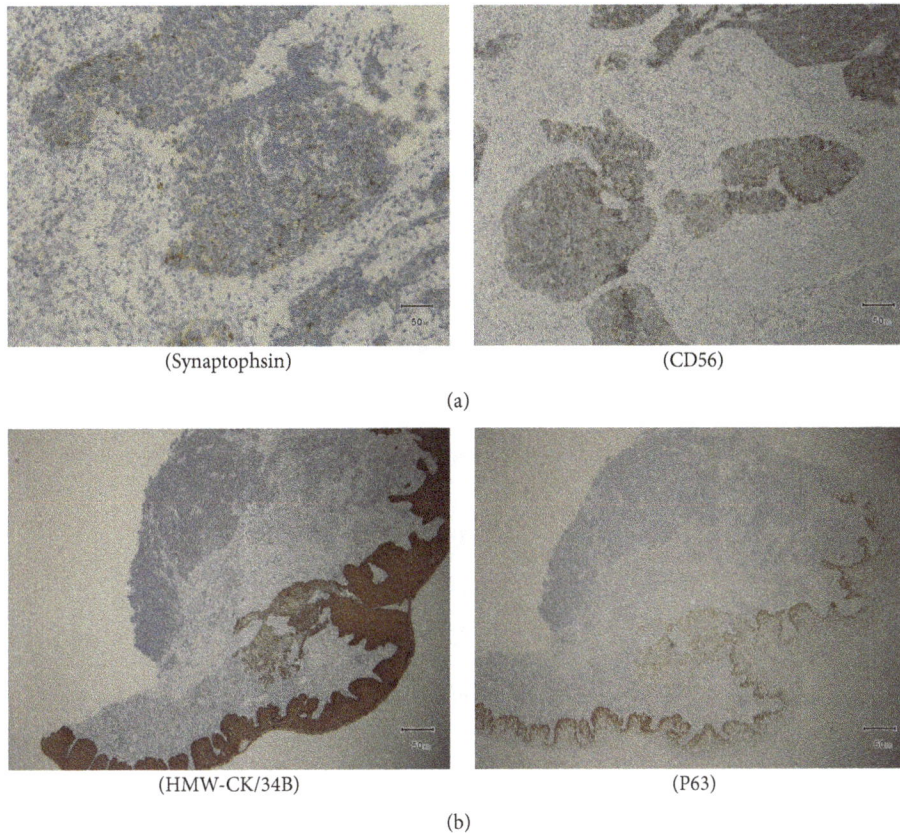

(Synaptophsin)   (CD56)

(a)

(HMW-CK/34B)   (P63)

(b)

FIGURE 5: (a) Immunohistochemical staining shows that the tumor cells are positive for synaptophysin and CD56 in SCC. (b) Immunohisto-chemical staining shows that the tumor cells are positive for HMW-CK/34B and P63 in SCC.

during pancytopenia after second chemotherapy. The leuko-cyte counts recovered on administrating of G-CSF and aspiration pneumonia was improved with the administration of antibiotics. The treatment effect was complete response both of primary tumor and of neck metastases.

The recurrence of the primary site occurred 6 months from the end of chemoradiotherapy with a diagnosis of pri-mary site biopsy (Figure 6). The volume of lymph node metastases was decreased and changed to resectable. Bilateral modified radical neck dissection and tumor resection of the floor of the mouth with reconstructive surgery of anterior lateral thigh (ALT) free flap were performed under general anesthesia. The pathological diagnosis was SCC without AC in the primary site (Figure 7). There were no metastases in the specimen of neck lymph nodes. Although the primary and neck tumor did not recur, the multiple lung metastases and mediastinum lymph node metastases were diagnosed with FDG PET at 6 months after surgery (Figure 8). The patient received best supportive care with chemotherapy of paclitaxel and cetuximab.

3. Discussion

NETs represent a rare, heterogeneous subset in the laryngeal malignancies and are classified into distinct groups and ranging from benign to highly malignant. The oral cavity is a rare site of a primary NET and only 12 cases were reported [2].

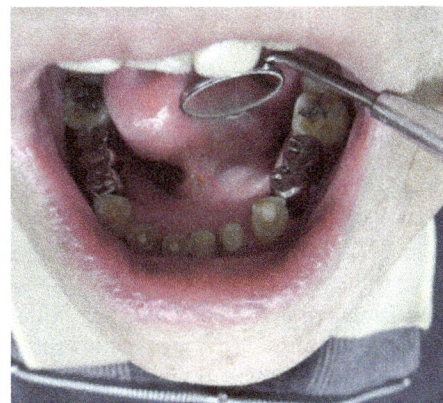

FIGURE 6: Intraoral examination 6 months after chemoradiotherapy shows small ulcer in the left floor of the mouth.

Neuroendocrine differentiation has recently been reported in SCC of the lung and esophagus. The occurrence and possible role of neuroendocrine differentiation in the head and neck SCC have not yet been analyzed [8]. It has been hypothesized that tumor cells with neuroendocrine characterization may produce peptides to stimulate tumor growth via autocrine or paracrine mechanisms [4]. Three previously reported SCC with AC of head and neck cases were larynx, maxillary sinus,

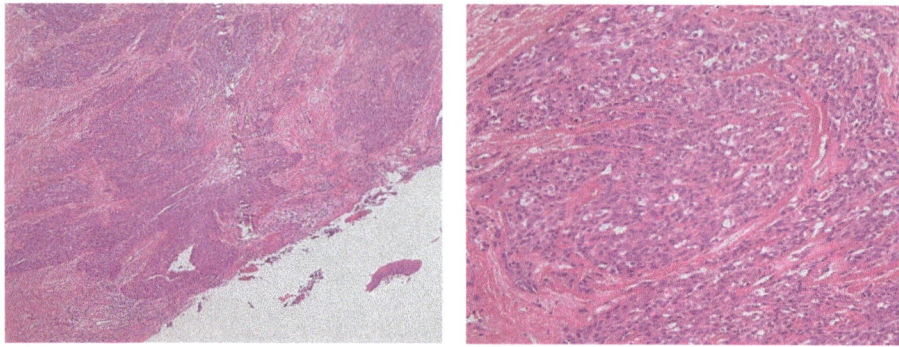

FIGURE 7: The histopathology of recurred resected specimen (HE ×40, ×100). Microscopically, the resected tumor of floor of mouth was SCC.

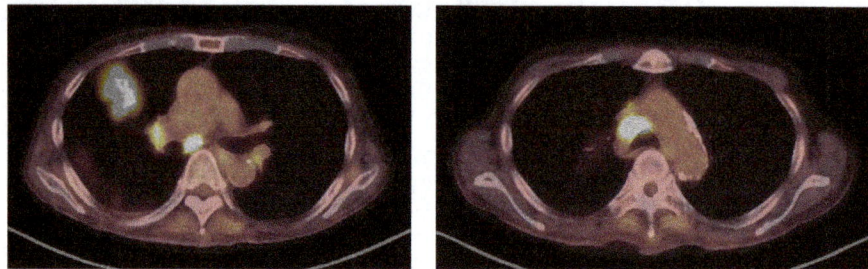

FIGURE 8: Lung metastasis and mediastinum lymph node metastases are depicted in the PET-CT.

and upper gingiva [5–7]. The present case was the first report represented on the floor of the mouth with a composite tumor consisting of SCC and AC. Although the composite tumor consisted of combined SCC and small cell carcinoma was reported sometimes, to our knowledge, our case is the fourth to document a composite tumor including AC [5, 7].

A capacity for multidirectional differentiation could arise from pluripotent stem cells. SCC and AC could have arisen from pluripotent cells that differentiated along two distinct paths or the AC could have differentiated secondarily from cells arising in SCC [5, 9]. Another hypothesis is that AC derived from pluripotential indifferent cells of either the squamous epithelium or the minor salivary gland [10]. In the present case, there was no transitional part between SCC and AC in the biopsy specimen, suggested to arise from pluripotent cells that differentiated along two distinct paths.

Immunohistochemically, NET frequently expresses chromogranin A, synaptophysin, and CD56. The tumor cells of NET component are positive for synaptophysin and CD56 in our case. The SCC component was negative for synaptophysin and CD56 and positive for HMW-CK/34B and P63. Nisman et al. reported neuroendocrine differentiation in SCC was associated with poor prognosis [3]. On the other hand, chromogranin A and synaptophysin expression were reported not to associate with advanced disease stage and not to affect patient survival [8]. More cases of this tumor need to accumulate to clarify biological behavior and prognosis.

The AC most occur in supraglottic submucosal in the sixth- and seventh-decade males (M : F, 3 : 1). The rate of metastases was reported 66.7% and the 5-year survival 46% [10]. There was no evidence for the treatment of head and neck AC. The primary treatment is reported to be the surgery

and the radiotherapy, with rare response in the chemotherapy [10]. However, AC is reported to be relatively resistant to chemotherapy and radiation therapy [11], and there is no proven optimal therapy for metastatic unresectable AC. Although surgical resection is usually recommended, patients did respond to radiotherapy and chemotherapy, suggesting a combined approach may be indicated in the larynx AC [12]. It was reported that the treatment of primary neoplasms consisting of more than one histological type is tailored to the most histologically aggressive tumor [7]. In our case, the clinical stage was advanced with bilateral multiple neck lymph node metastasis and the chemoradiotherapy was selected because of unresectable and aggressive tumor feature.

Treatment regimens showing efficacy in pulmonary carcinoid were reported to include octreotide-based therapies (10% response rate (RR), 70% disease control rate (DCR)), etoposide (VP-16) + platinum (23% RR, 69% DCR), and temozolomide-based therapies (14% RR, 57% DCR) [13]. The regimen for our case was selected as etoposide + platinum, because platinum is standard regimen for SCC and both effective for SCC and effective for AC. Fortunately the chemotherapy with CDDP and VP-16 and radiotherapy were effective and achieved complete response. The side effect for CDDP and VP-16 of grade 4 leukocytopenia occurred after chemotherapy and the aspiration pneumonia occurred during pancytopenia. This chemotherapy was tolerable because the leukocyte counts recovered on administrating of G-CSF and aspiration pneumonia was improved with antibiotics.

Although the treatment effect was complete response, the recurrence of the primary site occurred 6 months from the end of chemoradiotherapy. The resected primary tumor was

SCC without AC, and there were no tumors in the lymph nodes. In the reported combined SCC and AC of the lung, intermediate-grade AC is considered as less aggressive than SCC. The rapid disease progression was suggested that SCC component contributes to the metastasis [14]. In the present case, the component of AC suggested to metastasize to the lymph nodes and to be sensitive to chemoradiotherapy. The component of SCC in primary site was not sensitive for chemoradiotherapy and recurred.

We experienced the first case of SCC with AC of the floor of mouth. More cases of this tumor need to accumulate to clarify biological behavior, treatment, and prognosis. Moreover the occurrence and possible role of SCC with AC have not yet been analyzed, and further research will be desired in the future.

Competing Interests

The authors declare that there is no conflict of interests regarding the publication of this paper.

References

[1] L. Barnes, *Tumours of the Hypopharynx, Larynx, and Trachea: Neuroendocrine Tumors*, IARC Press, Lyon, France, 2005.

[2] B.-Z. Wu, Y. Gao, and B. Yi, "Primary neuroendocrine carcinoma in oral cavity: two case reports and review of the literature," *Journal of Oral and Maxillofacial Surgery*, vol. 72, no. 3, pp. 633–644, 2014.

[3] B. Nisman, N. Heching, H. Biran, V. Barak, and T. Peretz, "The prognostic significance of circulating neuroendocrine markers chromogranin A, pro-gastrin-releasing peptide and neuron-specific enolase in patients with advanced non-small-cell lung cancer," *Tumor Biology*, vol. 27, no. 1, pp. 8–16, 2006.

[4] A. Yuan, J. Liu, Y. Liu, and G. Cui, "Chromogranin a-positive tumor cells in human esophageal squamous cell carcinomas," *Pathology and Oncology Research*, vol. 13, no. 4, pp. 321–325, 2007.

[5] Y. Mochizuki, K. Omura, K. Sakamoto et al., "A case of primary combined neuroendocrine carcinoma with squamous cell carcinoma in the upper gingiva," *Oral Surgery, Oral Medicine, Oral Pathology, Oral Radiology, and Endodontology*, vol. 109, no. 4, pp. e34–e39, 2010.

[6] A. Franchi, D. Rocchetta, A. Palomba, D. R. D. Innocenti, F. Castiglione, and G. Spinelli, "Primary combined neuroendocrine and squamous cell carcinoma of the maxillary sinus: report of a case with immunohistochemical and molecular characterization," *Head and Neck Pathology*, vol. 9, no. 1, pp. 107–113, 2015.

[7] C. R. Davies-Husband, P. Montgomery, D. Premachandra, and H. Hellquist, "Primary, combined, atypical carcinoid and squamous cell carcinoma of the larynx: a new variety of composite tumour," *Journal of Laryngology and Otology*, vol. 124, no. 2, pp. 226–229, 2010.

[8] V. H. Schartinger, C. Falkeis, K. Laimer et al., "Neuroendocrine differentiation in head and neck squamous cell carcinoma," *Journal of Laryngology and Otology*, vol. 126, no. 12, pp. 1261–1270, 2012.

[9] K.-J. Cho, J.-J. Jang, S.-S. Lee, and J.-I. Zo, "Basaloid squamous carcinoma of the oesophagus: a distinct neoplasm with multi-potential differentiation," *Histopathology*, vol. 36, no. 4, pp. 331–340, 2000.

[10] A. Ferlito, K. O. Devaney, and A. Rinaldo, "Neuroendocrine neoplasms of the larynx: advances in identification, understanding, and management," *Oral Oncology*, vol. 42, no. 8, pp. 770–788, 2006.

[11] R. Hage, A. B. de la Rivière, C. A. Seldenrijk, and J. M. M. van den Bosch, "Update in pulmonary carcinoid tumors: a review article," *Annals of Surgical Oncology*, vol. 10, no. 6, pp. 697–704, 2003.

[12] A. Gillenwater, J. Lewin, D. Roberts, and A. El-Naggar, "Moderately differentiated neuroendocrine carcinoma (atypical carcinoid) of the larynx: a clinically aggressive tumor," *Laryngoscope*, vol. 115, no. 7, pp. 1191–1195, 2005.

[13] C. R. Chong, L. J. Wirth, M. Nishino et al., "Chemotherapy for locally advanced and metastatic pulmonary carcinoid tumors," *Lung Cancer*, vol. 86, no. 2, pp. 241–246, 2014.

[14] M. Okazaki, Y. Sano, Y. Soga et al., "Combined atypical carcinoid tumour and squamous cell carcinoma of the lung," *Internal Medicine*, vol. 54, no. 11, pp. 1385–1388, 2015.

Nondestructive Microcomputed Tomography Evaluation of Mineral Density in Exfoliated Teeth with Hypophosphatasia

Sachiko Hayashi-Sakai,[1] Takafumi Hayashi,[1] Makoto Sakamoto,[2] Jun Sakai,[3] Junko Shimomura-Kuroki,[4] Hideyoshi Nishiyama,[1] Kouji Katsura,[1] Makiko Ike,[1] Yutaka Nikkuni,[1] Miwa Nakayama,[1] Marie Soga,[1] and Taichi Kobayashi[1]

[1]*Division of Oral and Maxillofacial Radiology, Niigata University Graduate School of Medical and Dental Sciences, 2-5274 Gakkocho-dori, Chuo-ku, Niigata 951-8514, Japan*
[2]*Department of Health Sciences, Faculty of Medicine, Niigata University, 2-746 Asahimachi-dori, Chuo-ku, Niigata 951-8514, Japan*
[3]*Department of System and Automotive Engineering, Niigata College of Technology, 5-13-7 Kamishinei-cho, Nishi-ku, Niigata 950-2076, Japan*
[4]*Department of Pediatric Dentistry, The Nippon Dental University, School of Life Dentistry at Niigata, 1-8 Hamaura-cho, Chuo-ku, Niigata 951-8580, Japan*

Correspondence should be addressed to Sachiko Hayashi-Sakai; sachipro@dent.niigata-u.ac.jp

Academic Editor: Sukumaran Anil

Most cases of hypophosphatasia (HPP) exhibit early loss of primary teeth. Results of microcomputed tomography (micro-CT) analysis of teeth with HPP have rarely been reported. The purpose of the present study was to describe the mineral density distribution and mapping of exfoliated teeth from an HPP patient using micro-CT. Four exfoliated teeth were obtained from a patient with HPP. Enamel and dentin mineral densities of exfoliated teeth were measured on micro-CT. The mean values of enamel and dentin mineral densities in mandibular primary central incisors with HPP were 1.61 and 0.98 g/cm^3, respectively. The corresponding values in the mandibular primary lateral incisors were 1.60 and 0.98 g/cm^3, respectively. Enamel hypoplasia was seen in the remaining teeth, both maxillary and mandibular primary canines and first and second molars. Micro-CT enables nondestructive, noninvasive evaluation and is useful for studying human hard tissues obtained from patients.

1. Introduction

Hypophosphatasia (HPP) is a rare congenital metabolic bone disease with autosomal dominant or recessive inheritance. The disorder of HPP is caused by mutations to the tissue-nonspecific alkaline phosphatase gene (TNSALP) and results in decreased serum alkaline phosphatase (ALP) levels and hard tissues with defective calcification. HPP is classified by the age at diagnosis into six clinical forms: (1) perinatal; (2) infantile; (3) childhood; (4) adult; (5) odonto-; and (6) a rare benign perinatal form [1–5]. The clinical picture shows a wide spectrum from dental abnormalities without skeletal manifestations in odonto-HPP to lethal skeletal hypomineralization in perinatal HPP [1, 2, 4].

A major dental feature of HPP is premature loss of dentition, which most commonly affects the incisors. In previous studies of HPP, hypoplasia of cementum tissue was found to be responsible for early primary tooth loss in childhood HPP [1, 2, 6, 7], but few reports have examined exfoliated teeth of childhood HPP patients.

Microcomputed tomography (micro-CT) uses X-ray attenuation to visualize the internal structure of objects. Since it enables three-dimensional analysis with nondestructive, noninvasive evaluation, it is a useful modality for studying human hard tissues [8]. Many studies have been conducted on the mineral density of dental hard tissues using commercial micro-CT systems. However, exfoliated teeth with HPP using the micro-CT analysis have not been reported.

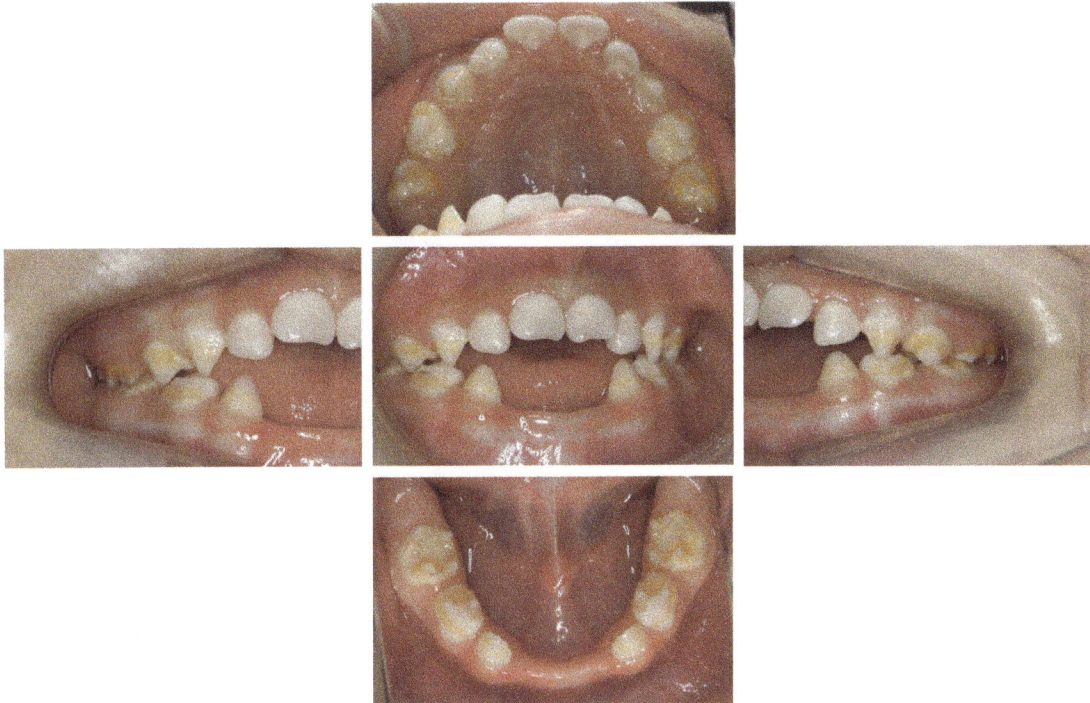

FIGURE 1: Clinical intraoral views at age of 3 years and 2 months.

The present study utilized micro-CT to describe the oral findings, mineral density distribution, and mapping of exfoliated teeth in HPP.

2. Case Presentation

2.1. Case Summary. A 1-year and 2-month-old Japanese female patient was referred to the Dental Clinic of Niigata University Medical and Dental Hospital by the pediatrician at our hospital for dental examination on admission.

The patient was delivered normally at 40 weeks of pregnancy. Her birth weight was 3,212 g, and her height was 49.0 cm. No abnormal symptoms were observed at birth. Her weight gain was poor at 1 month old, and she was admitted to hospital for medical investigation and treatment at 2 months. She was subsequently diagnosed with infantile HPP by means of gene analysis. She was found to be a compound heterozygote carrying the genotype H32IR/c.1559delT *ALPL* gene encoding TNSALP. At 8 months of age, she joined a clinical trial for a new enzyme replacement therapy drug.

At the first visit to our clinic, the patient's weight was 10.3 kg, and her height was 86.3 cm. Intraoral examination showed that the mandibular primary central incisors (71 and 81) had started to erupt. She continued to undergo clinical testing for the new enzyme replacement therapy drug. Four primary teeth were lost early during dental follow-up (Figures 1 and 2). Since enamel hypoplasia was found in both maxillary and mandibular primary canines and first and second molars from eruption, glass ionomer cement fillings were performed on eight primary molars to

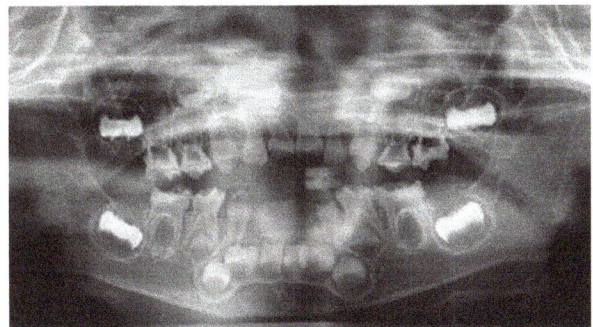

FIGURE 2: Panoramic radiographic appearance at age of 3 years and 2 months.

prevent dental caries. Furthermore, the patient had received regular oral hygiene instruction and topical application of fluoride. The patient's oral hygiene was good, and she had no caries to date. Although she was too young to wear a partial denture, we considered using one with later development.

Radiographic examination revealed enlarged pulp chambers and abnormal alveolar bone resorption (Figure 2). As the four germs of permanent second premolars were not found at the age of 3 years and 2 months, retarded development or congenitally missing teeth germs were suspected.

2.2. Age at Teeth Exfoliation. The age at teeth exfoliation is shown in Table 1. Four primary anterior teeth had exfoliated spontaneously or been extracted because of marked mobility

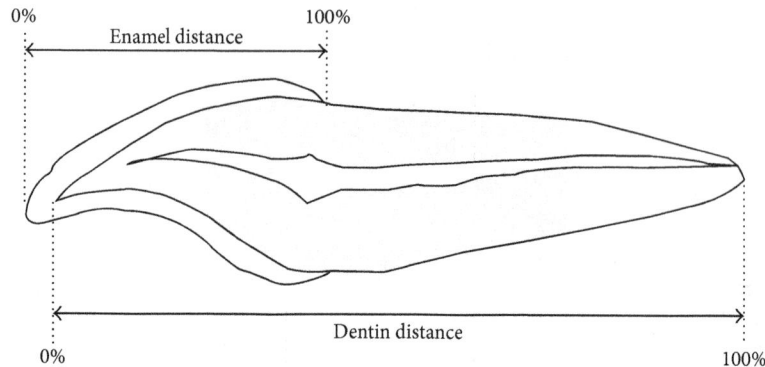

FIGURE 3: Schematic representation of enamel and dentin distance.

TABLE 1: Age at which teeth exfoliated spontaneously or were extracted because of the marked mobility in the present case. Four exfoliated anterior teeth were used as samples.

	Left	Right
Mandibular		
Primary central incisor (71, 81)	1 y and 4 m	1 y and 9 m
Primary lateral incisor (72, 82)	2 y and 6 m	2 y and 9 m

between the ages of 1 year and 2 months at the first visit to our clinic and 3 years and 2 months (Figures 1 and 2).

2.3. Sample Preparation. The four exfoliated teeth were immersed in Teeth Keeper Neo® (Neo Dental Chemical Products Co., Ltd., Tokyo, Japan) at 4°C because the patient's parents wished that we keep them at our clinic (Table 1). All teeth were used after obtaining informed consent from the donating patient's parents.

The findings of exfoliated teeth with incomplete root formation could not be compared with those of teeth with complete root formation. Consequently, for comparison of mineral densities with healthy teeth, mandibular primary central incisors ($n = 2$) that had been completely luxated due to trauma at the same age were used as controls. The study was performed according to a protocol approved by the Institutional Review Board of the Faculty of Dentistry, Niigata University (approval number: 26-R30-10-09).

2.4. Mineral Density Analysis of Exfoliated Teeth. Measurements were performed using a micro-CT compact desktop system, SkyScan-1174 (Bruker Micro-CT, Kontich, Belgium). Images were scanned at a pixel size of 32 μm. Cross sections were reconstructed using software (NRecon, Version 1.6.6.0, Bruker Micro-CT) provided by the scanner manufacturer. Data analysis was performed from the edge to the apex in each tooth sample. For quantitative measurements of enamel and dentin mineral densities, the software package CT Analyzer was used. Two hydroxyapatite phantoms with different mineral densities (0.25 and 0.75 g/cm^3) were used as calibration standards. For each sample, regions of interest

(ROIs) were drawn on the enamel and dentin of each sample, and the obtained datasets were extracted from the data for the whole teeth. Grey values were detected, and mineral densities could be calculated. In the present study, the edge was defined as 0% and the cementoenamel junction was defined as 100% of the distance on the enamel, and the dentinoenamel junction was defined as 0% and the apex was defined as 100% of the distance on the dentin (Figure 3). Each mineral density on each scanned image was plotted in a scatter diagram. The reconstructed dataset was imported into DataViewer (Version 1.4.4, Bruker Micro-CT) and false colored for visualization.

2.5. Result of Mineral Density Analysis. The mineral density distribution in enamel and dentin is shown in Figures 4(a) and 4(b). The number of data for mandibular primary central incisors was 266. The maximum enamel mineral density was 2.01 g/cm^3, and the minimum value was 1.03 g/cm^3 (mean value 1.61 g/cm^3) in mandibular primary central incisors. A cubic regression curve was obtained ($y = 1E - 06x^3 - 0.0002x^2 + 0.0068x + 1.7917$) using the least squares method. For the mandibular primary lateral incisors, the number of data was 289, the maximum value was 1.98 g/cm^3, and the minimum value was 1.07 g/cm^3 (mean value 1.60 g/cm^3). A cubic regression curve was obtained ($y = 5E - 07x^3 - 0.0001x^2 + 0.0003x + 1.86$). The number of data was 256, and the corresponding values for controls were 1.84 g/cm^3, 1.19 g/cm^3, and 1.61 g/cm^3. A cubic regression curve was obtained ($y = 7E - 07x^3 - 0.0002x^2 + 0.0065x + 1.7096$).

As for the dentin mineral density, the number of data for mandibular primary central incisors was 517. The maximum value was 1.55 g/cm^3, the minimum value was 0.71 g/cm^3, and the mean value was 0.98 g/cm^3 for the mandibular primary central incisors. A cubic regression curve was obtained ($y = -2E - 06x^3 - 0.0003x^2 + 0.0268x + 1.547$) using the least squares method. For the mandibular primary lateral incisors, the number of data was 684, the maximum value was 1.59 g/cm^3, the minimum value was 0.63 g/cm^3, and the mean value was 0.98 g/cm^3. A cubic regression curve was obtained ($y = -4E - 06x^3 + 0.0006x^2 + 0.037x + 1.5936$). The number of data was 555, and the corresponding values for controls were

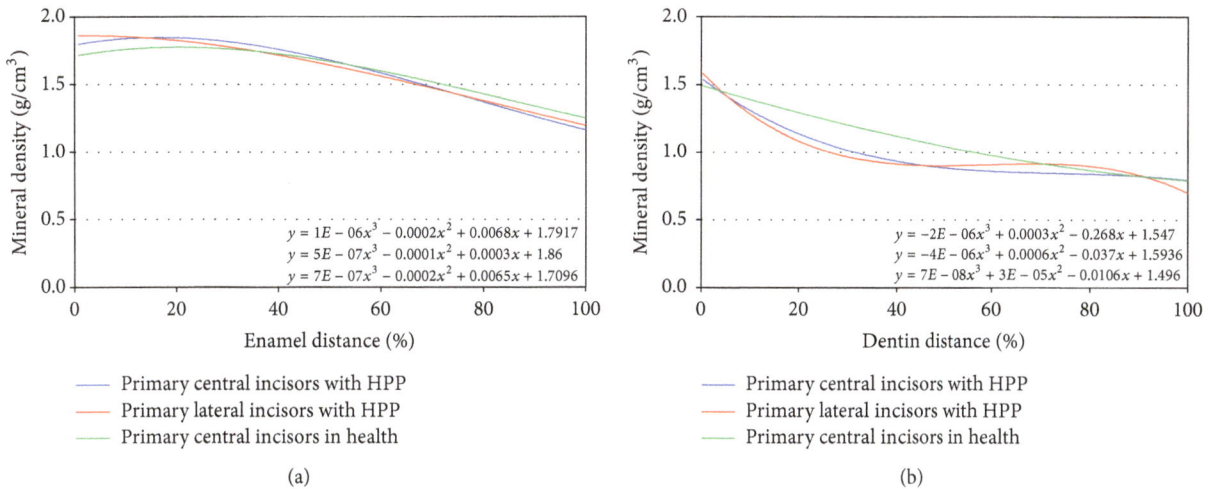

$$y = 1E - 06x^3 - 0.0002x^2 + 0.0068x + 1.7917$$
$$y = 5E - 07x^3 - 0.0001x^2 + 0.0003x + 1.86$$
$$y = 7E - 07x^3 - 0.0002x^2 + 0.0065x + 1.7096$$

(a)

—— Primary central incisors with HPP
—— Primary lateral incisors with HPP
—— Primary central incisors in health

$$y = -2E - 06x^3 + 0.0003x^2 - 0.268x + 1.547$$
$$y = -4E - 06x^3 + 0.0006x^2 - 0.037x + 1.5936$$
$$y = 7E - 08x^3 + 3E - 05x^2 - 0.0106x + 1.496$$

(b)

—— Primary central incisors with HPP
—— Primary lateral incisors with HPP
—— Primary central incisors in health

FIGURE 4: Mineral density distribution in (a) enamel and (b) dentin. The cubic regression curves were obtained using the least squares methods.

$1.50\,\text{g/cm}^3$, $0.68\,\text{g/cm}^3$, and $1.18\,\text{g/cm}^3$. A cubic regression curve was obtained ($y = 7E - 08x^3 + 3E - 05x^2 + 0.0106x + 1.496$).

The mineral density distribution on enamel in HPP was higher than in control samples at the edge region of both primary central and lateral incisors. Although some HPP values were higher than control samples, approximately 60%, HPP values were decreased compared to the control samples, approximately 60% to the cementoenamel junction. All teeth tended to show a peak around 20% in the enamel distance and a decrease in gradient towards the cementoenamel junction (Figure 4(a)).

On the other hand, there were differences between HPP and controls in terms of mineral density distribution in dentin. The gradient and laniary in control teeth decreased from the dentinoenamel junction to the apex without an apparent peak. However, HPP values decreased rapidly to approximately 40% dentin distance and then leveled off at around 50% dentin distance. The mineral density of the mandibular primary lateral incisors decreased before the apex to roughly 90% (Figure 4(b)).

The mineral density distribution mapping in the left primary central incisor is shown in Figure 5. These findings were also seen in the visualized mapping of mineral densities.

3. Discussion

Hypophosphatasia is a congenital error of metabolism in which those affected show defective calcification of hard tissues such as bone and teeth. There are various clinical dental symptoms of HPP, and the disease frequency is low. In the present case, it was possible to describe the clinical oral findings in terms of mineral density. Although the patient's parents consented to examination of the exfoliated teeth, they were not willing to accept destructive testing. Therefore, measurement and analysis of the exfoliated teeth were performed by nondestructive micro-CT imaging. Based on the

general phase of root formation, the mandibular left primary central incisor appeared to have exfoliated just prior to the completion of root formation, while the other teeth exfoliated after root completion [9].

It was not possible to compare the mineral density analysis data from the exfoliated teeth with incomplete root formation with those of teeth with complete root formation, because enamel matures after eruption. Therefore, the data were compared with those of controls, sound mandibular primary central incisors of children of similar age.

The enamel mineral densities in HPP were similar to those of controls in the present case, even though the distribution of dentin mineral densities differed from controls. The gradient and laniary in controls decreased from the dentinoenamel junction to the apex with no apparent peak, but HPP values decreased rapidly to around 40% dentin distance and then leveled off at around 50%. On mapping of mineral densities, mineral density distribution was clearly visible. Since there was enamel hypoplasia in both mandibular and maxillary primary canines and first and second molars, enamel hypoplasia might overlap HPP. Enzyme replacement therapy has recently been developed as treatment for HPP, which the present patient underwent. Further studies may help determine the effects of enzyme replacement therapy on permanent teeth.

Since patients with HPP present with various symptoms and hypomineralization levels, the results of this study on primary teeth size and mineral densities may not be generalizable to all HPP patients. As the patient was too young, her general bone mineral density was not investigated. It is also necessary to study the correlation between bone mineral density and tooth mineral density. A positive correlation would suggest that prediction of general bone mineral density could be possible in cases of premature exfoliation of teeth.

Recently, an increasing number of patients and their parents ask to have their extracted teeth returned. The high degree of attention being paid to the management of oral

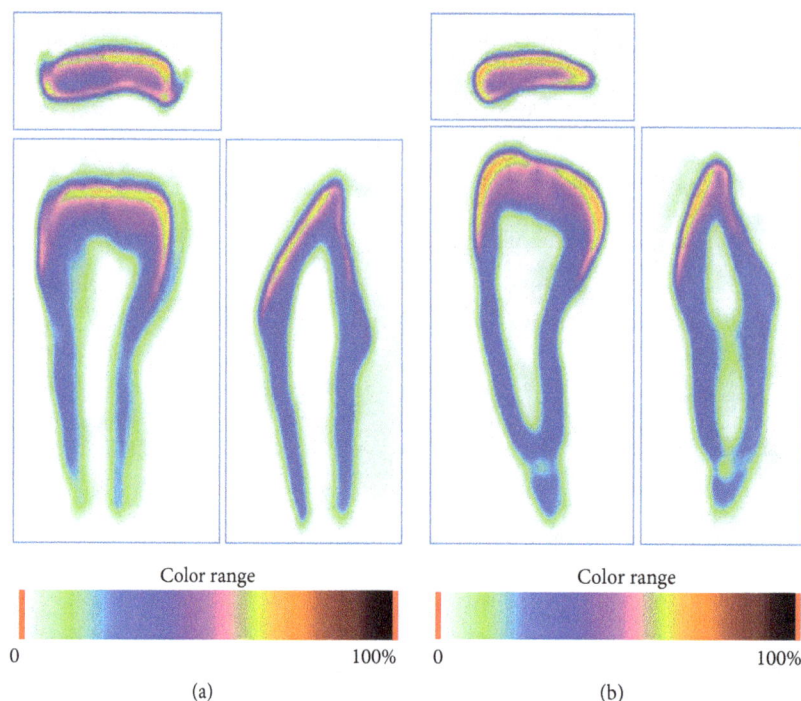

FIGURE 5: Mineral density mapping of incisal, labial, and mesial views in HPP and on (a) mandibular primary left central incisor (71) and (b) mandibular primary left lateral incisor (82). Color range represents the relative values of attenuation coefficient. Here, 100% is equal to $3.0\,g/cm^3$.

health and the declining birthrate have led to difficulty in obtaining teeth, especially primary teeth, for experimental purposes. As a result, dental researchers have difficulty collecting and using human hard tissues from patients. Though experimental animals are an alternative source of materials, human tissues should be used as much as possible to assure that the results will be clinically applicable. Hence, micro-CT was used in the present study. Studies using micro-CT make it easy to obtain data from donated experimental teeth because of the nondestructive nature of the procedure and the fact that the teeth can be returned after micro-CT scanning. Since micro-CT was helpful in resolving the above problem, we believe that micro-CT imaging is a suitable tool for studying hard tissues.

4. Conclusion

HPP is a rare inherited disorder in which most cases show early loss of primary teeth. However, there is almost no information regarding the dental symptoms. Therefore, the clinical oral findings and mineral densities of exfoliated teeth in HPP were described in this report. Enamel mineral densities were similar in HPP and controls, but the distribution of dentin mineral density differed in HPP from that of controls.

Enamel hypoplasia was found in both maxillary and mandibular primary canines and first and second molars. Micro-CT is a suitable tool to study human hard tissues from patients since it enables nondestructive, noninvasive imaging for subsequent evaluation.

Competing Interests

The authors declare that there is no conflict of interests regarding the publication of this paper.

Acknowledgments

The authors would like to acknowledge the patient and her parents for their kind cooperation. This study was supported in part by a Grant-in-Aid for Scientific Research (C) (no. 26462835) from the Ministry of Education, Culture, Sports, Science, and Technology of Japan.

References

[1] M. P. Whyte, *The Metabolic and Molecular Bases of Inherited Diseases*, McGraw-Hill, New York, NY, UAS, 8th edition, 2001.

[2] E. Mornet, "Hypophosphatasia," *Orphanet Journal of Rare Diseases*, vol. 2, article 40, 2007.

[3] M. P. Whyte, "Physiological role of alkaline phosphatase explored in hypophosphatasia," *Annals of the New York Academy of Sciences*, vol. 1192, pp. 190–200, 2010.

[4] E. Mornet, "Genetics of hypophosphatasia," *Clinical Reviews in Bone and Mineral Metabolism*, vol. 11, no. 2, pp. 71–77, 2013.

[5] K. Oda, N. N. Kinjoh, M. Sohda, K. Komaru, and N. Amizuka, "Tissue-nonspecific alkaline phosphatase and hypophosphatasia," *Clinical Calcium*, vol. 24, no. 2, pp. 233–239, 2014 (Japanese).

[6] T. Van den Bos, G. Handoko, A. Niehof et al., "Cementum and dentin in hypophosphatasia," *Journal of Dental Research*, vol. 84, no. 11, pp. 1021–1025, 2005.

[7] K.-W. Wei, K. Xuan, Y.-L. Liu et al., "Clinical, pathological and genetic evaluations of Chinese patients with autosomal-dominant hypophosphatasia," *Archives of Oral Biology*, vol. 55, no. 12, pp. 1017–1023, 2010.

[8] W. Zou, N. Hunter, and M. V. Swain, "Application of polychromatic μcT for mineral density determination," *Journal of Dental Research*, vol. 90, no. 1, pp. 18–30, 2011.

[9] I. Schour and M. Massler, "The development of the human dentition," *The Journal of the American Dental Association*, vol. 28, pp. 1153–1160, 1941.

23

World's First Clinical Case of Gene-Activated Bone Substitute Application

I. Y. Bozo,[1,2,3] R. V. Deev,[2,4] A. Y. Drobyshev,[1] A. A. Isaev,[2] and I. I. Eremin[5]

[1]*Department of Maxillofacial and Plastic Surgery, A.I. Evdokimov Moscow State University of Medicine and Dentistry, Moscow, Russia*
[2]*Human Stem Cells Institute, Moscow, Russia*
[3]*Department of Maxillofacial Surgery, A.I. Burnazyan Federal Medical Biophysical Center, Moscow, Russia*
[4]*I.P. Pavlov Ryazan State Medical University, Ryazan, Russia*
[5]*Central Clinical Hospital with Outpatient Health Center of the Business Administration for the President of the Russian Federation, Moscow, Russia*

Correspondence should be addressed to I. Y. Bozo; bozo.ilya@gmail.com

Academic Editor: Luis M. J. Gutierrez

Treatment of patients with large bone defects is a complex clinical problem. We have initiated the first clinical study of a gene-activated bone substitute composed of the collagen-hydroxyapatite scaffold and plasmid DNA encoding vascular endothelial growth factor. The first patient with two nonunions of previously reconstructed mandible was enrolled into the study. Scar tissues were excised; bone defects (5–14 mm) between the mandibular fragments and nonvascularized rib-bone autograft were filled in with the gene-activated bone substitute. No adverse events were observed during 12 months of follow-up. In 3 months, the average density of newly formed tissues within the implantation zone was 402.21 ± 84.40 and 447.68 ± 106.75 HU in the frontal and distal regions, respectively, which correlated with the density of spongy bone. Complete distal bone defect repair with vestibular and lingual cortical plates formation was observed in 6 and 12 months after surgery; thereby the posterior nonunion was successfully eliminated. However, there was partial resorption of the proximal edge of the autograft entailed to relapse of the anterior nonunion. Thus, the first clinical data on the safety and efficacy of the gene-activated bone substitute were obtained. Given a high complexity of the clinical situation the treatment, results might be considered as promising. NCT02293031.

1. Introduction

The treatment of patients with skeletal bone pathology requires frequently the use of bone substitutes, which replace the lost volumes of bone tissue and accelerate reparative osteogenesis [1]. The methods of bone grafting and the choice of bone substitute depend on the size of bone defect or bone atrophy region, coexisting disorders, and patient's age. Wide range of bone substitutes from conventional materials, such as allogenic and xenogenic bone matrix [2], hydroxyapatite [3], calcium phosphates [4], silicates [5], organic polymers [6], and their combinations, to vascularized bone autografts is available for surgery [7]. However, most of bone substitutes approved for clinical use are not effective for large bone defects repair as they could not overcome "osteogenic insufficiency" specific for such defects [8]. Therefore, physicians almost have no choice for this category of medical indications other than using bone autografts, which are characterized by a number of known limitations and drawbacks (donor site morbidity, an increased risk of complications, and a prolonged surgical intervention) [7, 8].

Different variants of "activated" bone substitutes have been developed when trying to provide an effective alternative to bone autografts [8]; these materials along with an *osteoconductive* matrix contain biological active components standardized under qualitative and quantitative parameters such as cells [9, 10], growth factors [11], or gene constructs [12, 13] which provide *osteoinduction* and/or *osteogenicity* of a bone substitute.

To date, a number of tissue-engineered bone grafts and bone substitutes with growth factors have been already approved for a clinical use. The analysis of published clinical data on their usage confirms the more efficacy compared with conventional bone substitutes [14]. However, their superiority over bone autografts remains doubtful.

Up to date, gene-activated bone substitutes have not been investigated in the clinical trials, although numerous results of experimental studies confirmed the safety and efficacy of the technological approach and individual variants of the materials [12, 13, 15–17].

We have developed a gene-activated bone substitute which consisted of two components: the collagen-hydroxyapatite scaffold and plasmid DNA encoding vascular endothelial growth factor (VEGF). This gene construct is an active substance of the drug "Neovasculgen" (PJSC Human Stem Cells Institute, Russia) which has been shown to be safe and highly effective in the treatment of patients with chronic lower limb ischemia (CLI) of stages 2a-3 and is approved for a clinical use in the territories of Russia and Ukraine [18].

The gene-activated bone substitute demonstrated an obvious osteoinductive effect in an experiment with the repair of cranial defects (with a diameter of 10 mm) in rabbits that manifested with the presence of focal reparative osteogenesis within the central defect part at 15 days after implantation. Complete restoration of bone integrity was observed in 120 days after implantation. This effect was not shown when using the same matrix without plasmid DNA: bone tissue was formed only in the periphery, from the side of bone defect edges, and there was no consolidation up to the final follow-up [19, 20].

Based on successful experimental results, we have initiated the world's first clinical trial of the gene-activated bone substitute to treat patients with maxillofacial bone defects and atrophy of alveolar ridges. The study protocol was approved by the interuniversity Ethics Committee and registered on the website https://clinicaltrials.gov/ (NCT02293031) in November of 2014.

This article describes the treatment results (safety and efficacy) for the first patient enrolled into the clinical study with 12-month follow-up.

2. Case Presentation

2.1. Patient Information. The patient, aged 37 years, a female, was admitted to the Department of Maxillofacial Surgery with complaints on the mandible mobility in the frontal and right distal regions when opening and closing the mouth and impaired mastication due to partial mandibular edentulism on the right side.

In 2011, in a clinic at place of the patient's residence, she was diagnosed to have fibrous dysplasia of the mandible on the right side, for which the patient underwent the resection of the lower jaw from the frontal region to the right ramus with external approach. Later on she had two surgeries of microsurgical mandibular reconstruction with the use of vascularized fibular bone autografts carried out in the regional clinical center. Unfortunately, the autotransplants were removed in both cases due to vascular anastomosis failure.

In May 2012, a reconstruction of the right mandible was done with a free nonvascularized rib autograft in our Department. Within a year after the surgery, the patient had retention of more than 90% of the autotransplant volume and the satisfactory function of mastication on the left side. However, no consolidation was observed and nonunions were diagnosed within the proximal and distal fixation areas that caused mobility and prevented any prosthetic treatment in the mandible on the right side. Therefore, reconstructive surgery with the resection of nonunions, bone grafting, and osteosynthesis was performed. Despite the surgical intervention, a control clinical and instrumental examination in 0.5 year after the operation detected slight mobility in the frontal region and within the right ramus and no radiological evidence of consolidation (Figure 1). The diastasis in the frontal mandible ranged from 5 mm on the upper edge to 14 mm on the lower one; the average tissue density between bone edges was 158.55 ± 116.29 HU; the separation between the transplant edge and the mandibular ramus on the vestibular surface achieved 9.2 mm, with the average tissue density in the nonunion area being 204.52 ± 97.84 HU.

Taking into account a potentially poor blood supply within the fixation of the autotransplant and the mandibular fragments due to numerous operations previously performed including two failed microsurgical ones as well as a prolonged smoking experience (more than 15 years), the patient was offered to undergo a surgical treatment with the use of the gene-activated bone substitute. Considering the patient's characteristics and anamnesis, the total score according to Nonunion Scoring System [21] was estimated to be 31, which corresponded with high risk of nonunion relapse and required more specialized care. Additionally, the nonunions were complicated being formed by nonvascularized bone autograft intended to be resorbed and replaced by newly generated bone tissue. The voluntary written informed consent was obtained.

2.2. Gene-Activated Bone Substitute. The gene-activated bone substitute we developed consists of two components. The first one is the composite scaffold of bovine collagen and synthetic hydroxyapatite (granules with diameter of 500–1000 μm) registered as a bone substitute (CJSC Polystom, Russia) and approved for clinical use in Russia, the second one is a supercoiled naked plasmid DNA with cytomegalovirus promoter and gene encoding VEGF which is the active substance of "Neovasculgen" [18]. We made the gene-activated bone substitute in the form of rectangular sponge-like matrix (size of 20 × 10 × 10 mm, weight of 200 ± 10 mg) containing 0.2 mg of the gene constructs. 5 units were used for clinical study. 5 plates were used for a surgical intervention (total amount of the scaffold: 1000 mg; total dose of the plasmid DNA: 1 mg).

2.3. Surgery. The standard surgical protocol with metal constructs removal, nonunions fibrous tissues excision, and approximated bone surfaces careful grinding was performed. Bone defects (5–14 mm in the frontal region; 7–9 mm in the distal region of the mandible) within the rib autograft, still present from previous interventions and mandibular

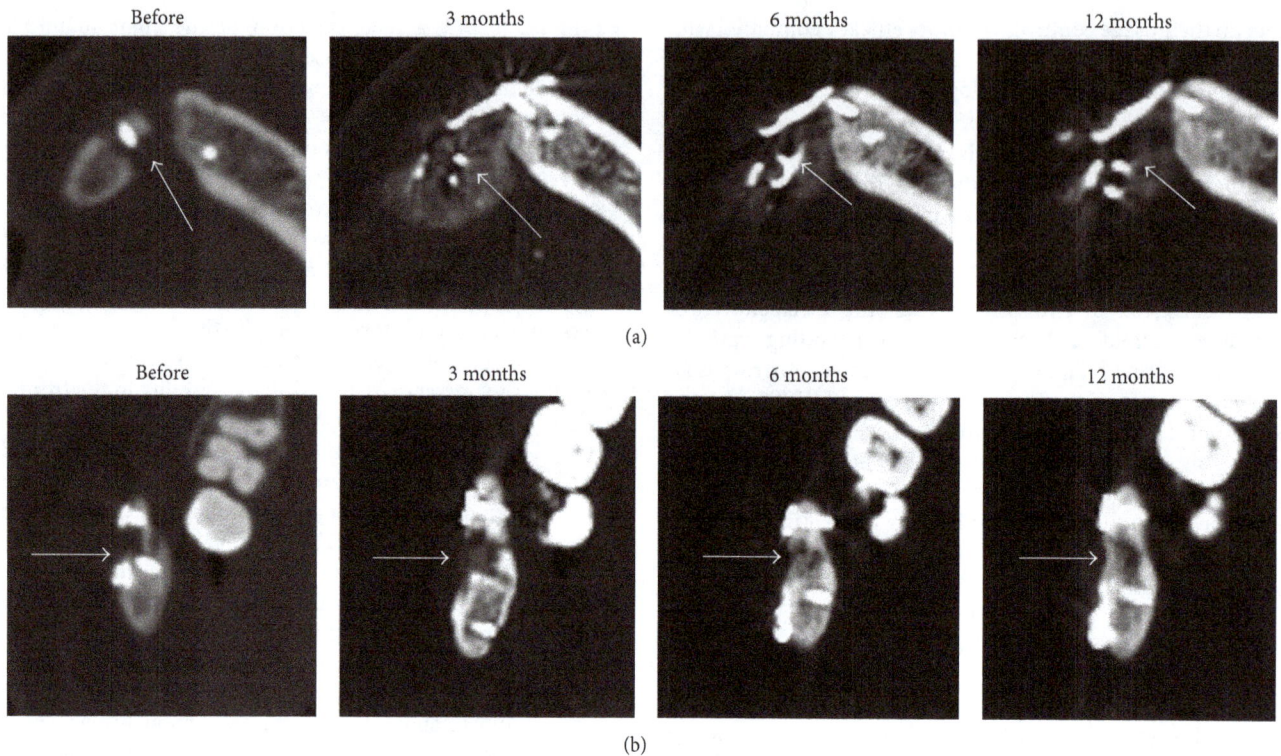

FIGURE 1: CT scans of the patient's mandible in the frontal region (a) and within the ramus on the right side (b) prior to the operation and 3, 6, and 12 months after surgery. Arrows indicate nonunions (before operation) and the sites of gene-activated bone substitute implantation.

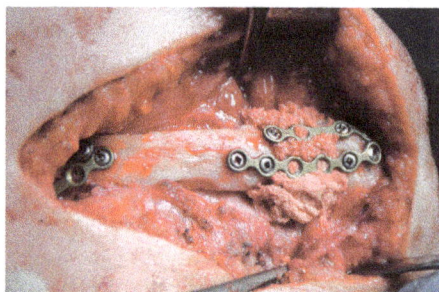

FIGURE 2: Intraoperative view: nonunions are removed; mandible fragments and rib autograft are fixed with miniplates; bone defects filled with gene-activated bone substitute.

fragments, were filled in with the gene-activated bone substitute (Figure 2). The autotransplant was fixed in the correct position with four straight miniplates and miniscrews.

In a postoperative period, a soft diet and conservative therapy including antibiotics, analgesics, and desensitizing and anti-inflammatory agents were prescribed to the patient.

2.4. Safety and Efficacy Evaluation.
To evaluate the treatment results, clinical and radiological diagnostic methods were used during the first 14 days of the postoperative period (in a hospital) and in 3, 6, and 12 months after surgery.

A pain level in the postoperative region was rated with the use of the Visual Analog Scale; edema was scored with the Numeric Rating Scale.

A control panoramic radiograph was made the next postoperative day; dental CT was done in 3, 6, and 12 months after surgery. A manual segmentation of the mandible was performed in the software 3D Slicer (Brigham, USA). The newly formed tissues within the bone substitute grafting were separately selected; their average density was calculated in Hounsfield units (HU) by using the "Label statistics" module. 3D bone reconstruction with volume rendering in the range of 250–2,000 HU was made, which complied with an optimal "bone window" with retention of spongy and lamellar bone in a model without metal constructs. A minimal size of diastases between mandibular fragments and rib autograft edges was determined with standard morphometry in the software Planmeca Romexis Viewer (Planmeca Oy, Finland).

2.5. Outcome.
Neither adverse events nor serious adverse events were observed. The postoperative pain score did not exceed 6 within the first three days after surgery; it was controlled with pain-relievers; an average score for the following four days was 3.5, no pain relief was required. Later on the patient did not notice any tenderness or discomfort within the postsurgical area. The maximal edema rated as 5 by the Numeric Rating Scale was observed on the third postoperative day. Then edema gradually decreased; its score was 3 by the end of the first week and remained at the same level for up to 14 days.

Based on the panoramic radiograph data (Figure 3) the autograft was fixed in a right position, the gene-activated bone substitute was located within bone defects, and its

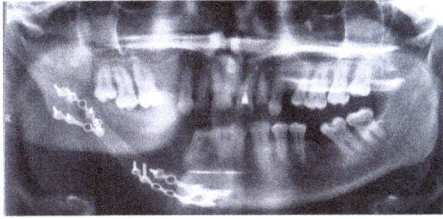

FIGURE 3: Panoramic radiography, next day after surgery.

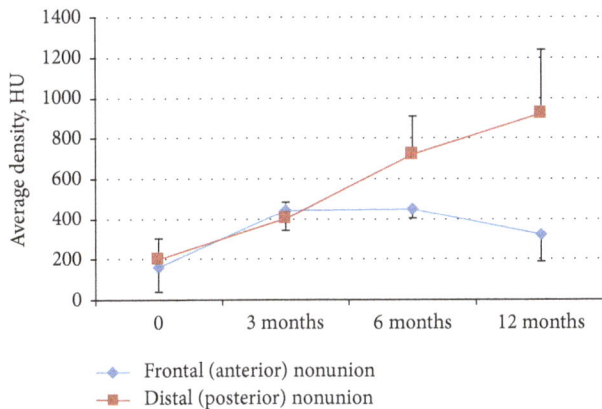

FIGURE 4: Average density in the regions of nonunions (0) and the sites of gene-activated bone substitute implantation in 3, 6, and 12 months after surgery.

radiodensity was approximately twice as less as that of the bone autograft.

No inflammation sings, edema, or pain was observed in the postsurgical area for 12 months after surgery. Control CT showed that the rib autograft and metal constructs were correctly positioned.

3 months after surgery, increased density regions were visualized in the zones of the distal and proximal autograft fixation and bone grafting (Figure 1). The average density of these areas was 402.21 ± 84.40 in the frontal fixation and 447.68 ± 106.75 HU within the distal fixation (Figure 4).

The diastasis sizes between the bone fragments were 4.8 mm on the upper edge and 12.5 mm on the lower one in the frontal surface and 6.2 mm on the vestibular surface without dissociations on the lingual one within the distal region. No defects in the zones of proximal and distal fixation of the autograft were detected using 3D reconstruction. Heteromorphic newly formed tissues were seen in these areas; the tissues overstretched the bone boarders of the reconstructed mandible outlining to a certain extent the substitute engrafted previously (Figure 5).

The newly formed tissues with average density about 400 HU within gene-activated bone substitute implantation area were observed in the frontal region 6 and 12 months after surgery (Figures 1 and 4). However, there was moderate partial resorption in the proximal edge of the bone auto-transplant which prevented consolidation and maintained a diastasis. Clinical examination identified the appearance

of minimal mandible mobility in the frontal region only 12 months after surgery, which corresponded with CT results.

Meanwhile, the distal edge of the rib autograft was completely integrated with adjacent mandibular ramus on both latest time points which did not allow distinguishing the borders between the mandible fragment, newly formed bone tissue, and rib autograft to segment these regions (Figure 5). Normotrophic bone callus with no defects was formed 6 months after surgery and fully mineralized later on revealing the average density of 921.51 ± 321.89 on the last time point. Moreover, we found the completed remodeling of newly formed bone tissue with distinguished vestibular (1028.67 ± 169.77 HU) and lingual (1528.78 ± 81.53) cortical plates and spongy bone between them in 12 months. No mandibular mobility was detected in this region.

3. Discussion

Complex clinical cases with bone defects characterized by "osteogenic insufficiency" (large ones, nonunions, etc.) [8] are the main indications for the use of activated bone substitutes as conventional ones will be suitable in less complicated settings.

Therefore, to study the safety and efficacy of the gene-activated bone substitute, we started with a very difficult clinical case when the main standard methods and materials used either resulted in specific complications or had limited efficacy. Four previous surgical interventions on the mandible resulted in scarring and impaired blood supply within the fixation areas of the bone autograft, which predisposed to the development of osteogenic insufficiency and as a consequence formation of nonunions with high score according to Nonunion Scoring System proposed by Calori et al. (2008) [21]. Moreover, one side of each nonunion was a nonvascularized bone autograft intended to be completely resorbed and simultaneously replaced by newly formed bone tissue. Such a feature has not been taken into account by current Nonunion Scoring System but obviously significantly increased a complexity of the clinical case.

Angiogenesis is known to be of critical importance for bone tissue formation [22], one of its main regulators being VEGF [23]. Moreover, in addition to affecting osteogenesis via blood vessel formation, VEGF also exerts a direct stimulating effect on cells of the osteoblastic line, enhancing their proliferation and differentiation [24]. Therefore, we used the plasmid DNA encoding *vegf* gene to make the gene-activated bone substitute. Reparative osteogenesis, as a clinical efficacy indicator, could be achieved both due to an obvious angiogenic effect of the gene construct [18–20] and owing to the direct VEGF effect on bone tissue cells.

In 3 months after surgery, newly formed tissues with an increased density equal to spongy bone were visualized within the both zones of gene-activated bone substitute grafting. The volume of those tissues correlated with that of the substitute implanted. It is known from the previous experimental studies that the gene-activated bone substitute investigated has a baseline density equal to 130 ± 350 HU. Collagen comprising 60% of the scaffold mass undergoes

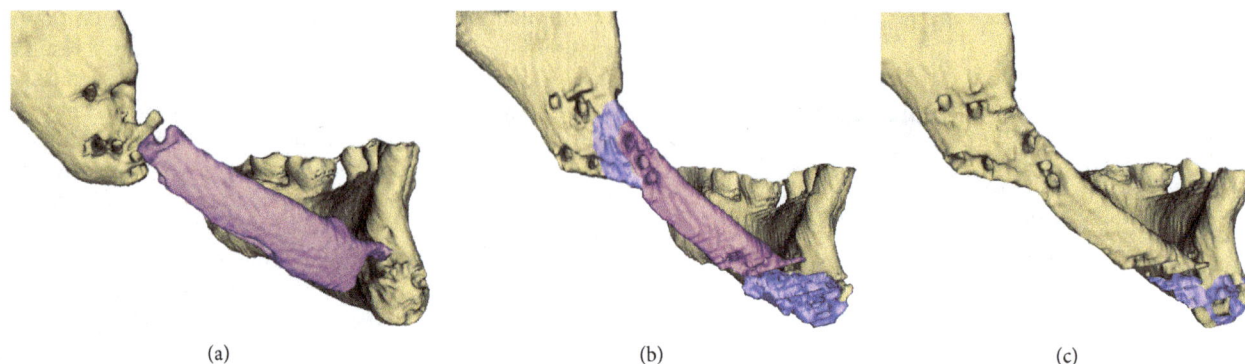

<table>
</table>

(a)   (b)   (c)

FIGURE 5: The patient's mandible in different time points after bone grafting with the gene-activated bone substitute: (a) before; (b) 6 months; (c) 12 months. Dental CT; 3D reconstruction with volume rendering 250–2000 HU (titanium constructs are excluded).

rapid biodegradation (within 1 month). Starting from 45 days after the operation, only single hydroxyapatite granules remain from the scaffold within the zone of a bone defect [19]. Therefore, considering a low standard deviation, bone tissue formation within the substitute implanted rather than the density of the remained scaffold fragments determined the high tissue density in the zone of bone grafting in 3 months.

The main encouraging result is that we showed that complete consolidation with normotrophic bone formation was achieved on the site of previously diagnosed distal nonunion. Bone remodeling process with cortical plates formation was completed in this area within 12 months after surgery. Unfortunately, the treatment of the other, more complex nonunion was not successful: although the gene-activated bone substitute stimulated bone formation preserved in the frontal region during the 12 months of follow-up, the partial resorption of the adjacent autotransplant edge contributed to the proximal nonunion relapse. Such a resorption of the rib bone is normal but expectedly increased in response of the surgical intervention. Basically, any nonvascularized bone autograft undergoes continuous bioresorption to be completely replaced by newly formed bone tissue. No bone substitute is able to stop this natural process. The only option for gene-activated bone substitute to provide a consolidation was to accelerate the reparative osteogenesis so highly to make it outrun the bioresorption rate. This bone formation activity was achieved in the distal nonunion site but was not enough in the proximal one. That prevents any prosthetic treatment and requires additional surgery in the frontal region with bone autografting and more rigid fixation (e.g., long custom-made titanium reconstructive plate).

Neither adverse events (hypersensitive reaction, abnormal pain, edema, inflammatory complications, development of local vascular malformations, tumors, etc.) nor serious adverse events (life-threatening conditions) were observed throughout the follow-up. Pain and edema levels in the postoperative region did not exceed the average values specific for postoperation periods of this type of surgical interventions, which confirms the substitute's safety. These clinical data on safety were expected because the gene-activated bone substitute components, the collagen-hydroxyapatite scaffold and plasmid DNA, separately were registered and approved

for clinical use previously in Russia as medical devise for bone grafting and drug for CLI treatment, respectively.

Thus, considering the complexity of the case, the results of the first clinical application of the gene-activated bone substitute which is composed of the collagen-hydroxyapatite scaffold and the plasmid DNA with the *vegf* gene are quite promising and indicate the safety but limited efficacy concerning a medical indications range. Possibly, the use of more osteoconductive scaffold (e.g., xenogenic bone matrix [19]) to make a gene-activated bone substitute could extend the medical indications where it might be effective. At any case we need more clinical trials and published data to assess the treatment options and opportunities gene-activated bone substitutes could provide.

Competing Interests

The authors declare that there are no competing interests regarding the publication of this paper. I. Y. Bozo, A. A. Isaev, and R. V. Deev are employees of the PJSC "Human Stem Cells Institute" marketing "Neovasculgen". A. A. Isaev and R. V. Deev are shareholders of the PJSC "Human Stem Cells Institute." NextGen Co. Ltd., a sponsor of the clinical trial NCT02293031, is a subsidiary company of PJSC "Human Stem Cells Institute."

References

[1] P. Garcia, D. Franz, and M. Raschke, "Bone substitutes—basic principles and clinical applications," *Zeitschrift für Orthopädie und Unfallchirurgie*, vol. 152, no. 2, pp. 152–160, 2014.

[2] G. I. Drosos, P. Touzopoulos, A. Ververidis, K. Tilkeridis, and K. Kazakos, "Use of demineralized bone matrix in the extremities," *World Journal of Orthopaedics*, vol. 6, no. 2, pp. 269–277, 2015.

[3] S. R. Dutta, D. Passi, P. Singh, and A. Bhuibhar, "Ceramic and non-ceramic hydroxyapatite as a bone graft material: a brief review," *Irish Journal of Medical Science*, vol. 184, no. 1, pp. 101–106, 2015.

[4] V. S. Komlev, S. M. Barinov, I. I. Bozo et al., "Bioceramics composed of octacalcium phosphate demonstrate enhanced biological behavior," *ACS Applied Materials and Interfaces*, vol. 6, no. 19, pp. 16610–16620, 2014.

[5] S. Wang, X. Wang, F. G. Draenert et al., "Bioactive and biodegradable silica biomaterial for bone regeneration," *Bone*, vol. 67, pp. 292–304, 2014.

[6] R. P. F. Lanao, A. M. Jonker, J. G. C. Wolke, J. A. Jansen, J. C. M. van Hest, and S. C. G. Leeuwenburgh, "Physicochemical properties and applications of poly(lactic-co-glycolic acid) for use in bone regeneration," *Tissue Engineering Part B: Reviews*, vol. 19, no. 4, pp. 380–390, 2013.

[7] C. Mauffrey, B. T. Barlow, and W. Smith, "Management of segmental bone defects," *Journal of the American Academy of Orthopaedic Surgeons*, vol. 23, no. 3, pp. 143–153, 2015.

[8] R. V. Deev, A. Y. Drobyshev, I. Y. Bozo, and A. A. Isaev, "Ordinary and activated bone grafts: applied classification and the main features," *BioMed Research International*, vol. 2015, Article ID 365050, 19 pages, 2015.

[9] V. L. Zorin, V. S. Komlev, A. I. Zorina et al., "Octacalcium phosphate ceramics combined with gingiva-derived stromal cells for engineered functional bone grafts," *Biomedical Materials*, vol. 9, no. 5, Article ID 055005, 2014.

[10] A. Y. Drobyshev, K. A. Rubina, V. Y. Sysoev et al., "Clinical trial of tissue-engineered construction based on autologous adipose-derived stromal cells in patients with alveolar bone atrophy of the upper and lower jaws," *Bulletin of Experimental and Clinical Surgery*, vol. 4, no. 4, pp. 764–772, 2011.

[11] W. F. McKay, S. M. Peckham, and J. M. Badura, "A comprehensive clinical review of recombinant human bone morphogenetic protein-2 (INFUSE® Bone Graft)," *International Orthopaedics*, vol. 31, no. 6, pp. 729–734, 2007.

[12] M. Kaipel, S. Schützenberger, A. T. Hofmann et al., "Evaluation of fibrin-based gene-activated matrices for BMP2/7 plasmid codelivery in a rat nonunion model," *International Orthopaedics*, vol. 38, no. 12, pp. 2607–2613, 2014.

[13] C. H. Evans, "Advances in regenerative orthopedics," *Mayo Clinic Proceedings*, vol. 88, no. 11, pp. 1323–1329, 2013.

[14] B. Fishero, N. Kohli, A. Das, J. Christophel, and Q. Cui, "Current concepts of bone tissue engineering for craniofacial bone defect repair," *Craniomaxillofacial Trauma and Reconstruction*, vol. 8, no. 1, pp. 23–30, 2015.

[15] M. Keeney, J. J. J. P. van den Beucken, P. M. van der Kraan, J. A. Jansen, and A. Pandit, "The ability of a collagen/calcium phosphate scaffold to act as its own vector for gene delivery and to promote bone formation via transfection with $VEGF_{165}$," *Biomaterials*, vol. 31, no. 10, pp. 2893–2902, 2010.

[16] S. Elangovan, S. R. D'Mello, L. Hong et al., "The enhancement of bone regeneration by gene activated matrix encoding for platelet derived growth factor," *Biomaterials*, vol. 35, no. 2, pp. 737–747, 2014.

[17] Y. Zhang, N. Cheng, R. Miron, B. Shi, and X. Cheng, "Delivery of PDGF-B and BMP-7 by mesoporous bioglass/silk fibrin scaffolds for the repair of osteoporotic defects," *Biomaterials*, vol. 33, no. 28, pp. 6698–6708, 2012.

[18] R. V. Deev, I. Y. Bozo, N. D. Mzhavanadze et al., "PCMV-vegf165 intramuscular gene transfer is an effective method of treatment for patients with chronic lower limb ischemia," *Journal of Cardiovascular Pharmacology and Therapeutics*, vol. 20, no. 5, pp. 473–482, 2015.

[19] R. V. Deev, A. Y. Drobyshev, I. Y. Bozo et al., "Construction and biological effect evaluation of gene-activated osteoplastic material with human vegf gene," *Cellular Transplantation and Tissue Engineering*, vol. 8, no. 3, pp. 78–85, 2013.

[20] R. Deev, A. Drobyshev, I. Bozo, and A. Isaev, "Angiogenic non-viral gene transfer: from ischemia treatment to bone defects repair," *Journal of Tissue Engineering and Regenerative Medicine*, vol. 8, supplement 1, pp. 64–65, 2014.

[21] G. M. Calori, M. Phillips, S. Jeetle, L. Tagliabue, and P. V. Giannoudis, "Classification of non-union: need for a new scoring system?" *Injury*, vol. 39, supplement 2, pp. S59–S63, 2008.

[22] Y.-Q. Yang, Y.-Y. Tan, R. Wong, A. Wenden, L.-K. Zhang, and A. B. M. Rabie, "The role of vascular endothelial growth factor in ossification," *International Journal of Oral Science*, vol. 4, no. 2, pp. 64–68, 2012.

[23] L. Coultas, K. Chawengsaksophak, and J. Rossant, "Endothelial cells and VEGF in vascular development," *Nature*, vol. 438, no. 7070, pp. 937–945, 2005.

[24] I. D'Alimonte, E. Nargi, F. Mastrangelo et al., "Vascular endothelial growth factor enhances in vitro proliferation and osteogenic differentiation of human dental pulp stem cells," *Journal of Biological Regulators and Homeostatic Agents*, vol. 25, no. 1, pp. 57–69, 2011.

24

Soft Tissue Schwannomas of the Hard Palate and the Mandibular Mentum

Cennet Neslihan Eroglu,[1] Serap Keskin Tunc,[1] and Omer Gunhan[2]

[1]Oral and Maxillofacial Surgery Department, Faculty of Dentistry, Yuzuncu Yil University, Van, Turkey
[2]Department of Pathology, Gulhane Military Medical Academy, Ankara, Turkey

Correspondence should be addressed to Cennet Neslihan Eroglu; neslihanakca2003@yahoo.com

Academic Editor: Darko Macan

Schwannomas are benign, slow growing, encapsulated tumours that originate from the Schwann cells. Intraoral schwannomas are rare, and most of these tumours involve the tongue. They are rarely located in the hard palate or in the facial soft tissue. Herein, we present the clinical and histological features as well as the prognoses of two male patients with schwannoma, one of which was localized to the hard palate and the other to the facial soft tissue around the mandibular mentum and caused swelling.

1. Introduction

Schwannomas, also called as neurilemmomas, were first reported in the early 20th century in the field of pathology. Schwannomas which arise from the Schwann cells of peripheral nerve sheaths can develop in any nerve trunk in the body as encapsulated lesions, with 25%–40% being located in the head and neck region. They primarily affect young-to middle-aged adults, especially females [1–3]. Although intraoral schwannoma is mainly located at the base of the tongue, it can be seen at the palate, buccal mucosa, gingiva, and lips [4]. Herein, we present the clinical findings, treatment, and prognoses of two cases of schwannomas encountered in the hard palate and in the facial soft tissue around the mentum of the mandible.

2. Case Presentation

2.1. Case 1. An intraoral mass was diagnosed incidentally in a 29-year-old male patient who was admitted to the hospital with tooth pain. The patient did not recall the time when the mass began to enlarge, since the mass caused no functional impairment. Physical examination revealed a painless, solid, asymptomatic mass, approximately 2 × 2 cm in size with a rough surface in the left palatal region (Figure 1(a)). There was no lymphadenopathy. Radiographic examination revealed no remarkable findings. The mass was enucleated

under local anaesthesia with a Y-shaped incision and primary closure was performed. The encapsulated material was sent for histopathological examination (Figure 1(b)).

Examination of the histological sections demonstrated that the tumour was composed of clusters of mesenchymal-like cells with oval fusiform nuclei, which were arranged in palisading pattern. Cellular atypia or mitotic activity was not observed (Figure 1(c)). The follow-up period (18 months) was uneventful (Figure 1(d)).

2.2. Case 2. A 33-year-old male patient was admitted with complaints of pain in his lower incisor and swelling at the tip of the mandible. On clinical examination, the painful, solid, and nonulcerated mass, which at first appeared to be soft tissue inflammation near the affected tooth, was observed to cause destruction in the neighbouring mandibular buccal cortex. There was no lymphadenopathy, and the patient had no systemic disease or notable medical or family history. Radiographic examination revealed a cyst-like radiolucency with a regular margin at the apex of the affected tooth (Figure 2(a)). After performing root canal treatment on the lower left lateral incisor, the encapsulated lesion was totally enucleated from the buccal soft tissue under local anaesthesia. It was observed that the lesion perforated both the buccal and lingual cortices and caused a mandibular cavity and that the lower lateral incisor was indirectly affected by the lesion and required treatment. On histological

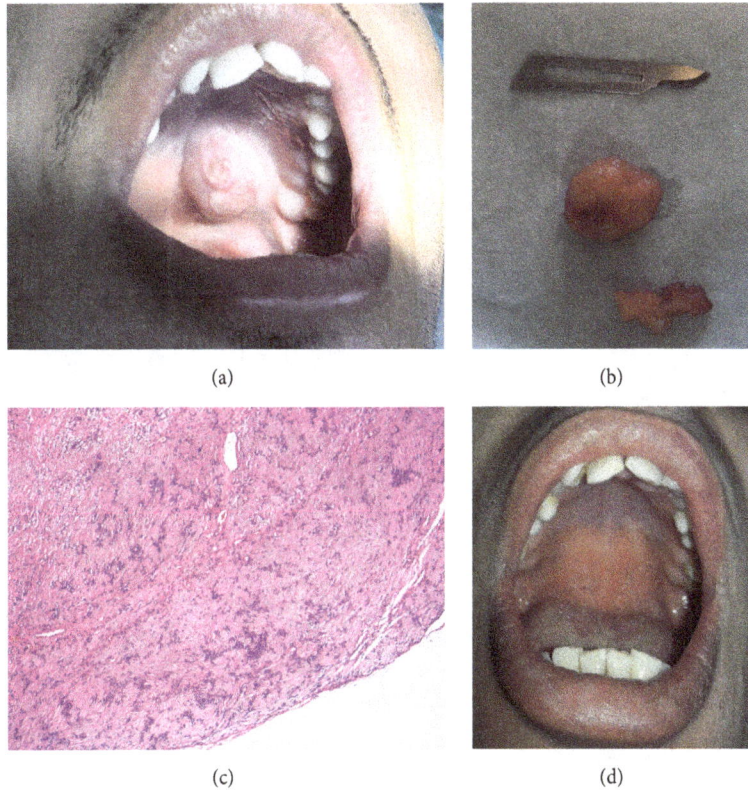

FIGURE 1: Images of the first case: (a) preoperative image of the oral cavity, (b) enucleated material, (c) schwannoma with massive cellular and fibrotic stroma (40x magnification), and (d) image of the oral cavity at the postoperative 18th month.

examination of the excised mass (Figure 2(b)), a collagenous lesion characterized by nonatypical cells with long, fusiform, and wavy nuclei arranged to form loose clusters was seen. There were occasional hyalinised vessels and aggregates of foamy macrophages. Cytologic atypia, high-mitotic activity, or necrosis was not observed (Figure 2(c)). The follow-up period of one year was uneventful (Figure 2(d)).

3. Discussion

Although it is known that schwannomas transform into tumours with the proliferation of Schwann cells, trauma is considered to be the likely unclear etiological cause [5, 6]. Intraoral schwannomas most commonly involve the tongue [7]. The currently presented cases of schwannomas are important since they were at uncommon locations. Particularly, the second case presented herein is unique and interesting in terms of its location and the type of destruction it caused. Baranović et al. [3] reported a case of schwannoma at the lingual mucosa of the mandible that caused secondary erosion of mandible. In that case, the erosion was beneath the mass, in direct contact; however, in our case, there was a healthy mucosal lining in the internal surface and at the anterior aspect of the mandible between the erosion and the lesion.

Since schwannoma is a slow-growing and painless tumour, it is very unlikely to detect schwannomas of small size. In general, patients become aware of the tumour when it reaches a size that causes functional or aesthetic problems. There may be paraesthesia in half of the schwannoma cases [8]. Although the first patient presented herein had a lesion at the hard palate, it was detected incidentally when the patient was admitted due to tooth pain. Interestingly, it caused no primary complaints, although it was in such a location that it might have caused problems in eating and swallowing. The second case was admitted with tooth pain due to the lesion and complained of facial swelling due to tooth-related abscess.

The different histopathological types of schwannomas include common, plexiform, epithelioid, cellular, and ancient schwannomas; however, mainly they have two distinct histological patterns: Antoni types A and B [1, 9]. Antoni type A areas are characterized by hypercellular proliferation of fusiform cells, while Antoni type B areas consist of a few fusiform cells in a myxoid stroma, in which not only degeneration areas, oedematous, necrotic, and haemorrhagic tissues, but also cystic formations are observed [10]. The cases presented herein were composed of Antoni type A structures without signs of degeneration.

Major pathologies, to which a number of authors recommend to pay particular attention in the differential diagnosis, include neurofibromas, traumatic neuroma, fibroma, benign salivary gland tumour, and granular cell tumour [11, 12].

Schwannomas are encapsulated tumours and, therefore, can be easily excised, and the risk of relapse is low. The rate of malignant transformation is low; however, extended

(a)

(b)

(c)

(d)

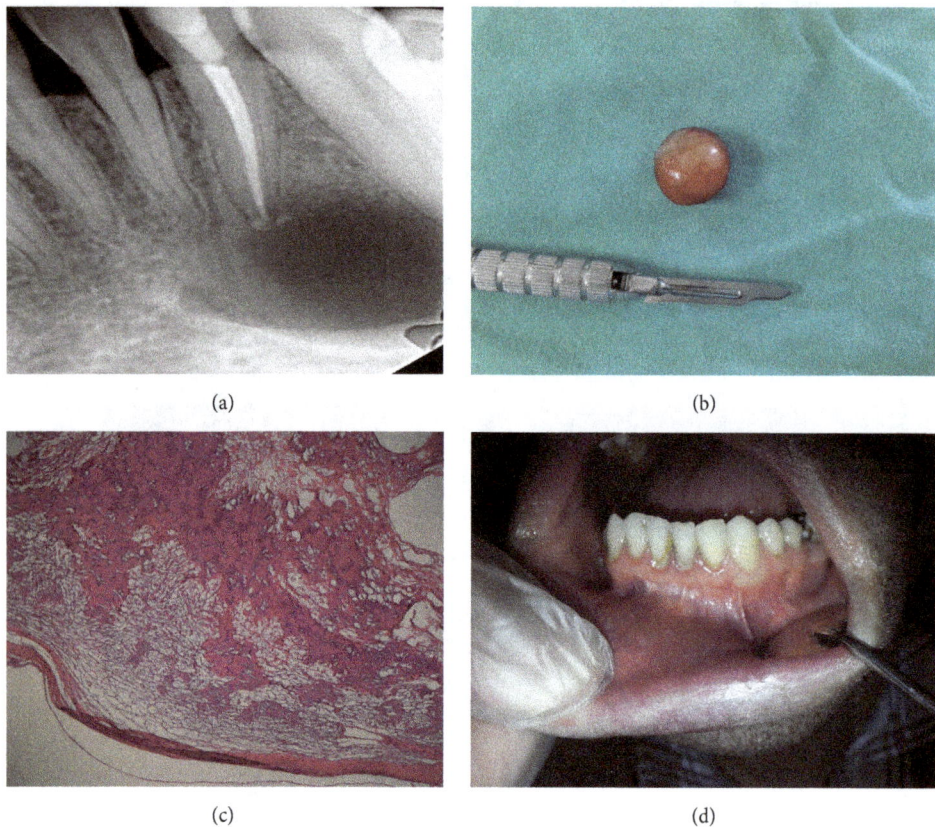

FIGURE 2: Images of the second case: (a) periapical radiographic image of the mandibular cavity that occurred secondary to schwannoma, (b) enucleated material, (c) fusiform mesenchymal cells forming cellular (Antoni type A) and loose (Antoni type B) areas (40x magnification), and (d) oral cavity at the postoperative 1st year.

dissection may be necessary in case of malignant transformation [13, 14]. In simple cases, conservative surgery performed by preserving the nerve of origin would be an adequate and appropriate treatment [15]. Although relapse is rare, the patient should be followed up for the possibility of relapse.

In conclusion, we think that schwannoma cases presented herein will contribute to the literature. Pathologies of soft tissues can lead to destructions on adjacent surfaces not only due to invasion but due to compression. Therefore, in addition to odontogenic factors, surrounding soft tissue should also be investigated by computerized tomography or magnetic resonance imaging while searching for primary tumour site in the oral cavity.

Competing Interests

The authors declare no competing interests.

References

[1] K. Bildirici, H. Cakli, C. Keçik, E. Dündar, and M. F. Agikalin, "Schwannoma (neurilemmoma) of the palatine tonsil," *Otolaryngology-Head and Neck Surgery*, vol. 127, no. 6, pp. 693–694, 2002.

[2] M. Enoz, Y. Suoglu, and R. Ilhan, "Lingual schwannoma," *Journal of Cancer Research and Therapeutics*, vol. 2, no. 2, pp. 76–78, 2006.

[3] M. Baranović, D. Macan, E. A. Begović, I. Lukšić, D. Brajdić, and S. Manojlović, "Schwannoma with secondary erosion of mandible: case report with a review of the literature," *Dentomaxillofacial Radiology*, vol. 35, no. 6, pp. 456–460, 2006.

[4] J. A. H. Jones and L. J. McWilliam, "Intraoral neurilemmoma (schwannoma): an unusual palatal swelling," *Oral Surgery, Oral Medicine, Oral Pathology*, vol. 63, no. 3, pp. 351–353, 1987.

[5] R. Pfeifle, D. A. Baur, A. Paulino, and J. Helman, "Schwannoma of the tongue: report of 2 cases," *Journal of Oral and Maxillofacial Surgery*, vol. 59, no. 7, pp. 802–804, 2001.

[6] P. López-Jornet and A. Bermejo-Fenoll, "Neurilemmoma of the tongue," *Oral Oncology Extra*, vol. 41, no. 7, pp. 154–157, 2005.

[7] W. J. Gallo, M. Moss, D. N. Shapiro, and J. V. Gaul, "Neurilemoma: review of the literature and report of 5 cases," *Journal of Oral Surgery*, vol. 35, no. 3, pp. 235–236, 1977.

[8] T. Nakasato, K. Katoh, S. Ehara et al., "Intraosseous neurilemmoma of the mandible," *American Journal of Neuroradiology*, vol. 21, no. 10, pp. 1945–1947, 2000.

[9] E. R. Mindell, "Parotis schwannoma," in *Enzinger and Weiss's Soft Tissue Tumors*, S. W. Weiss and J. R. Goldblum, Eds., pp. 1146–1167, Mosby, St. Louis, Mo, USA, 4th edition, 2001.

[10] H. Zhang, C. Cai, S. Wang, H. Liu, Y. Ye, and X. Chen, "Extracranial head and neck schwannomas: a clinical analysis of 33 patients," *Laryngoscope*, vol. 117, no. 2, pp. 278–281, 2007.

[11] K. W. Lollar, N. Pollak, B. D. Liess, R. Miick, and R. P. Zitsch III, "Schwannoma of the hard palate," *American Journal of*

Otolaryngology—Head and Neck Medicine and Surgery, vol. 31, no. 2, pp. 139–140, 2010.

[12] J. C. Hatziotis and H. Asprides, "Neurilemoma (schwannoma) of the oral cavity," *Oral Surgery, Oral Medicine, Oral Pathology*, vol. 24, no. 4, pp. 510–526, 1967.

[13] T. K. Das Gupta and R. D. Brasfield, "Solitary malignant schwannoma," *Annals of Surgery*, vol. 171, no. 3, pp. 419–428, 1970.

[14] J. Conley and I. P. Janecka, "Neurilemmoma of the head and neck," *Transactions of the American Academy of Ophthalmology and Otolaryngology: Otolaryngology Section*, vol. 80, no. 5, pp. 459–464, 1975.

[15] H. Isildak, M. Yilmaz, M. Ibrahimov, M. Aslan, E. Karaman, and O. Enver, "Schwannoma of the hard palate," *Journal of Craniofacial Surgery*, vol. 21, no. 1, pp. 276–278, 2010.

25

Autogenous Tooth Fragment Adhesive Reattachment for a Complicated Crown Root Fracture: Two Interdisciplinary Case Reports

Antonello Francesco Pavone,[1] Marjan Ghassemian,[2,3,4] Manuele Mancini,[1] Roberta Condò,[1] Loredana Cerroni,[1] Claudio Arcuri,[1] and Guido Pasquantonio[1]

[1]*Department of Clinical and Translational Medicine, University of Rome "Tor Vergata", Rome, Italy*
[2]*University of Sydney, Sydney, NSW, Australia*
[3]*Catholic University of the Sacred Heart, Rome, Italy*
[4]*Unit of Oral Surgery and Implant-Prosthetic Rehabilitation, Rome, Italy*

Correspondence should be addressed to Manuele Mancini; manuele.mancini@uniroma2.it

Academic Editor: H. Cem Güngör

Trauma of anterior teeth is quite a common occurrence in both children and adults. Various degrees of trauma leading to fracture may affect teeth in different ways depending on the age of the patient and extent of fracture and other factors that will be discussed. Guidelines have been given as to how each of these situations should be treated. In the past, often more aggressive restorations were performed to restore fractured teeth. However improved and more efficient adhesion may affect the type of treatment we decide to carry out, leading to more conservative therapies through an increased preservation of tooth structures.

1. Introduction

Traumatic injuries to teeth and their supporting tissues usually occur in young people aged 6–13 years, and damage may vary from enamel fracture to avulsion, with or without pulpal involvement or bone fracture [1]. A crown root fracture (CRF) is a type of dental trauma, usually resulting from a horizontal impact, which involves enamel, dentin, and cementum, often occurring below the gingival margin and depending on whether pulp involvement is present or absent, which may be classified as complicated or uncomplicated [2]. Most of these injuries occur in permanent maxillary incisors before complete root formation and cause pulp inflammation or necrosis [1, 2]. Treatment of complicated crown root fractures is often challenging due to difficulty in achieving isolation with a rubber dam for a dry operating field, which might compromise the hermetic seal. Furthermore, dentoalveolar trauma during the maturation of permanent teeth may result in incomplete root formation [3–6]. The nature and depth of the fracture will often dictate the type of treatment that is required. In order to provide predictable esthetics, function, structure, and biologic health, it is imperative that an interdisciplinary treatment approach is followed. This is especially true if the fracture extends into the attachment apparatus or below the osseous crest [4]. The first question the clinician must consider when treatment planning the traumatic fracture is whether the tooth/teeth can be saved. If the fracture extends so far apically that whichever treatment is provided, the resulting crown-to-root ratio is unfavorable, or the amount of coronal tooth structure will not allow restoration, extraction of the tooth and placement of an endosseous implant remains the treatment of choice. The use of natural tooth fragments is an excellent biological approach for restoring fractured anterior teeth [7], when the fragment is available, especially since adhesion technology has improved [8, 9] and further loss of tooth structure can be avoided [10, 11]. Biological restoration using autogenous tooth fragment requires minimal healthy tooth preparation, is esthetic and faster than a complete composite restoration [12], and has a psychological benefit to the patient that his own tooth has been retained [13]. This article addresses the available treatment alternatives when treating complicated fractures. In addition, a step-by-step guide to decision making in order to provide the most predictable results is presented. Two cases will be illustrated using an adhesive approach for the restoration when the tooth is in violation of biologic width to avoid further loss of tooth structure.

2. Epidemiology of Fractures

Anterior teeth fractures as a result of traumatic injury are frequently seen in dental practice. A high prevalence is noted in children between 7 and 12 years of age [14, 15]. Often maxillary anterior teeth are affected, and of them 80% are maxillary central incisors, followed by maxillary lateral incisors and mandibular incisors [14, 15]. Average incidence of injuries to anterior teeth reported in literature ranges from 4 to 46%, with 11 to 30% in primary dentition and 6 to 29% in permanent dentition. Epidemiological statistics revealed that crown root fractures represent 5% of dental injuries [14, 15], and the main causes of dental injuries are falls and collisions, sporting activities, violence, and traffic accidents.

3. Classification of Fractures

The position and the circumferential extent of the fracture are of considerable importance in treatment planning. However, the severity of the fracture in a subgingival direction is probably the most important factor influencing the treatment plan. With this respect, teeth with subgingival fractures may be classified into four categories [16] (Figure 1).

4. Diagnosis of Fractures

The first step in the process of determining if the teeth should be saved or extracted is to locate the most apical extent of the fracture. Traumatically fractured maxillary anterior teeth generally have an oblique fracture angle with the most apical portion located on the palatal or on the labial depending on the impact direction. For a palatal fracture the cause is usually the external direct force resulting from the impact on the maxillary central, whereas for a labial fracture the cause is the lower incisor impacting on the palatal of the upper incisor [17]. Often the extent and acuteness of the fracture angle may be challenging to identify where it ends radiographically. Thus, it is vital to locate the extent of the fracture clinically (Figures 2 and 3). Though it has been shown in the literature that one of the most important factors in the predictable restoration of endodontically treated teeth is having an adequate ferrule [18, 19]. The following are also significant factors which determine the treatment option and the prognosis of the fractured tooth: patient's age, dental eruption and stage of the root formation, location of the line fracture: palatal or labial, location of the line fracture in relation to the biological width, alveolar bone fracture, pulp exposion or proximity to the pulp, periodontal involvement, soft-tissue injuries, presence/absence of fractured tooth fragment,

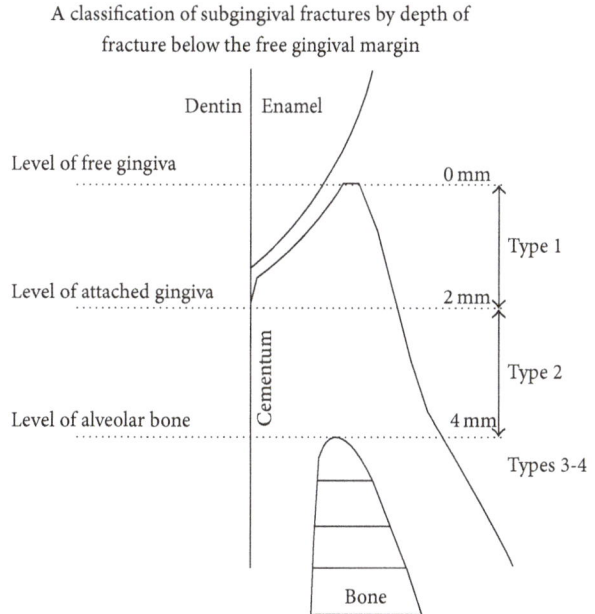

A classification of subgingival fractures by depth of fracture below the free gingival margin

FIGURE 1

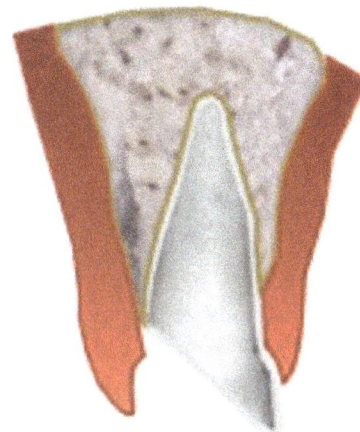

FIGURE 2

amount of remaining tooth structure, secondary traumatic injuries, occlusion, and aesthetics [3, 5].

5. Treatment of Fractures

Treatments of fractures are often interdisciplinary [3]. In fact, CRF always involve periodontal tissue, external tooth structures (enamel and dentine), and sometimes pulpal tissues. Therefore, treatment alternatives can be divided into six different approaches:

(1) Endotreatment + fragment reattachment

(2) Endotreatment + periodontal surgery + fragment reattachment

(3) Endotreatment + orthodontic extrusion + restoration of the teeth

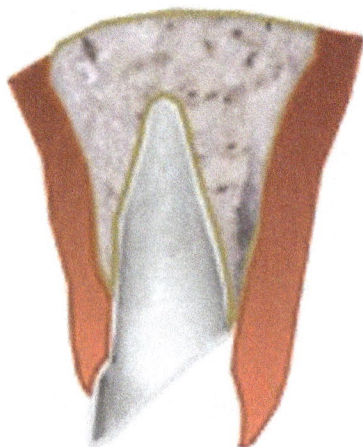

FIGURE 3

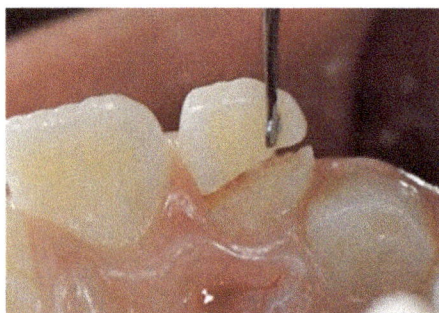

FIGURE 4

(4) Fragment removal and direct or indirect restoration

(5) Endotreatment + post and core + periodontal surgery + prosthetic restoration

(6) Extraction + implant

6. Case Reports

6.1. Case 1. An 11-year-old patient presented following a complicated CRF trauma to tooth 2.2 (Figure 4). The treatment involved root canal treatment since there was pulp exposure (Figure 5). Due to the subgingival extent of the labial fracture line a flap was raised to expose the fracture margin (Figure 6). Following the root canal therapy and correct isolation, the fractured fragment (Figure 7) was cleaned, etched, and adhesively recemented using a heated composite, and then the flap was sutured (Figure 8). A few years later orthodontic therapy was carried out to resolve orthodontic problems, and the reattached fragment was still in place, showing normal periodontal maturation of the tissues and aesthetic and restorative integration (Figures 9 and 10). Five years since the initial treatment the restoration continues to maintain successful functional, aesthetic, and biologic parameters (Figure 11).

6.2. Case 2. A 28-year-old man presented following a complicated CRF trauma of the 11 and less severe dentin-enamel

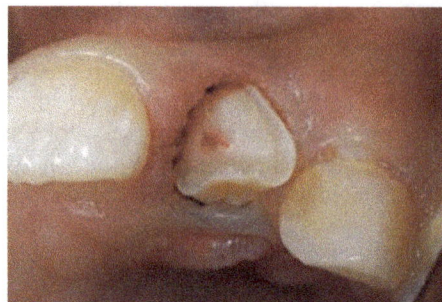

FIGURE 5

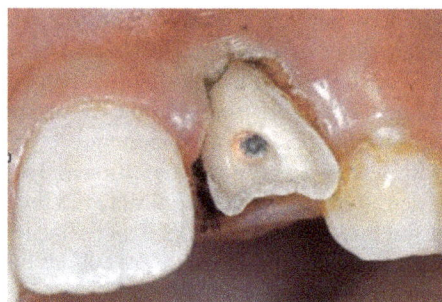

FIGURE 6

fracture of the 21 (Figures 12 and 13). Removal of the fragment of the 11 revealed an almost complete detachment of the clinical crown with a deep palatal fracture line (Figures 14 and 15). Root canal therapy was required (Figure 16) and a flap was raised to surgically expose the palatal fracture margin through osteotomy (Figure 17). Following root canal therapy the tooth fragment was prepared with mechanical retention, cleaned, etched (Figure 18), and adhesively recemented using a heated composite. Once gingival healing was obtained, three months after trauma, it was decided to restore the two teeth with minimal preparation porcelain veneers to strengthen the labial surfaces (Figure 19), as well as to improve aesthetics in masking the labial fracture of the two teeth (Figure 20) which were placed (Figure 21), and after 18 months the papilla had reached full maturation and optimum aesthetic result (Figure 22).

7. Discussion

Conventional approaches to rehabilitating fractured anterior teeth include composite restorations and post-core-supported prosthetic restorations when the tooth has had pulpal exposure and extensive fracture of the crown [1, 3, 4]. The fractured segment is usually removed and post-core and crown restoration is done after root canal therapy. However, disadvantages of these two alternatives may be the reduced aesthetic results (both immediately and in the long term) due to discoloration of composite resin restorations and aggressiveness of post-core full crowns. The use of tooth fragment reattachment technique to preserve the fractured segment of a tooth has been in the literature for decades [11, 20] and offers better short- [21, 22] and

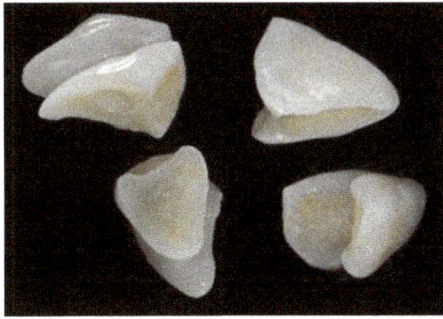

FIGURE 7

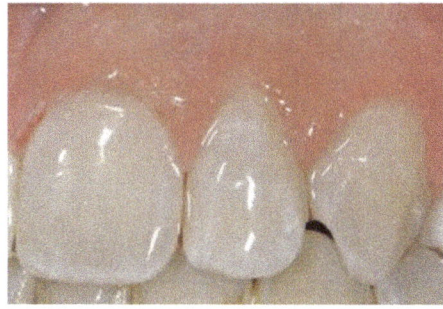

FIGURE 11

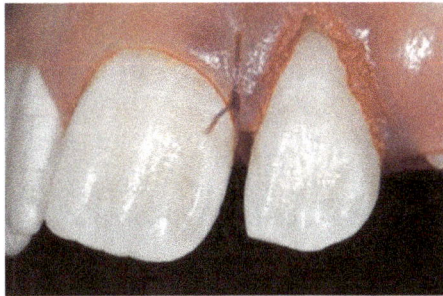

FIGURE 8

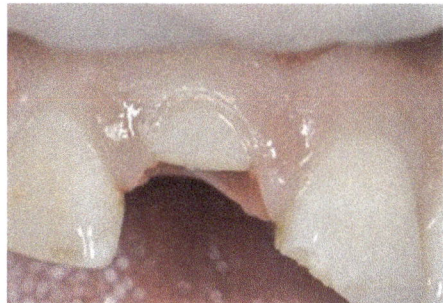

FIGURE 12

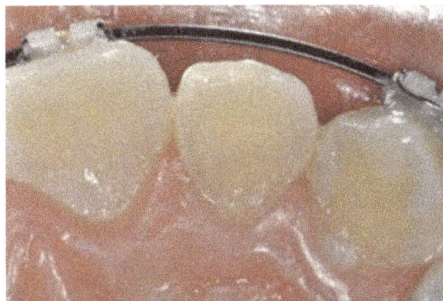

FIGURE 9

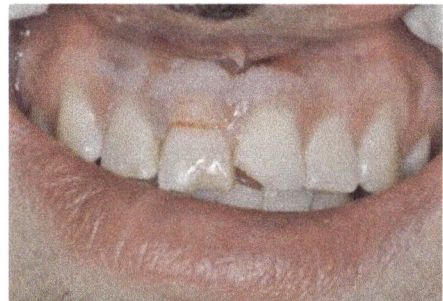

FIGURE 13

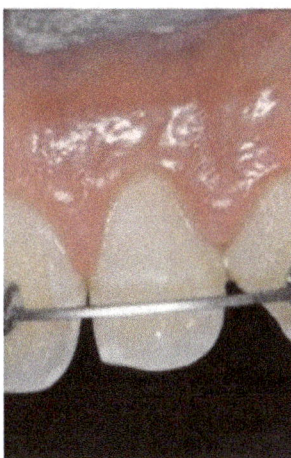

FIGURE 14

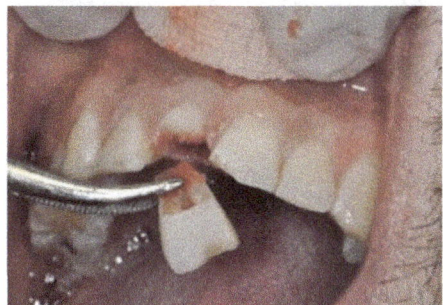

FIGURE 10

medium-term [23] results compared to resin composite restorations. This technique is more so encouraged nowadays due to the improvement of newer adhesives and especially in the case of younger patients. It is an optimal approach for restoring fractured anterior teeth, when the fragment is available [7, 10, 23]. The fractured fragment has been proposed as a favorable crown repair material due to its superior morphology, conservation of structure, and patient

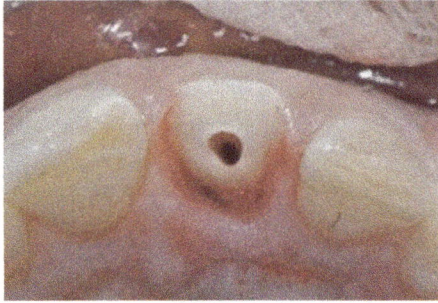

FIGURE 15

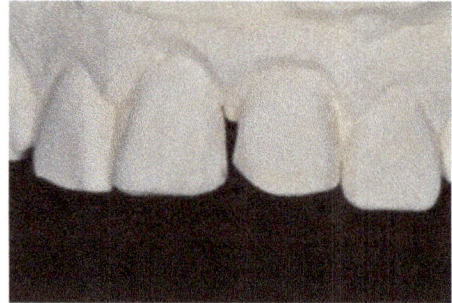

FIGURE 19

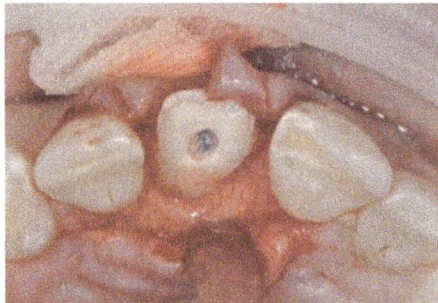

FIGURE 16

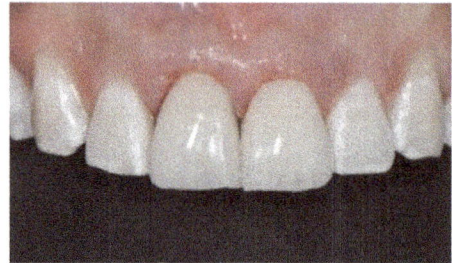

FIGURE 20

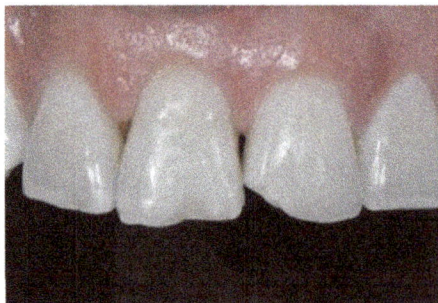

FIGURE 17

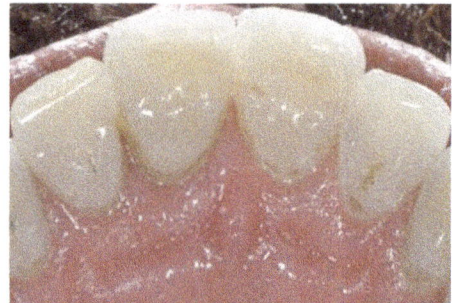

FIGURE 21

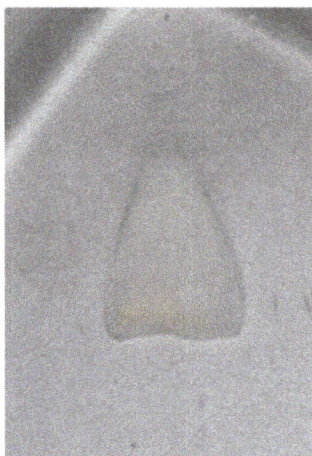

FIGURE 18

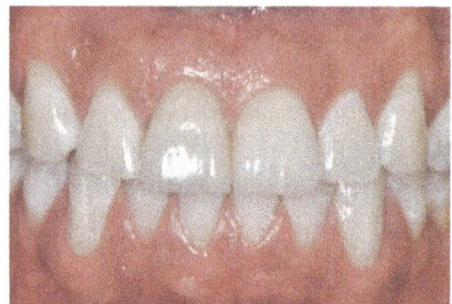

FIGURE 22

acceptance [10]. It requires minimal preparation of the tooth, is more esthetic and faster to reattach than a composite resin restoration, and has a psychological benefit to the patient that his own tooth has been retained. This is regardless as to whether root canal treatment is required or not. Loss of vitality followed by proper endodontic therapy proved to affect tooth biomechanical behavior only to a limited extent.

Whether it is because of caries or restorative procedures, tooth strength is reduced in proportion to coronal tissue loss. Therefore, the key strategies to restore endodontically treated teeth are to minimize the removal of tooth structure, especially in the cervical region to maximize the ferrule effect, to use adhesive procedures at both radicular and coronal levels to strengthen remaining tooth structure, and to optimize restoration stability and retention and use post and core materials with physical properties similar to those of natural dentin, because of the limitations of current adhesive procedures [24]. The concepts that support this therapeutic option are similar to that of endocrowns [25, 26] but with the original tooth fragment as the ideal material, avoiding the use of artificial materials which require further tooth demolition and preparation to obtain mechanical retention, deep posts, and ferrule for conventional restorations. The use of cast metal cores was associated with wedge effect which may lead to tooth fracture [19], whereas adhesion of prefabricated posts has limited long-term stability [27, 28]. Alternatively, maintaining as much enamel as possible is an advantage when using endocrowns, porcelain veneers, or tooth fragments due to increased bond strength of adhesives on enamel [8, 9]. In both case reports showed in this manuscript, conventional treatment may have led to post-core crowns or even extraction and implant placement. But in making the more conservative choice of treatment, the authors have taken into consideration other important factors like the patient's age, the irretrievability of the restoration in case of failure, and the possibility of postponing more aggressive treatment without any negative implications in the meantime. The key to this type of treatment was to immediately expose the fracture margin to allow an ideal isolation with rubber dam placement. In the first case the depth of the labial fracture margin presented an esthetic challenge; however given the young age of the patient and the incomplete eruptive phase of the tooth and gingiva, following a minimal gingivectomy and osteotomy, the cementation of the fragment and resulting aesthetics were obtained satisfactorily, whereas, in the second case, the palatal location of the deep fracture margin permitted the exposure with a palatal flap elevation and osteotomy and minimal labial involvement of the gingival tissues and papillae. Subsequently, given the patients age, it was decided to further increase the esthetic final result and the ferrule effect and thus the durability of the treatment with porcelain veneers [29, 30].

8. Conclusion

The authors consider the immediate reattachment of the tooth fragment not a temporary or transitory alternative but a reliable and long-term treatment alternative, considering the efficacy of current adhesive systems. This type of treatment is immediate, uses the ideal restorative material, and eliminates the need for aggressive and complex restorations [30, 31].

Competing Interests

The authors deny any conflict of interests. They affirm that they have no financial affiliation (e.g., employment, direct payment, stock holdings, retainers, consultantships, patent licensing arrangements, or honoraria) or involvement with any commercial organization with direct financial interest in the subject or materials discussed in this manuscript, nor have any such arrangements existed in the past three years. Any other potential conflict of interests is disclosed.

References

[1] N. Zerman and G. Cavalleri, "Traumatic injuries to permanent incisors," *Endodontics & Dental Traumatology*, vol. 9, no. 2, pp. 61–64, 1993.

[2] P. Delivanis, H. Delivanis, and M. M. Kuftinec, "Endodontic-orthodontic management of fractured anterior teeth," *The Journal of the American Dental Association*, vol. 97, no. 3, pp. 483–485, 1978.

[3] J. O. Andreasen and F. M. Andreasen, *Textbook and Color Atlas of Traumatic Injuries to the Teeth*, Blackwell, Oxford, UK, 4th edition, 2007.

[4] S. R. Potashnick and E. S. Rosenberg, "Forced eruption: principles in periodontics and restorative dentistry," *The Journal of Prosthetic Dentistry*, vol. 48, no. 2, pp. 141–148, 1982.

[5] S. Olsburgh, T. Jacoby, and I. Krejci, "Crown fractures in the permanent dentition: pulpal and restorative considerations," *Dental Traumatology*, vol. 18, no. 3, pp. 103–115, 2002.

[6] A. Robertson, F. M. Andreasen, J. O. Andreasen, and J. G. Norén, "Long-term prognosis of crown-fractured permanent incisors. The effect of stage of root development and associated luxation injury," *International Journal of Paediatric Dentistry*, vol. 10, no. 3, pp. 191–199, 2000.

[7] V. Badami and S. K. Reddy, "Treatment of complicated crown-root fracture in a single visit by means of rebonding," *Journal of the American Dental Association*, vol. 142, no. 6, pp. 646–650, 2011.

[8] J. De Munck, K. Van Landuyt, M. Peumans et al., "A critical review of the durability of adhesion to tooth tissue: methods and results," *Journal of Dental Research*, vol. 84, no. 2, pp. 118–132, 2005.

[9] M. Peumans, P. Kanumilli, J. De Munck, K. Van Landuyt, P. Lambrechts, and B. Van Meerbeek, "Clinical effectiveness of contemporary adhesives: a systematic review of current clinical trials," *Dental Materials*, vol. 21, no. 9, pp. 864–881, 2005.

[10] D. P. Lise, L. C. C. Vieira, É. Araújo, and G. C. Lopes, "Tooth fragment reattachment: the natural restoration," *Operative Dentistry*, vol. 37, no. 6, pp. 584–590, 2012.

[11] T. N. Tennery, "The fractured tooth reunited using the acid-etch bonding technique," *Texas Dental Journal*, vol. 96, no. 8, pp. 16–17, 1978.

[12] D. Dietschi, T. Jacoby, J. M. Dietschi, and J. P. Schatz, "Treatment of traumatic injuries in the front teeth: restorative aspects in crown fractures," *Practical Periodontics and Aesthetic Dentistry*, vol. 12, no. 8, pp. 751–760, 2000.

[13] F. A. Hamilton, F. J. Hill, and P. J. Holloway, "An investigation of dento-alveolar trauma and its treatment in an adolescent population. Part 1: the prevalence and incidence of injuries and the extent and adequacy of treatment received," *British Dental Journal*, vol. 182, no. 3, pp. 91–95, 1997.

[14] J. L. Gutmann and M. S. Gutmann, "Cause, incidence, and prevention of trauma to teeth," *Dental Clinics of North America*, vol. 39, no. 1, pp. 1–13, 1995.

[15] S. Sharma and R. Dua, "Prevalence, causes, and correlates of traumatic dental injuries among seven-to-twelve-year-old school children in Dera Bassi," *Contemporary Clinical Dentistry*, vol. 3, no. 1, pp. 38–41, 2012.

[16] G. S. Heithersay and A. J. Moule, "Anterior subgingival fractures: a review of treatment alternatives," *Australian Dental Journal*, vol. 27, no. 6, pp. 368–376, 1982.

[17] J. O. Andreasen, S. S. Ahrensburg, and G. Tsilingaridis, "Tooth mobility changes subsequent to root fractures: a longitudinal clinical study of 44 permanent teeth," *Dental Traumatology*, vol. 28, no. 5, pp. 410–414, 2012.

[18] W. J. Libman and J. I. Nicholls, "Load fatigue of teeth restored with cast posts and cores and complete crowns," *The International Journal of Prosthodontics*, vol. 8, no. 2, pp. 155–161, 1995.

[19] A. S. Fernandes and G. S. Dessai, "Factors affecting the fracture resistance of post-core reconstructed teeth: a review," *International Journal of Prosthodontics*, vol. 14, no. 4, pp. 355–363, 2001.

[20] R. J. Simonsen, "Restoration of a fractured central incisor using original tooth fragment," *The Journal of the American Dental Association*, vol. 105, no. 4, pp. 646–648, 1982.

[21] A. D. Loguercio, J. Mengarda, R. Amaral, A. Kraul, and A. Reis, "Effect of fractured or sectioned fragments on the fracture strength of different reattachment techniques," *Operative Dentistry*, vol. 29, no. 3, pp. 295–300, 2004.

[22] A. Reis, A. D. Loguercio, A. Kraul, and E. Matson, "Reattachment of fractured teeth: a review of literature regarding techniques and materials," *Operative Dentistry*, vol. 29, no. 2, pp. 226–233, 2004.

[23] F. M. Andreasen, J. G. Norén, J. O. Andreasen, S. Engelhardtsen, and U. Lindh-Strömberg, "Long-term survival of fragment bonding in the treatment of fractured crowns: a multicenter clinical study," *Quintessence International*, vol. 26, no. 10, pp. 669–681, 1995.

[24] D. Dietschi, O. Duc, I. Krejci, and A. Sadan, "Biomechanical considerations for the restoration of endodontically treated teeth: a systematic review of the literature. Part II (Evaluation of fatigue behavior, interfaces, and in vivo studies)," *Quintessence International*, vol. 39, no. 2, pp. 117–129, 2008.

[25] P. Magne, A. O. Carvalho, G. Bruzi, R. E. Anderson, H. P. Maia, and M. Giannini, "Influence of no-ferrule and no-post buildup design on the fatigue resistance of endodontically treated molars restored with resin nanoceramic CAD/CAM crowns," *Operative Dentistry*, vol. 39, no. 6, pp. 595–602, 2014.

[26] F. Zarone, R. Sorrentino, D. Apicella et al., "Evaluation of the biomechanical behavior of maxillary central incisors restored by means of endocrowns compared to a natural tooth: a 3D static linear finite elements analysis," *Dental Materials*, vol. 22, no. 11, pp. 1035–1044, 2006.

[27] S. Mazzoleni, F. Graf, E. Salomon, F. Simionato, C. Bacci, and E. Stellini, "Influence of root canal posts on the reattachment of fragments to endodontically treated fractured incisors: an in vitro experimental comparison," *Journal of Esthetic and Restorative Dentistry*, vol. 28, no. 2, pp. 92–101, 2016.

[28] A. Ramírez-Sebastià, T. Bortolotto, M. Cattani-Lorente, L. Giner, M. Roig, and I. Krejci, "Adhesive restoration of anterior endodontically treated teeth: influence of post length on fracture strength," *Clinical Oral Investigations*, vol. 18, no. 2, pp. 545–554, 2014.

[29] M. C. Cagidiaco, C. Goracci, F. Garcia-Godoy, and M. Ferrari, "Clinical studies of fiber posts: a literature review," *International Journal of Prosthodontics*, vol. 21, no. 4, pp. 328–336, 2008.

[30] P. Magne and W. H. Douglas, "Porcelain veneers: dentin bonding optimization and biomimetic recovery of the crown," *International Journal of Prosthodontics*, vol. 12, no. 2, pp. 111–121, 1999.

[31] P. Magne and W. H. Douglas, "Optimization of resilience and stress distribution in porcelain veneers for the treatment of crown-fractured incisors," *International Journal of Periodontics and Restorative Dentistry*, vol. 19, no. 6, pp. 543–553, 1999.

26

Cholesterol Granuloma in Odontogenic Cyst: An Enigmatic Lesion

Mala Kamboj, Anju Devi, and Shruti Gupta

Department of Oral Pathology and Microbiology, Postgraduate Institute of Dental Sciences,
Pt. BD Sharma University of Medical Sciences, Rohtak, Haryana, India

Correspondence should be addressed to Mala Kamboj; malskam@gmail.com

Academic Editor: Roberto Sacco

Cholesterol granuloma (CG) is the outcome of the foreign body type of response to the accumulation of cholesterol crystals and is frequently present in conjunction with chronic middle ear diseases. Recently, cases of CG in jaws have been reported, but still, very few cases have been found of CG in dental literature. This article presents three rare cases of CG in the wall of odontogenic cysts emphasizing on its possible role in expansion of the associated lesion and bone erosion. It also lays stress on the fact that more cases of CG should be reported so that its nature and pathogenesis in the oral cavity become more perceivable.

1. Introduction

Cholesterol granuloma (CG) is a histopathological entity that is characterized by collection of numerous cholesterol clefts, which are associated with foreign body giant cells, foam cells, and hemosiderin filled macrophages [1]. Most common site of occurrence of CG is middle ear (generally associated with chronic middle ear diseases). Lungs, brain, kidneys, mastoid process, breast, sella turcica, pontocerebelline angle, testis, and apex of temporal bone pyramid are the other sites where CG can occur [2]. Recently, it was reported that CG could also occur in the facial skeleton, maxillary antrum and frontal bone being the two common sites [3]. The clinical symptoms are nonspecific and depend on the localization and extent in each individual case [1]. Very few cases of CG occurring in jaws have been reported in the English literature. We report three unique cases where the odontogenic cysts were secondarily inflamed and showed expansion and associated bone destruction due to CG formation.

2. Case Series

2.1. Case 1. A 45-year-old male reported to the institute with the complaint of swelling in the posterior tooth region of right maxilla since one month. Patient gave a history for the extraction of 17, 18 (with grade II mobility) for the same in private dental clinic but after extraction the swelling persisted. On palpation, swelling was soft and fluctuant in nature extending from the buccal vestibule till midline of the hard palate. FNAC was attempted but the mass bled profusely. CT scan revealed a huge expansile, well demarcated, and osteolytic mass extending from maxilla into the maxillary sinus. A provisional diagnosis of keratocystic odontogenic tumor (KCOT) was made. Surgical enucleation of the cyst was performed and the tissue was sent for histopathological examination. The sections revealed proliferation of cystic odontogenic epithelial lining with palisaded hyperchromatic columnar nuclei, stellate reticulum like areas, and sheets of abundant ghost cells. Surrounding connective tissue stroma showed mature collagen bundles. Abundant hemorrhagic areas and fibrin deposits were evident both in fibrous wall and in cystic lumen. Also visible both in the connective tissue and in cystic lumen were abundant cholesterol clefts and hemorrhagic areas. Focal areas of ghost cell formation were also visible in the stroma surrounded by foreign body giant cells and hemosiderin pigmentation. Thus, based on this a final diagnosis of *calcifying odontogenic cyst with cholesterol granuloma* was made (Figure 1).

2.2. Case 2. A 38-year-old female complained of swelling since 6 months at right side posterior mandible. Patient stated

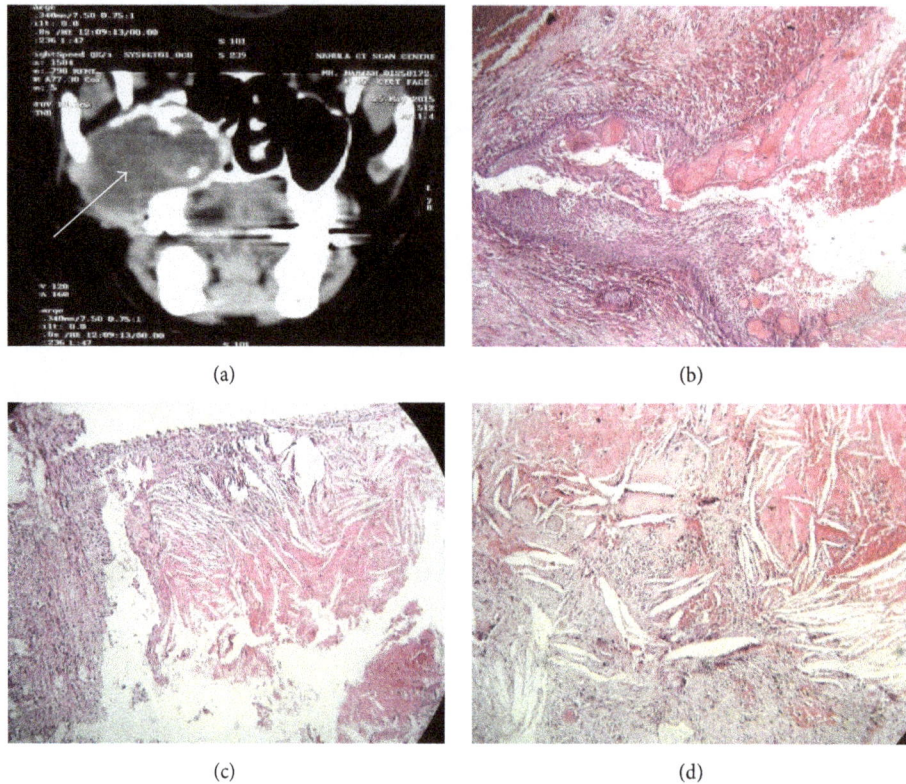

(a)

(b)

(c)

(d)

FIGURE 1: (a) CT scan image showing huge expansile, well demarcated, and osteolytic mass extending from maxilla into the maxillary sinus on right side; (b) proliferation of cystic odontogenic epithelial lining with palisaded hyperchromatic columnar nuclei, stellate reticulum like areas, and sheets of abundant ghost cells (H/E 4x); (c) cholesterol clefts in cystic wall (H/E 4x); (d) cholesterol clefts in cystic wall (H/E 10x).

that the swelling gradually increased in size with pus discharge and no pain. Intraorally, the swelling was 3 × 2 cm in size at right angle region with missing 48. Overlying mucosa appeared smooth, nonerythematous and nontender on palpation. A well-defined radiolucency in relation to crown of 48 was seen in the orthopantomography. A provisional diagnosis of dentigerous cyst and keratocystic odontogenic tumor (KCOT) was made. The cyst was surgically enucleated and the histopathology revealed nonkeratinized stratified squamous cystic epithelial lining, 2-3-cell layer thick, which showed proliferation in few areas associated with underlying inflammation. In the connective tissue cystic capsule, mixed inflammatory cell infiltrates with areas of hemorrhage were evident. A part of the tissue revealed abundant cholesterol clefts in the cystic capsule in association with multinucleated giant cells. Based on this a diagnosis of *dentigerous cyst with cholesterol granuloma* was made (Figure 2).

2.3. Case 3. A 47-year-old male reported with complaint of pain in lower left posterior mandible for past two days. He gave history of swelling on this side since two months. Mild swelling was present on left side of mandible, which was hard on palpation and nontender. Intraorally the swelling was soft in consistency and painful with a slight opening present on crest region through which yellowish green color discharge

was noticed. Computed tomography revealed a well-defined radiolucency (30 × 14 mm in size) present on left angle of mandible region with 38 displaced near the inferior border of the mandible. Incisional biopsy was sent for histopathological evaluation which revealed cystic lining of varying thickness, nonkeratinized stratified squamous in nature with few areas of mucus metaplasia. Connective tissue capsule was fibrocellular with vascular channels and mild inflammatory cell infiltrate and a diagnosis of dentigerous cyst was made. After this the excised tissue was sent which after repeated regrossing and tissue sectioning did not show any cystic lining. The connective tissue stroma was ectomesenchymal and fibrocellular with abundant cholesterol clefts and chronic inflammatory cell infiltrate (Figure 3).

3. Discussion

CG histopathologically depicts a large collection of longitudinal cholesterol clefts that are formed at the site of cholesterol crystals because of dissolution of crystals at the time of tissue processing and is embedded in fibrous granulation tissue with surrounding foreign body type of multinucleated giant cells and macrophages filled with hemosiderin [4]. After an extensive survey, six cases of CG have been found in the oral cavity, in which only three cases of CG occurring in the wall of

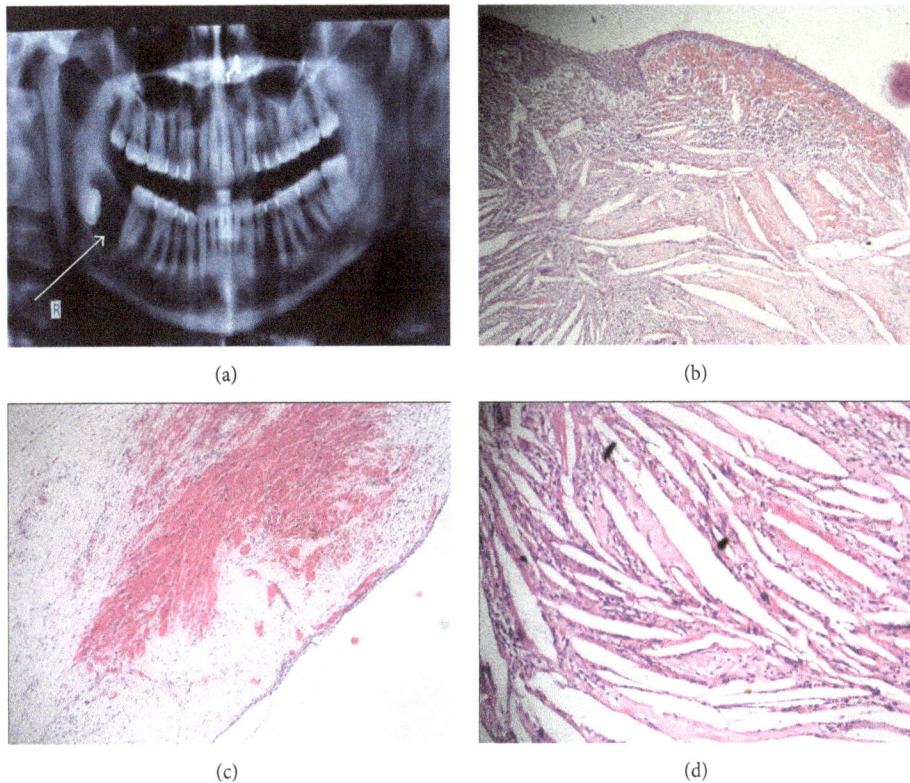

FIGURE 2: (a) An OPG showing a well-defined radiolucency in relation to crown of 48; (b) nonkeratinized stratified squamous cystic epithelial lining which showed proliferation in few areas associated with underlying cholesterol clefts and extravasated RBCs in the cystic wall (H/E 4x); (c) cystic lining with abundant area of hemorrhage in the cystic wall (H/E 4x); (d) cholesterol clefts in cystic wall (H/E 20x).

odontogenic cyst have been reported so far [3–7]. We report additional three cases of CG occurring in wall of odontogenic cysts (Table 1).

An ambiguity has always persisted regarding the terminology of CG in the oral cavity, as Bhaskar, Wood, and Goaz described a lesion in the jaw with similar histopathological features but termed it cholesteatoma [3]. Stating that cholesterol was the main component of tumor the term "cholesteatoma" was introduced in 1838 by Muller [7]. Cholesteatoma describes those cystic cavities lined by keratinized squamous epithelium and surrounded by stroma of variable thickness. The microscopic diagnosis depends entirely on the presence and identification of squamous epithelium and/or laminated keratinized material [3]. The main difference between histogenesis of CG and cholesteatoma is that no epithelium is involved in formation of CG. Transition of CG into cholesteatomas has not been observed, although the two anomalies may occur simultaneously [7]. Thus, use of the term cholesteatoma for a mass of connective tissue with numerous cholesterol crystals but without epithelial components and keratin is inappropriate and misleading [3].

CG should be considered in clinical-radiographic differential diagnoses of odontogenic cysts or tumors. Netto et al. reported a case of mandibular CG mimicking a dentigerous cyst [8].

The cholesterol crystals are reported to occur more commonly in inflammatory cysts, especially in radicular cysts. Lowest incidence was reported in noninflammatory cysts such as odontogenic keratocyst [5]. In all of our cases, CG is seen in the wall of cysts with developmental background.

The pathogenesis of CG is controversial as many possible mechanisms have been proposed to explain it but no clear consensus has been made. CG is formed due to irritant effect of accumulated cholesterol crystals as a result of the breakdown of blood, inflammatory tissue, or exudate. They attract foreign body giant cells and thus cause fibrosis [7]. Our cases also seem to reflect similar mechanism. In the middle ear, formation of CG could be attributed to the obstruction of ear drainage. Secondary to absorption of air into mucosa a negative pressure is created within the air cavity because of disturbance of air drainage. As a result, mucosal edema and hemorrhage develop. Hematoma from the mucosal bleeding would not be absorbed, resulting in its conversion to cholesterol crystals. However this cannot be a possible cause of CG occurring in the mandible due to the absence of intrabony cavities or drainage pathways [4].

The buildup of cholesterol crystals in the cyst wall and cystic fluid could result from the disintegrating red blood cells of stagnant blood vessels within the lesion, circulating plasma lipids, or fatty degeneration of connective tissue in a cavity blocked by inflammation [6]. Our cases reported abundant

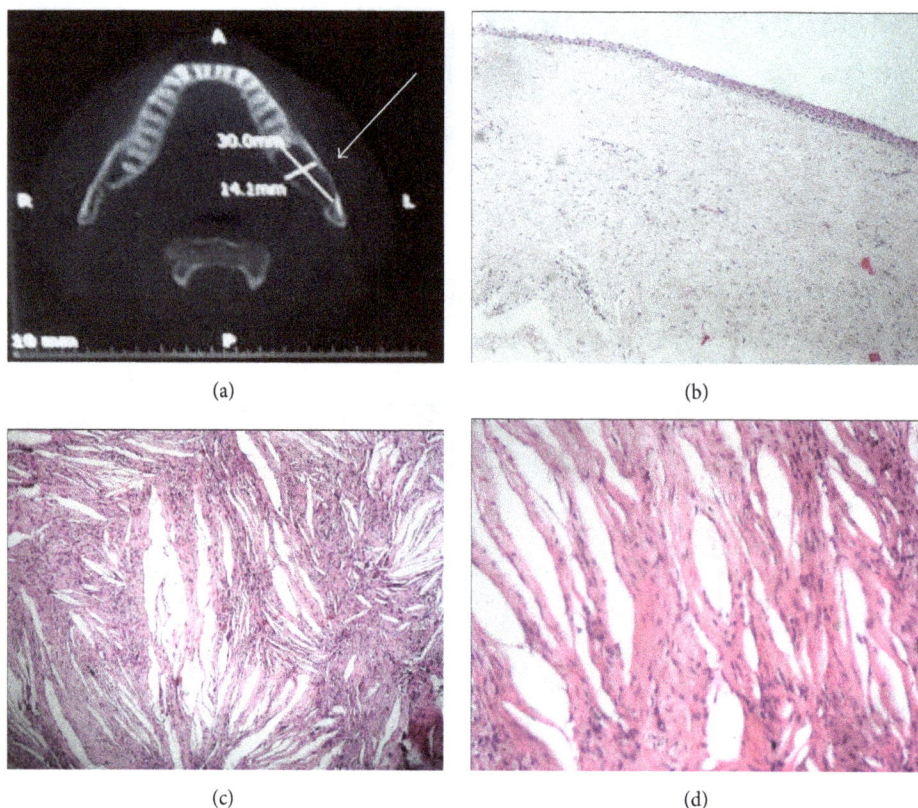

(a)

(b)

(c)

(d)

Figure 3: (a) CT scan revealed a well-defined radiolucency (30 × 14 mm in size) present on left angle of mandible region; (b) on incisional biopsy, 2-3-cell layer thick nonkeratinized stratified squamous cystic epithelial lining which showed proliferation in few areas associated with underlying inflammation (H/E 4x); (c) on excisional biopsy cholesterol clefts in cystic wall (H/E 10x); (d) cholesterol clefts in cystic wall (H/E 40x).

Table 1: Reported cases of cholesterol granuloma in association with odontogenic cyst.

Author	Year	Age/sex	Site	Associated with
Lee et al. [4]	2010	68/male	Right anterior to posterior mandible	Dentigerous cyst
Bhullar et al. [5]	2012	43/male	Left posterior mandible	Dentigerous cyst
Aparna et al. [6]	2013	68/female	Right posterior mandible	Ameloblastomatous calcifying odontogenic cyst
Case 1	2016	45/Male	Right posterior maxilla	Calcifying odontogenic cyst
Case 2	2016	38/Female	Right posterior mandible	Dentigerous cyst
Case 3	2016	47/Male	Left posterior mandible	Dentigerous cyst

areas of hemorrhage, which could be the cause of formation of CG. However, little is currently known about the molecular mechanism for CG formation in the cyst wall. A recent study by Yamazaki et al. suggested that formation of CG could be related to the presence of abundant perlecan (a basement membrane heparan sulfate proteoglycan) in the cyst wall of immature granulation tissue [9].

CG could lead to expansion of the lesion with which it is associated. Almada et al. [10] reported that there are chances of primarily or secondarily inflamed odontogenic lesions that exhibit foreign body reaction to cholesterol crystals in their capsule and could extend to maxillary sinuses due to anatomical continuity. Yamazaki et al. [9] reported that CG seems to be one of the driving forces for growth of jaw cysts, especially those with inflammatory background. They suggested that

low density lipoprotein entrapped by perlecan is accumulated and oxidized in the extracellular space and that oxidized-low density lipoprotein is scavenged by macrophages and is primarily deposited intracellularly; then the macrophages are converted into lipid-laden foamy cells. These foamy cells may originally rupture and release lipids concentrated in their cytoplasm into the extracellular space. Following this, concentrated free cholesterol results in crystallization. Cholesterol crystals in turn cause foreign body reactions to extend inflammatory reactions for cystic growth. Bone erosion may be seen in cholesterol granuloma showing expansive growth [1]. Nair PN et al. stated that macrophages change the hydrophobic cholesterol crystals into a soluble form by incorporating it into lipoprotein vehicle. However, the large cholesterol crystals resist internalization by macrophages and circumfuse to form multinucleated giant cells. Although they persist for prolonged periods, the phagocytes failed to degrade cholesterol and release inflammatory and bone resorptive mediators that cause further loss of bone and extension of lesion [6].

4. Conclusion

CG is considered as a nonspecific histopathological reaction to cholesterol crystals rather than a clinical or pathological entity. As its clinical and radiographic characteristics are nonspecific, it should be considered in differential diagnosis of odontogenic cyst and tumors and histopathological analysis is essential for a correct final diagnosis of CG. Due to paucity of the intraoral reported CG cases the true nature and pathogenesis are still ambiguous. There also persists confusion on the terminologies and distinctiveness of CG reported in the oral cavity and ear. More CG cases of the oral cavity should be brought to light so that their unique identity could be revealed and elaborated upon.

Competing Interests

The authors declare that there is no conflict of interests regarding the publication of this paper.

References

[1] A. Alkan, O. Etoz, C. Candirli, M. Ulu, and E. H. Dayisoylu, "Cholesterol granuloma of the jaws: report of two cases," *Journal of the Pakistan Medical Association*, vol. 64, no. 1, pp. 86–88, 2014.

[2] S. Singh, S. Chhabra, P. Gupta, P. Malik, and S. Singh, "Cholesterol granuloma: An uncommon clinical entity of the maxillary sinus," *Head and Neck Oncology*, vol. 6, no. 1, 2014.

[3] A. Hirshberg, D. Dayan, A. Buchner, and A. Freedman, "Cholesterol granuloma of the jaws," *International Journal of Oral and Maxillofacial Surgery*, vol. 17, no. 4, pp. 230–231, 1988.

[4] J. H. Lee, M. S. Alrashdan, K. M. Ahn, M. H. Kang, S. P. Hong, and S. M. Kim, "Cholesterol granuloma in the wall of a mandibular dentigerous cyst: a rare case report," *Journal of Clinical and Experimental Dentistry*, vol. 2, no. 2, pp. e88–e90, 2010.

[5] R. K. Bhullar, S. Kler, A. Bhullar, M. S. Kamat, K. Singh, and S. Kaur, "Cholesterol granuloma in the wall of dentigerous cyst," *Indian Journal of Dentistry*, vol. 3, no. 2, pp. 106–109, 2012.

[6] M. Aparna, M. Gupta, N. Sujir et al., "Calcifying odontogenic cyst: a rare report of a non-neoplastic variant associated with cholesterol granuloma," *Journal of Contemporary Dental Practice*, vol. 14, no. 6, pp. 1178–1182, 2013.

[7] I. Kaffe, M. M. Littner, A. Buchner, and M. Friedman, "Cholesterol granuloma embedded in an odontoma of the maxilla," *Journal of Oral and Maxillofacial Surgery*, vol. 42, no. 5, pp. 319–322, 1984.

[8] A. C. M. Netto, J. A. R. Brito, C. N. A. de Oliveira, R. R. Arruda, R. S. Gomez, and R. A. Mesquita, "Mandibular cholesterol granuloma mimicking a dentigerous cyst," *International Journal of Oral and Maxillofacial Pathology*, vol. 5, no. 3, pp. 21–23, 2014.

[9] M. Yamazaki, J. Cheng, N. Hao et al., "Basement membrane-type heparan sulfate proteoglycan (perlecan) and low-density lipoprotein (LDL) are co-localized in granulation tissues: a possible pathogenesis of cholesterol granulomas in jaw cysts," *Journal of Oral Pathology and Medicine*, vol. 33, no. 3, pp. 177–184, 2004.

[10] C. B. M. Almada, D. R. Fonseca, R. R. Vanzillotta, and F. R. Pires, "Cholesterol granuloma of the maxillary sinus," *Brazilian Dental Journal*, vol. 19, no. 2, pp. 171–174, 2008.

27

Treatment of Class III Malocclusion: Atypical Extraction Protocol

Fernando Pedrin Carvalho Ferreira,[1] **Maiara da Silva Goulart,**[2]
Renata Rodrigues de Almeida-Pedrin,[3] **Ana Claudia de Castro Ferreira Conti,**[3]
and Maurício de Almeida Cardoso[3]

[1]*Cora-Vilhena, Vilhena, RO, Brazil*
[2]*Sagrado Coração University, Bauru, SP, Brazil*
[3]*Department of Orthodontics, Sagrado Coração University, Bauru, SP, Brazil*

Correspondence should be addressed to Maiara da Silva Goulart; maiara_goulart@hotmail.com

Academic Editor: Andrea Scribante

The treatment of Angle Class III malocclusion is rather challenging, because the patient's growth pattern determines the success of long-term treatment. Early diagnosis and treatment are still highly discussed issues in orthodontic literature. This type of early intervention has been indicated more frequently in order to eliminate primary etiological factors and prevent an already present malocclusion from becoming severe. However, when a patient is diagnosed in adulthood, manipulation of the bone bases becomes extremely limited, as there is no longer any potential for growth. Treatments are restricted to dental compensations when possible or orthognathic surgery. However, owing to the high cost and inherent risk of the surgical procedure, this treatment option is often denied by the patient; in such a case, the orthodontist has little choice but to perform, where possible, compensatory treatments to restore a functional occlusion and improve facial esthetics. This article reports a case of Class III malocclusion in a patient who opted for compensatory treatment with lower molar extraction that allowed for correction of the midline and the overjet. Good facial esthetics and functional normal occlusion were achieved at the end of the treatment.

1. Introduction

Angle Class III malocclusion is the least common malocclusion. Its prevalence varies according to the surveyed area and is higher in Asian countries like Japan and Korea [1, 2]. Its prevalence in the general population in China is 15,69% [1] while that in Europe is only 2–6% [2]. It has a strong genetic component and is one of the most challenging malocclusions to treat.

When compared with normal occlusion, the lower posterior teeth occlude mesially in relation to the upper teeth, in Class III malocclusion cases. The anterior region also presents this discrepancy in the anteroposterior direction, seen as a reversal of the horizontal overlap of the incisors, with the incisal edges of the lower teeth located in front of those of the

upper. The bone bases reflect a sagittal skeletal discrepancy between the maxilla and the mandible. Development of the malocclusion can include skeletal retrusion of the maxilla, skeletal protrusion of the mandible, or a combination of these two factors [3, 4]. According to Guyer et al. [5], in a study with 5- to 15-year-old Class III patients, 57% had maxillary retrusion, irrespective of whether or not they presented with mandibular prognathism. Studies on the multifactorial etiology of Class III malocclusions show that maxillary retrognathism is as common as mandibular prognathism [3, 5].

Individuals with Class III malocclusion may present, as standard features of growth, excessive cranial prominence, mid-facial deficiency, lower lip prominence, and mandibular body that is often rotated forward and upward [4, 6]. Those

TABLE 1: Cephalometric analysis (USP-standard).

Measurement	Norm	Initial	Final	Control (2 years)
SNA	82.0°	82.39°	82.53°	83.53°
SNB	80.0°	82.27°	81.84°	84.13°
ANB	2.0°	0.13°	0.69°	0.60°
SN-MP	32.0°	44.17°	43.42°	42.05°
1.NA	22.0°	24.08°	27.14°	27.79°
1.NB	25.0°	17.62°	13.35°	14.78°
1.1	131.0°	138.17°	138.82°	138.02°

patients often face the possibility of undergoing orthosurgical treatment when craniofacial growth is finished, since the face tends to reveal an unfavorable growth pattern over time. The choice of treatment is even more limited and challenging when a late diagnosis is made. For some patients, orthognathic surgery is the best option. It is a corrective procedure for the skeletal discrepancy, and if favored when the bone deformity is severe and excessively affects the facial appearance of the patient [7]. However, in borderline cases, compensatory orthodontic treatment may be opted for, since the esthetic balancing of the face is not always the major motive for treatment.

Some authors recommended extraction, orthodontic protocol, as one of the most common ways to treat these cases. Traditionally, the extraction of four premolars is the most common choice. Others reported alternative extractions for the treatment of Class III malocclusion [8, 9]. According to De Oliveira Ruellas et al. [10], when the third molars are present, the extraction of the first molar might be a good option to solve the problems of anterior-inferior crowding and vertical growth, as well as to attain a Class I molar relationship. Other authors, such as Capelozza Filho et al. [11], have treated this malocclusion with bonding and orthodontic brackets with specific angles to achieve compensation whenever possible.

The purpose of this clinical report is to present the case of an adult male patient with Class III malocclusion, with no complaints regarding facial esthetics, treated by an atypical extraction protocol of the lower molars, in order to achieve a stable and functional occlusion as similar to a natural compensation as possible.

2. Materials and Methods

2.1. Diagnosis and Etiology.
A male Caucasian patient sought orthodontic treatment for functional and esthetic complaints regarding his smile. Diagnostic tests were conducted to identify the problem and seek out possible treatment alternatives. Frontal facial analysis showed a decreased zygomatic projection, an increased vertical growth in the lower face, and an asymmetrical appearance (deviation to the right side), without lip sealing (Figure 1). In the lateral view, a concave profile was evident, with an increased chin-neck line, protrusion of the lower lip, and an inadequate zygomatic projection (Figure 1). The lateral face radiograph confirmed the findings of the facial analysis: a vertical growth pattern, protruded mandible, proclined upper incisors, and

upright lower incisors, pointing towards compensation (Figure 2).

Cephalometric analysis showed a skeletal Class I malocclusion (ANB, 0.13°), with a well-positioned maxilla, a slight mandibular protrusion (SNA, 82.39°; SNB, 82.27°), and a hyperdivergent growth pattern (SN-MP, 44.17°). The angle between the upper incisors and the N-A line was 24.0°, and the angle between the latter and the lower incisors was 17.62°, verifying the lingual mandibular incisors. This position was confirmed by the reduction in the value of IMPA (73.96°). The interincisal angle was 138.1° (Table 1).

The panoramic radiograph showed the presence of all permanent teeth except 18 and 48 (Figure 2). The oral examination confirmed a Class III relationship of the molars and the canines that was more severe on the left side, with an inferior, midline deviation to the right, and an anterior cross-bite (Figure 1).

After radiological and facial evaluation, the patient was diagnosed with a Class III malocclusion, presenting a dolichofacial, asymmetrical, concave profile, with maxillary deficiency and a slightly increased mandibular growth. The etiology of skeletal Class III malocclusion in most cases is multifactorial, and therefore, the individuals affected by this anomaly demonstrate a combination of dental and skeletal factors [12, 13].

2.2. Therapeutic Options.
Two different therapeutic approaches could have been followed for the treatment of the malocclusion: orthosurgical treatment or compensatory treatment. Orthognathic surgery was proposed for correction of the bone bases, but the patient refused relying on the lack of esthetic complains. Based on that, an orthodontic corrective treatment plan was indicated with the objective of dental compensation.

2.3. Objectives of the Treatment.
The treatment aimed at (1) reestablishing a functional occlusion through dental compensation, (2) solving the sagittal imbalance, (3) correcting the midline deviation, and (4) improving the facial esthetics.

2.4. Treatment Progress.
Fixed orthodontic treatment was initiated with self-ligating straight-wire brackets only in the upper arch. A decision to extract tooth 36 was made because of its destruction, which aided the treatment by correcting the inferior midline and reducing the dental mass, thus solving the anterior edge-to-edge bite (Figure 3).

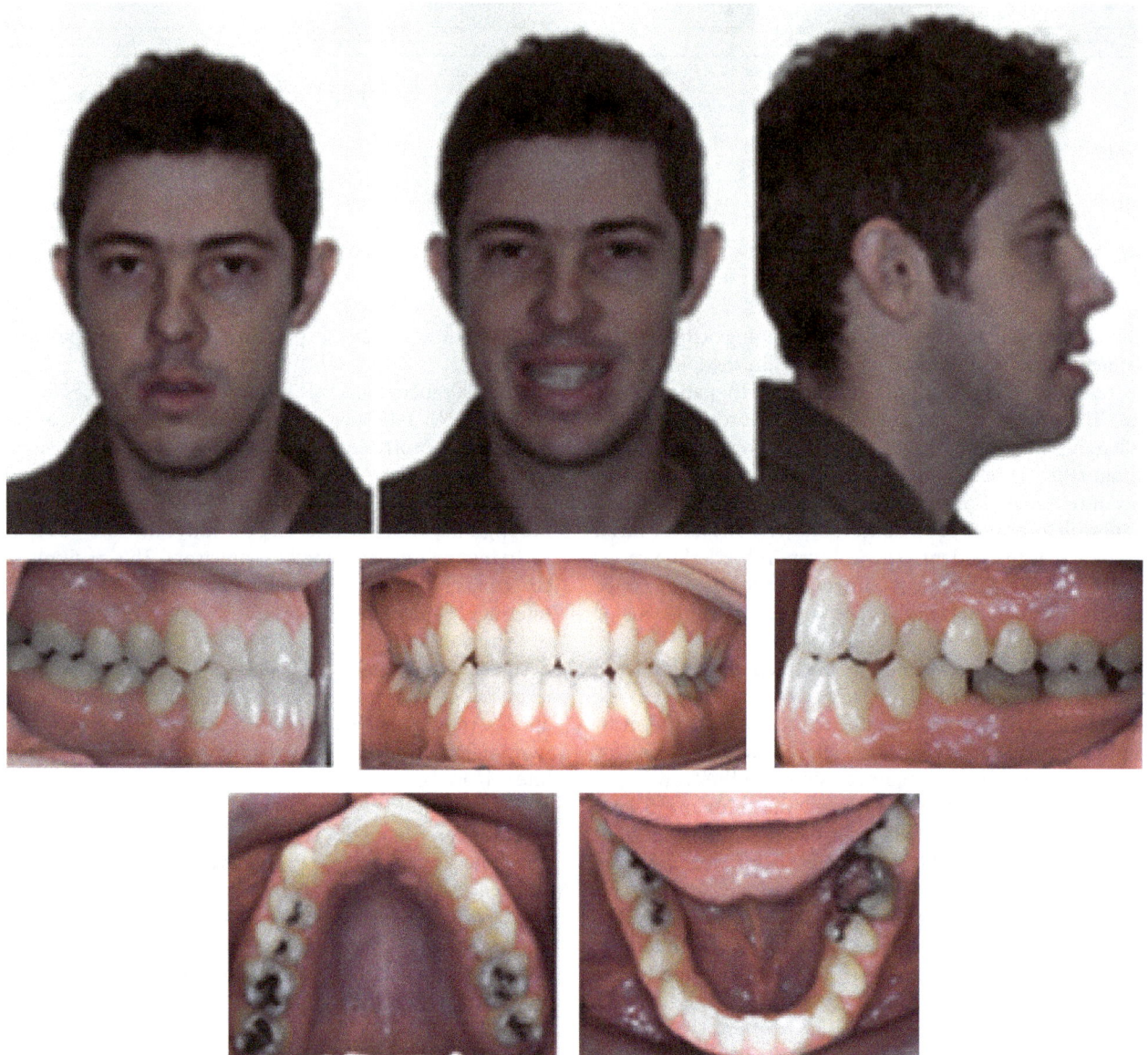

FIGURE 1: Pretreatment facial and intraoral photographs.

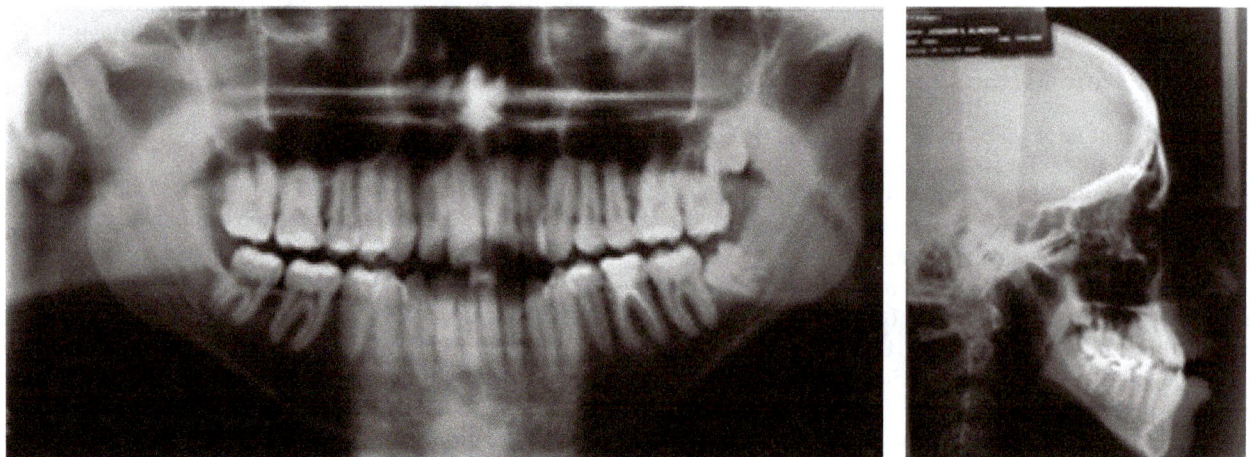

FIGURE 2: Pretreatment panoramic and cephalometric radiographs.

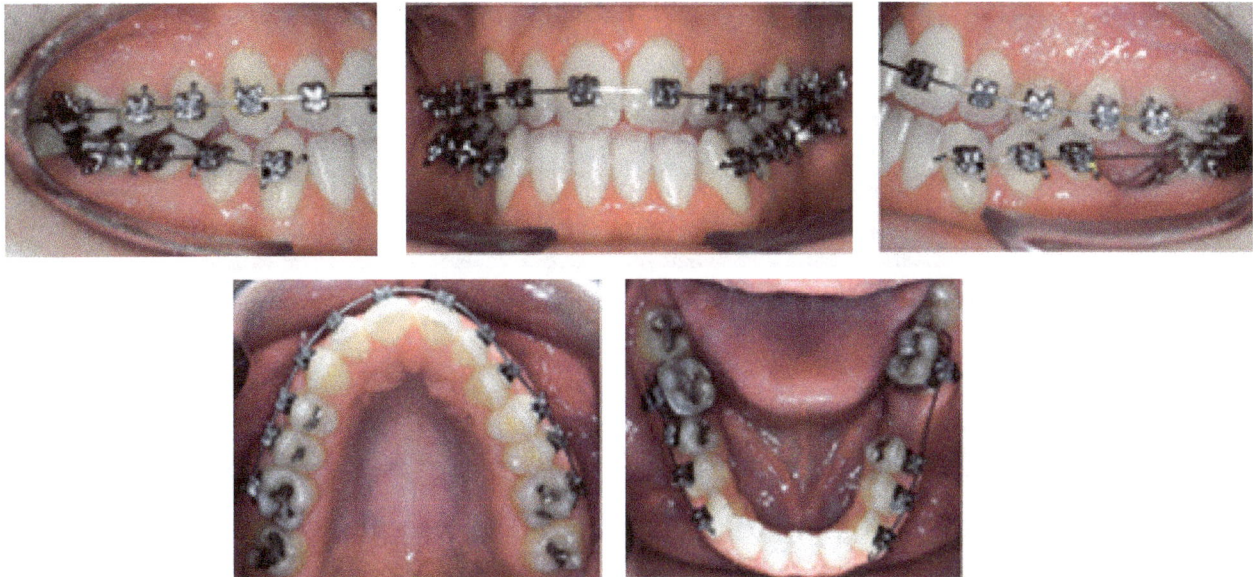

FIGURE 3: Intraoral views of treatment. Start of leveling, extraction of tooth 36, and segmented arch in the lower arch.

The wire sequence adopted for alignment and leveling was 0.014″ NiTi, 0.016″ NiTi, and 0.016″ stainless steel wire. The lower brackets were also bonded on molars and premolars only at this point and after the installation of the 0.017″ × 0.025″ TMA wire, the lower anterior retraction was performed, only to the left side where tooth 36 was extracted (Figure 3). The use of Class III elastics was indicated at the same time, to facilitate the correction of overjet. In the upper arch, 0.016″ × 0.022″ NITI wire was used, followed by 0.018″ and 0.020″ bowflex steel arch to expand the left side for transverse adjustment. After achieving sufficient room for the incisors alignment, the lower anterior teeth were bonded (Figure 4). In order to close the extraction space and to correct the midline deviation retraction loops were applied (Figure 5). With the 0.019″ × 0.025″ stainless steel wire, an elastic chain was used for the mesialization of tooth 37. Tooth 38 was subsequently bonded, and the remaining spaces were closed with an elastic chain (Figure 6). The total treatment duration was 30 months.

3. Results

At the end of treatment, a good occlusal relationship was achieved, with the correction of the overjet, coincidence of the midlines, and the correction of Angle Class III malocclusion, without the need for orthognathic surgery. It was also observed in the facial lateral view, passive lip sealing, and great improvement of facial esthetics (Figure 7).

New records were obtained 2 years after final treatment, last follow-up, and evaluation of the occlusion revealed Angle Class I molar relationship. The occlusion was stable and functional (Figure 8).

Final cephalometric analysis showed values for ANB, 0,69°; SNA, 82.53°; SNB, 81.84°; and a SN-MP, 43.42° defining the hyperdivergent growth pattern. It was observed an increase in the angle between the upper incisors and the N-A line from 24.0° to 27,14°, and for the lower incisors from 13,35° to 17.62°. A reduction in the value of IMPA from 73.96° to 68,1° was also noted. The interincisal angle was 138.8° (Table 1).

4. Discussion

Studies on the multifactorial etiology of Class III malocclusion show that maxillary retrognathism is as common as mandibular prognathism. Previous research has reported that 32–63% of the patients with skeletal Class III malocclusion have a maxillary deficiency or its combination with excessive mandibular growth [3, 5].

Most authors agree that an early intervention is the best option for Class III malocclusion treatment, because of the possibility of orthopedic management through face-mask therapy, after maxillary expansion. This would redirect growth, making the malocclusion correction possible [14, 15].

Treatment options at later stages are limited, restricted to orthosurgical approach to correct bone discrepancies or orthodontic treatment aimed at correcting malocclusion through dental compensation. Frequently, the treatment plan includes extractions, and the use of intermaxillary elastics. This, however, has no impact on the facial esthetics, since the skeletal problem remains uncorrected [13, 16, 17]. Even considering this advantage, some authors still have reported success performing the compensatory treatment protocol [4, 16–20].

Despite being the most indicated treatment option in these cases, the inherent risk and high cost of the orthosurgical procedures make patients reluctant to accept it [6, 17, 21, 22].

In this case the patient also opted for orthodontic treatment without orthognathic surgery. In order to make possible the lower compensation and midline correction, extraction

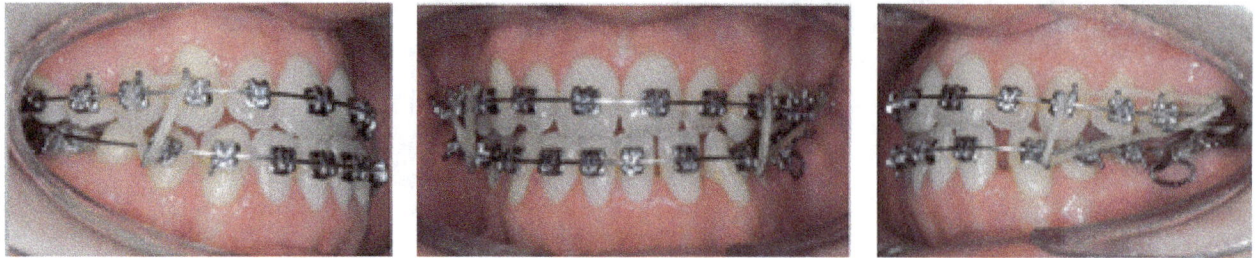

FIGURE 4: Intraoral views of treatment. Bonding the lower incisor, intermaxillary elastics, and loop to start closure extraction space.

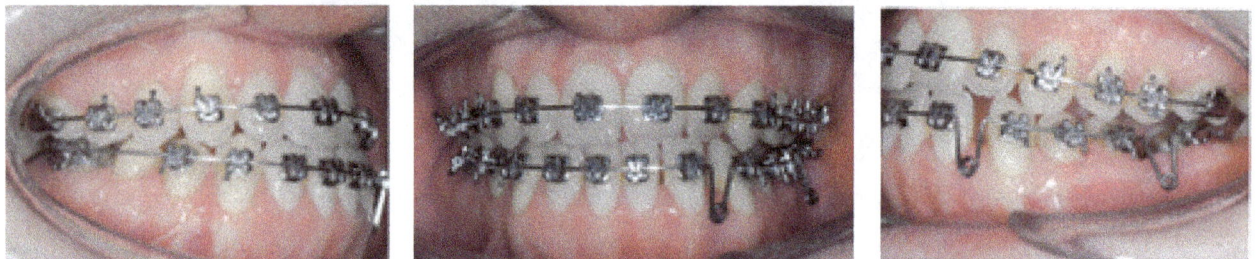

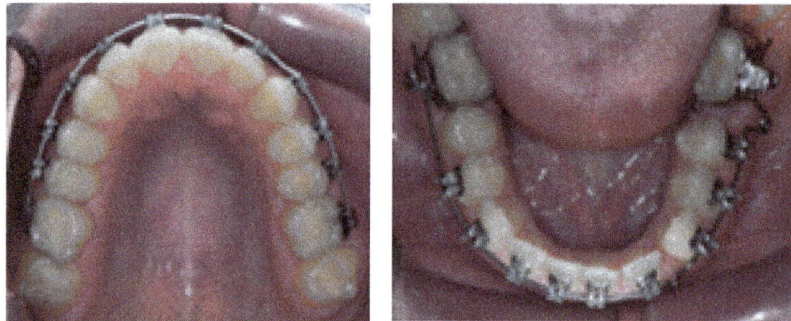

FIGURE 5: Intraoral views of treatment. End of leveling $0.017'' \times 0.025''$ stainless steel wire and retraction loops applied to close the extraction space and to correct the midline deviation.

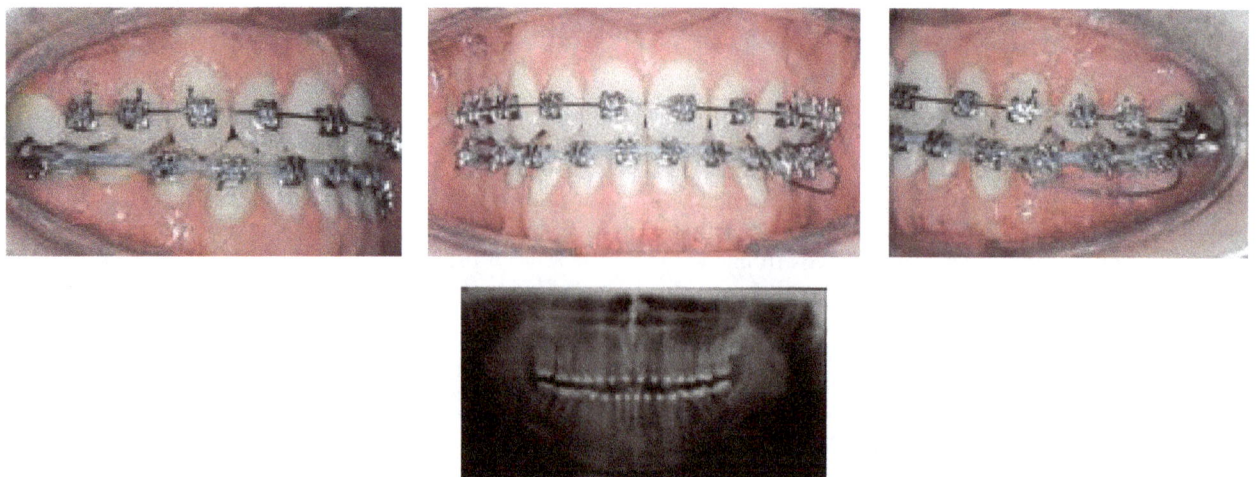

FIGURE 6: Intraoral views of treatment and panoramic radiograph. Bonding tooth 38, cantilever applied to upright tooth 37, and elastic chain to close the remaining spaces. Panoramic radiograph showing uprighted good position of tooth 38.

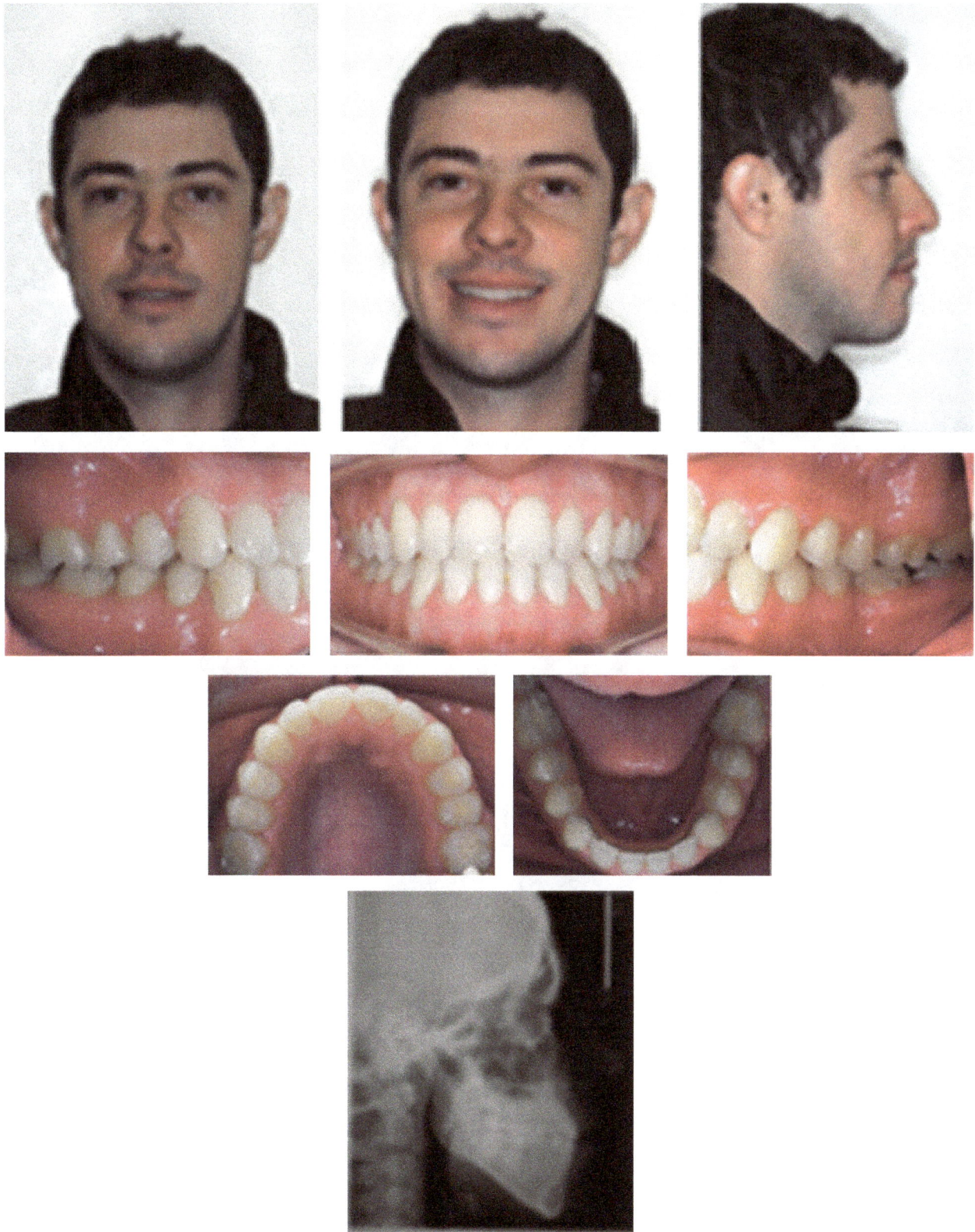

FIGURE 7: Posttreatment facial and intraoral photographs, and cephalometric radiograph.

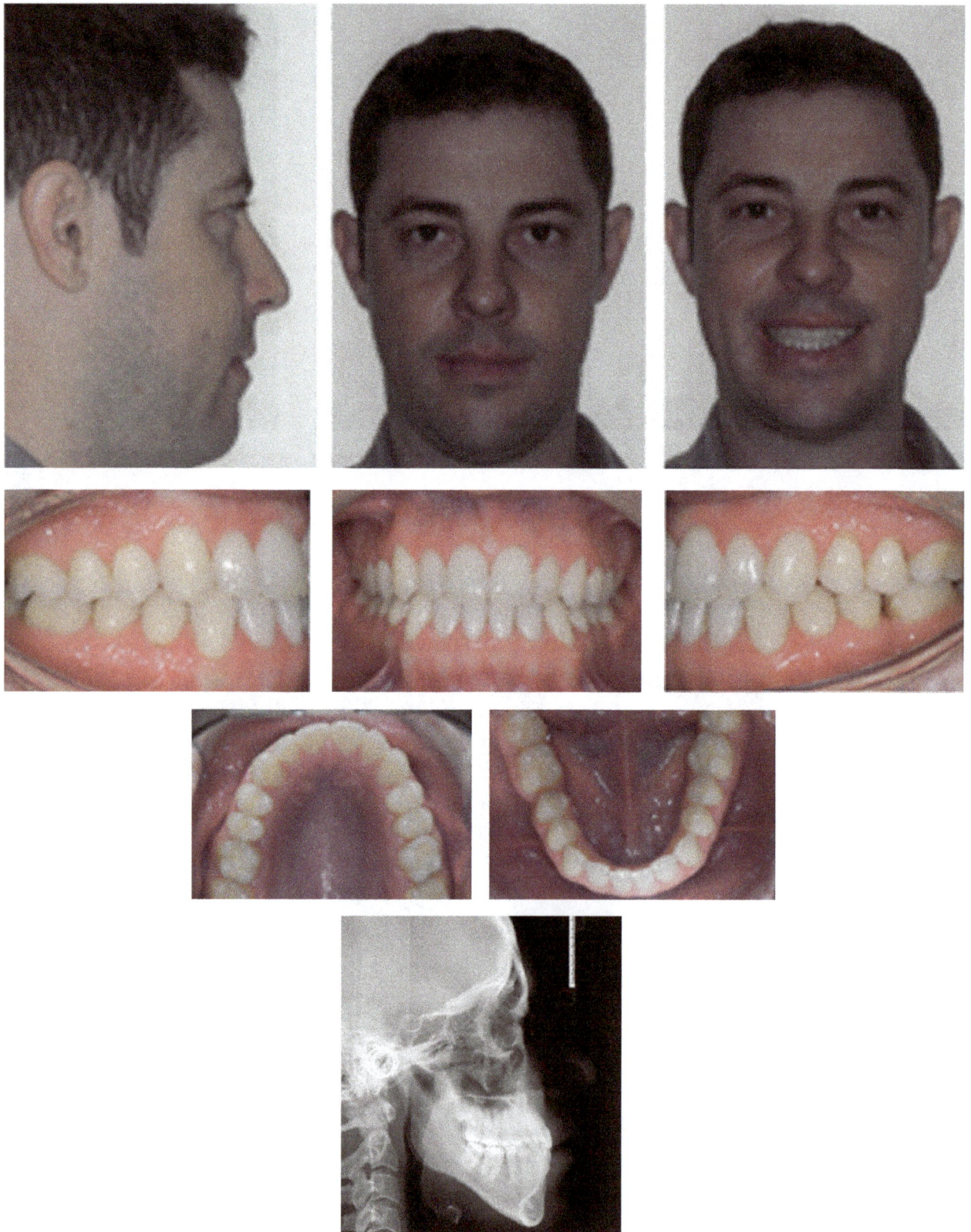

FIGURE 8: Posttreatment facial and intraoral photographs, and cephalometric radiograph (2 years after treatment completion).

of tooth 36 was necessary. De Oliveira Ruellas et al. [10] and Sandler et al. [23] indicated the extraction of the first molars as a feasible treatment option in the presence of extensive caries, apical pathologies, significant restorations, severe crowding in the posterior region or anterior open bite. The option to extract the first molar depends on the presence and position of the third molar.

For the correction of anterior cross-bite and the normalization of the molar relationship, Lin and Gu [24] suggested the extraction of the second molar as the best option, as long as the patient had the third molar. This was in concurrence with a previous report by M. E. Richardson and A. Richardson [25], supporting the idea that the third molar can take the place of the second molar.

The contraindication for lower molar extraction is the difficulty in closing the space [10]. However, in the case described here, most of the space was used for the retraction of the anterior teeth, midline correction, and obtaining an adequate overjet.

The treatment options for orthodontic compensation in such patients include multiple extraction patterns. The extraction of the lower incisors is a good option for moderate Class III cases or edge-to-edge bite [26]. Some authors may suggest premolar extraction [10, 24]. The extraction of four premolars is not indicated in cases of severe malocclusion, or when the upper and lower teeth are well aligned, or when the lower crowding is not severe, since it can handicap the development of the jaw. The extraction of the third molars can be an alternative in these situations. However, the space created with the extraction of the third molars is limited, compared to that with the second molar extractions, which can be critical for the correction of the molar relationship and the anterior cross-bite [22].

A common strategy for orthodontic compensation with or without extraction is the use of intermaxillary Class III elastics, causing mesial movement of the upper teeth and distal movement of the lower teeth, with proclination of the upper teeth and retroclination of the lower teeth [9, 27, 28]. In our case, since the use of elastics was indicated for this patient, they were utilized as an adjunct to mechanics.

In this case the retraction in the lower arch was performed with the aid of a segmented arch with retraction loop [29] only on the left side to promote overjet and midline deviation correction. A better control of the force moment generated by the retraction loop caused an adequate space closure and a good occlusion. The segmented mechanics was also indicated for the lower arch in order to prevent a protrusion of the lower incisors, which in this Class III case was not recommended. Based on that, the incisors were bonded only when enough room for their alignment was provided.

Overall, the straight-wire mechanics associated with segmented arches in this case report achieved a good occlusion.

5. Conclusion

The Class III malocclusion was successfully treated by atypical extraction of only one lower molar. This less invasive approach was a feasible option for the patient who declined the orthosurgical alternative. The excellent esthetic and functional treatment outcome was possible, in large part, by the patient compliance.

Consent

The patient hereby grants all rights to publish photographs or other images of them in the manuscript where they appear as a patient or subject without payment of any kind. The patient has been informed that any images of them that do appear may be modified.

Competing Interests

The authors have no competing interests to disclose.

References

[1] K. K. Lew, W. C. Foong, and E. Loh, "Malocclusion prevalence in an ethnic Chinese population," *Australian Dental Journal*, vol. 38, no. 6, pp. 442–449, 1993.

[2] R. Burgersdijk, G. J. Truin, F. Frankenmolen, H. Kalsbeek, M. van't Hof, and J. Mulder, "Malocclusion and orthodontic treatment need of 15–74-year-old Dutch adults," *Community Dentistry and Oral Epidemiology*, vol. 19, no. 2, pp. 64–67, 1991.

[3] J. A. McNamara Jr., "An orthopedic approach to the treatment of Class III malocclusion in young patients," *Journal of Clinical Orthodontics*, vol. 21, no. 9, pp. 598–608, 1987.

[4] P. Ngan and W. Moon, "Evolution of class III treatment in orthodontics," *American Journal of Orthodontics and Dentofacial Orthopedics*, vol. 148, no. 1, pp. 22–36, 2015.

[5] E. C. Guyer, E. E. Ellis 3rd, J. A. Jr. McNamara, and R. G. Behrents, "Components of class III malocclusion in juveniles and adolescents," *The Angle orthodontist*, vol. 56, no. 1, pp. 7–30, 1986.

[6] N. Hamanci, G. Basaran, and S. Sahin, "Nonsurgical correction of adult skeletal class III and open-bite malocclusion," *The Angle Orthodontist*, vol. 76, no. 3, pp. 527–532, 2006.

[7] S. G. Arslan, J. D. Kama, and S. Baran, "Correction of a severe class III malocclusion," *American Journal of Orthodontics and Dentofacial Orthopedics*, vol. 126, no. 2, pp. 237–244, 2004.

[8] J. L. Seddon, "Extraction of four first molars: a case for a general practitioner?" *Journal of Orthodontics*, vol. 31, no. 2, pp. 80–85, 2004.

[9] J. Lin and Y. Gu, "Preliminary investigation of nonsurgical treatment of severe skeletal class III malocclusion in the permanent dentition," *Angle Orthodontist*, vol. 73, no. 4, pp. 401–410, 2003.

[10] A. C. De Oliveira Ruellas, C. Baratieri, M. B. Roma et al., "Angle Class III malocclusion treated with mandibular first molar extractions," *American Journal of Orthodontics and Dentofacial Orthopedics*, vol. 142, no. 3, pp. 384–392, 2012.

[11] L. Capelozza Filho, O. G. Silva Filho, T. O. Ozawaka, and A. O. Cavassan, "Brackets individualization in straight-wire technique: concepts review and suggestions for prescribed use," *Revista Dental Press de Ortodontia e Ortopedia Facial*, vol. 4, no. 4, pp. 78–106, 1999.

[12] C. B. Staudt and S. Kiliaridis, "Different skeletal types underlying Class III malocclusion in a random population," *American Journal of Orthodontics and Dentofacial Orthopedics*, vol. 136, no. 5, pp. 715–721, 2009.

[13] B. A. Troy, S. Shanker, H. W. Fields, K. Vig, and W. Johnston, "Comparison of incisor inclination in patients with class III malocclusion treated with orthognathic surgery or orthodontic camouflage," *American Journal of Orthodontics and Dentofacial Orthopedics*, vol. 135, no. 2, pp. 146.e1–146.e9, 2009.

[14] D. Merwin, P. Ngan, U. Hagg, C. Yiu, and S. H. Wei, "Timing for effective application of anteriorly directed orthopedic force to the maxilla," *American Journal of Orthodontics and Dentofacial Orthopedics*, vol. 112, no. 3, pp. 292–299, 1997.

[15] T. Baccetti, F. Lorenzo, and I. Tollaro, "Sketelal effects of early treatmente of class III malocclusion with maxillary expansion and face-mask therapy," *American Journal of Orthodontics and Dentofacial Orthopedics*, vol. 113, no. 3, pp. 333–343, 1998.

[16] T. Yanagita, S. Kuroda, T. Takano-Yamamoto, and T. Yamashiro, "Class III malocclusion with complex problems of lateral open bite and severe crowding successfully treated with miniscrew anchorage and lingual orthodontic brackets," *American Journal of Orthodontics and Dentofacial Orthopedics*, vol. 139, no. 5, pp. 679–689, 2011.

[17] A. T. Moullas, J. M. Palomo, J. R. Gass, B. D. Amberman, J. White, and D. Gustovich, "Nonsurgical treatment of a patient with a class III malocclusion," *American Journal of Orthodontics and Dentofacial Orthopedics*, vol. 129, no. 4, supplement, pp. S111–S118, 2006.

[18] H. Maruo, I. T. Maruo, A. Y. Saga, E. S. Camargo, O. Guariza Filho, and O. M. Tanaka, "Orthodontic-prosthetic treatment of an adult with a severe Class III malocclusion," *American Journal of Orthodontics and Dentofacial Orthopedics*, vol. 138, no. 6, pp. 820–828, 2010.

[19] J. E. Bilodeau, "Nonsurgical treatment of a Class III patient with a lateral open-bite malocclusion," *American Journal of Orthodontics and Dentofacial Orthopedics*, vol. 140, no. 6, pp. 861–868, 2011.

[20] M. E. Hiller, "Nonsurgical correction of Class III open bite malocclusion in an adult patient," *American Journal of Orthodontics and Dentofacial Orthopedics*, vol. 122, no. 2, pp. 210–216, 2002.

[21] T. Deguchi, H. Kurosaka, H. Oikawa et al., "Comparison of orthodontic treatment outcomes in adults with skeletal open bite between conventional edgewise treatment and implant-anchored orthodontics," *American Journal of Orthodontics and Dentofacial Orthopedics*, vol. 139, no. 4, pp. s60–s68, 2011.

[22] H. Hu, J. Chen, J. Guo et al., "Distalization of the mandibular dentition of an adult with a skeletal Class III malocclusion," *American Journal of Orthodontics and Dentofacial Orthopedics*, vol. 142, no. 6, pp. 854–862, 2012.

[23] T. J. Sandler, R. Atkson, and A. M. Murray, "For four sixes," *American Journal of Orthodontics and Dentofacial Orthopedics*, vol. 117, no. 4, pp. 418–434, 2000.

[24] J. Lin and Y. Gu, "Lower second molar extraction in correction of severe skeletal class III malocclusion," *Angle Orthodontist*, vol. 76, no. 2, pp. 217–225, 2006.

[25] M. E. Richardson and A. Richardson, "Lower third molar development subsequent to second molar extraction," *American Journal of Orthodontics and Dentofacial Orthopedics*, vol. 104, no. 6, pp. 566–574, 1993.

[26] J. A. Canut, "Mandibular incisor extraction: indication and long-term evaluation," *European Journal of Orthodontics*, vol. 16, pp. 187–201, 1996.

[27] S. He, J. Gao, P. Wamalwa, Y. Wang, S. Zou, and S. Chen, "Camouflage treatment of skeletal Class III malocclusion with multiloop edgewise arch wire and modified Class III elastics by maxillary mini-implant Anchorage," *Angle Orthodontist*, vol. 83, no. 4, pp. 630–640, 2013.

[28] I. Saito, M. Yamaki, and K. Hanada, "Nonsurgical treatment of adult open bite using edgewise appliance combined with high-pull headgear and class III elastics," *Angle Orthodontist*, vol. 75, no. 2, pp. 277–283, 2005.

[29] S. Braun and M. R. Marcotte, "Rationale of the segmented approach to orthodontic treatment," *American Journal of Orthodontics and Dentofacial Orthopedics*, vol. 108, no. 1, pp. 1–8, 1995.

A Novel Procedure for the Immediate Reconstruction of Severely Resorbed Alveolar Sockets for Advanced Periodontal Disease

Mario Aimetti, Valeria Manavella, Luca Cricenti, and Federica Romano

Department of Surgical Sciences, Periodontology Section, CIR Dental School, University of Turin, Via Nizza 230, 10126 Turin, Italy

Correspondence should be addressed to Mario Aimetti; mario.aimetti@unito.it

Academic Editor: Gerardo Gómez-Moreno

Background. Several clinical techniques and a variety of biomaterials have been introduced over the years in an effort to overcome bone remodeling and resorption after tooth extraction. However, the predictability of these procedures in sockets with severely resorbed buccal/lingual plate due to periodontal disease is still unknown. *Case Description.* A patient with advanced periodontitis underwent extraction of upper right lateral and central incisors. The central incisor exhibited complete buccal bone plate loss and a 9 mm vertical bone deficiency on its palatal side. The alveolar sockets were filled with collagen sponge and covered with a nonresorbable high-density PTFE membrane. Primary closure was not attained and any rigid scaffold material was not used. Histologic analysis provided evidence of new bone formation. At 12 months a cone-beam computed tomographic scan revealed enough bone volume to insert two conventional dental implants in conjunction with minor horizontal bone augmentation procedures. *Clinical Implications.* This case report would seem to support the potential of the proposed reconstructive approach in changing the morphology of severely resorbed alveolar sockets, minimizing the need for advanced bone regeneration procedures during implant placement.

1. Introduction

Alveolar ridge resorption is a physiologic process initiated immediately after extraction leading to an average 40–60% decrease in the horizontal and vertical dimensions of the alveolar ridge during the first year [1]. Different ridge preservation techniques have been advocated to reduce the amount of bone resorption, using different bone grafting materials alone or in conjunction with barrier membranes [2]. Clinical and histologic studies reported favorable outcomes when the socket preservation therapy included sockets with intact four-wall configuration or buccal dehiscence/fenestration defects while maintaining the interdental bone peaks [3, 4].

In advanced periodontitis patients alveolar sockets often exhibit severely resorbed facial/lingual bone plate and loss of interproximal attachment level and require bone reconstruction procedures. In such patients the extraction sockets morphology often is not space maintaining. The resorption of the interproximal bone peaks as well as the inadequate soft tissue volume makes it difficult to ensure graft material stability and to obtain primary wound closure. This may

jeopardize the hard tissue volume reconstruction. Therefore, the aim of the present case report is to describe the clinical and histologic outcomes of a novel procedure for the immediate reconstruction of severely resorbed alveolar sockets for advanced periodontal disease.

2. Case Presentation

2.1. Patient and Alveolar Socket Reconstruction. A healthy, nonsmoker 48-year-old male presented with the chief complaint of gingival bleeding. The comprehensive periodontal examination and full-mouth periapical radiographs revealed a generalized severe chronic periodontitis. After etiological periodontal treatment was completed, the right maxillary incisors exhibited persistent suppuration, tooth number 7 had mobility grade II/III, and tooth number 8 had mobility grade III. Both teeth were extruded and tooth number 8 exhibited pathologic migration with a midline diastema of 2-3 mm (Figures 1(a)–1(c)). A combined approach consisting of regenerative periodontal surgery and orthodontic therapy was proposed to the patient as ideal treatment plan to try

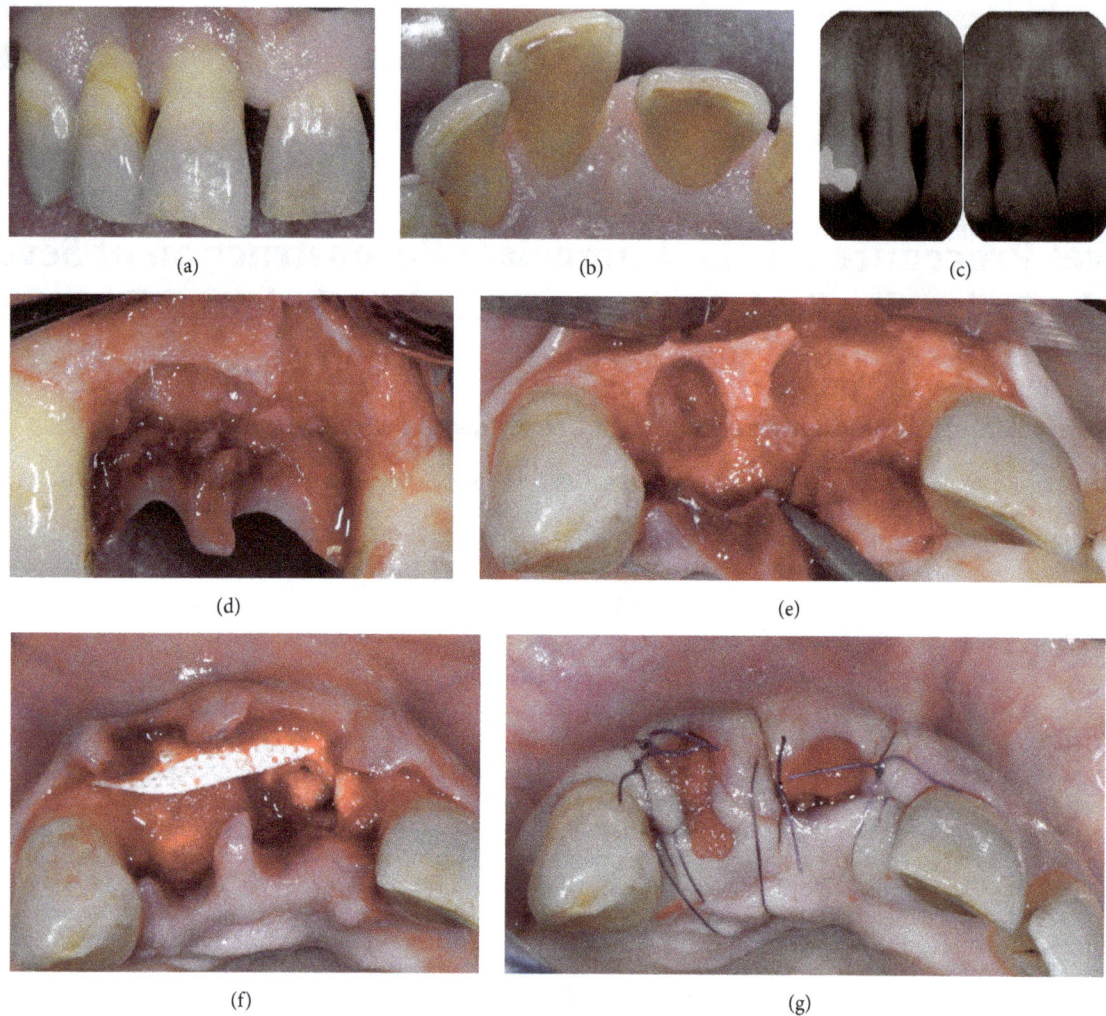

FIGURE 1: Maxillary right central and lateral incisors before extraction (a). Note extrusion of central and lateral incisors, migration of central incisor, and persistent inflammation (b). Preoperative radiographs showing severe interdental bone loss and widening of the residual periodontal ligament space as a consequence of the occlusal trauma (c). Intraoperative view following teeth removal (d). Occlusal view showing vertical bone resorption and partial nonspace maintaining defect at central incisor (e). After placement of a nonresorbable d-PTFE membrane to replace the missing buccal bony wall, the gap between the membrane and the residual palatal wall was filled with the collagen sponge (f). Flaps were repositioned and the membrane was left partially exposed and protected with the collagen sponge (g).

to retain compromised teeth. Given the unwillingness of the patient to undergo an orthodontic treatment, the achievement of clinical outcomes compatible with a good long-term prognosis was considered unpredictable. The patient was made aware of the consequences associated with his decision and of risks of retaining severely compromised teeth and consented to an implant-supported fixed rehabilitation. The extractions of tooth number 7 and tooth number 8 were scheduled together with the alveolar ridge reconstruction procedure. The patient signed informed consent.

At the time of tooth extraction, mucoperiosteal buccal and palatal flaps were reflected without vertical releasing incisions. The reflection of the palatal flap was limited to the most coronal portion of the alveolar crest. Minimally traumatic extractions were performed. The analysis of the alveolar sockets morphology confirmed the complete buccal bone wall deficiency at tooth number 8 and a vertical bone height deficiency of about 9 mm on its palatal side (Figures 1(d)-1(e)). The sockets were thoroughly debrided to remove the granulation tissue and to enhance vascular supply by opening the trabecular bony spaces.

A 25×30 mm textured high-density polytetrafluoroethylene (d-PTFE) nonresorbable membrane (Cytoplast GBR-200 singles, Osteogenics Biomedical, Lubbock, TX) was trimmed and placed under the buccal flap to replace completely the missing bony wall. A commercially available bioabsorbable sponge of equine lyophilized type I collagen (Gingistat, GABA, Italy) was used to fill the gap between the membrane and the residual palatal wall (Figure 1(f)). Afterwards, the membrane was tucked under the palatal flap taking care to keep the edge of the membrane a minimum of 1 mm away from the adjacent roots. The flaps were repositioned without periosteal incisions and secured with vertical and horizontal mattress sutures (Vicryl, Ethicon, Johnson

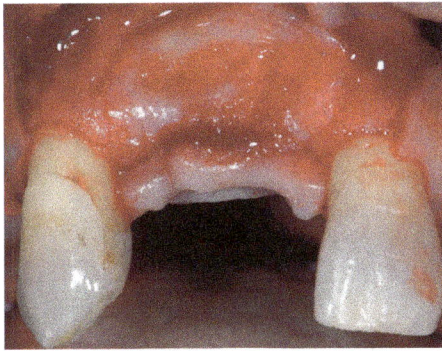

FIGURE 2: At 4 months the extraction sockets were completely filled by uniform radiodense bone tissue. Note the ridge morphology mimicking the space created beneath the membrane.

& Johosn, Sint-Stevens-Woluwe, Belgium). Intentional primary closure was not attempted and the membrane was left partially exposed and protected by the collagen sponge (Figure 1(g)). Postoperative care comprised 0.12% chlorhexidine mouthrinse three times daily for 2 weeks, systemic amoxicillin (1 g twice a day) for 6 days, and ibuprofen (600 mg twice a day) for 5 days. Sutures were removed after 14 days. A removable transparent acetate mask replacing upper incisors was used as provisional restoration to avoid any pressure on the underlying tissue.

At week 6 the membrane was gently removed from the tissue bed without flap elevation by means of a tissue forcep. Beneath the membrane a dense and highly vascularized connective tissue was detected. Three months later a corrective plastic surgery was carried out at the area of ridge reconstruction to increase soft tissue volume and so to obtain a more natural prosthetic emergence profile. After flap elevation, bone formation was observed with a ridge morphology mimicking the space created beneath the membrane (Figure 2). Before placing the palatal connective tissue over the recipient site, two approximately 5 mm long sample cores of newly formed tissue were collected for histologic examination from the central region of the former tooth sockets by using the bone chip extractor with a 2.9 mm internal diameter (9126 Komet srl, Italy). Native bone was not included. Specimens were marked to identify the coronal and apical ends. Paraffin blocks were sectioned in the apicocoronal plane to obtain 4 μm thick sections and stained with hematoxylin-eosin. The sections were evaluated by light microscopy to quantify bone content. Computer-assisted histomorphometric measurements of the newly formed bone were obtained using image analysis software (QWin, Leica Microsystems, Buffalo Grove, IL) on four to six fields for each section.

2.2. Clinical and Histologic Outcomes. During the 12 months of observation no signs of infection were noted. At 12 months postoperatively a cone-beam computed tomographic scan (CT) was taken in order to plan the implant-supported fixed prosthesis. Resolution of the alveolar bone deficiencies on tooth number 8 and limiting of the physiologic ridge

reduction were attained (Figure 3). The edentulous ridge had a vertical dimension between 13 mm and 14 mm and a horizontal dimension of 5 mm on its proximal sides and of 4.3 mm on the center of the former lateral incisor socket below the most coronal part of the crest. The final ridge dimensions allowed for insertion of two conventional dental implants in conjunction with a minor horizontal bone augmentation procedure to increase the buccopalatal crestal bone width. Unfortunately, the patient refused implant placement for unexpected incoming financial reasons and consented to replace the missing teeth with a conventional removable rehabilitation.

Histologic analysis revealed new bone formation through the entire length of the specimens without signs of inflammation. The newly formed bone was well structured with intense osteoblastic activity and it consisted of 100% living trabecular bone. The connective tissue was free of inflammation and well vascularized in all the examined sections. The overall mean percentage of newly formed bone was 49.3% ± 4.7% and was composed mostly by lamellar bone (33.2% ± 3.6%) (Figure 4). In the crestal region the mineralized fraction amounted to 47.1% ± 3.9%, and in the most apical part of the specimens it was 51.0% ± 6.2%.

3. Discussion

This case report describes a novel treatment approach in the immediate alveolar reconstruction of severely resorbed extraction sites due to periodontal disease. In the literature several data are available on the use of the guided bone regeneration (GBR) procedures to reconstruct alveolar ridge defects prior to or in conjunction with osseointegrated implants placement [5]. However, GBR techniques, in presence of severe atrophy, are complex and technically demanding. The most important factor limiting the amount of new bone formation is the early membrane exposure and infection.

In this case report, two maxillary incisors were atraumatically extracted, and the sockets were filled with a collagen sponge and covered with a nonresorbable d-PTFE membrane. Primary closure was not attained and any rigid scaffold material was not used. At 12 months the radiographic bone volume was enough to insert two implants in conjunction with a minor horizontal bone augmentation procedure. Histologically, the mean percentage of newly formed bone was 49.3% ± 4.7%. These findings are encouraging when considering the unfavorable anatomy of the alveolar socket on tooth number 8 which displayed complete loss of the buccal bone wall and a 9 mm vertical bone deficiency on its palatal aspect. It is reasonable to assume that such residual alveolar crest would undergo more contraction compared with a 4-wall extraction socket defect when is left to heal spontaneously. Tooth extraction without the use of grafting materials leads to percentage of horizontal dimensional changes of 29–63% after 6-7 months. Such bone remodeling is further complicated if the buccal bone wall is lost as a result of inflammatory processes or the extraction itself. Lee et al. observed a mean decrease of about 60% in the horizontal dimensions

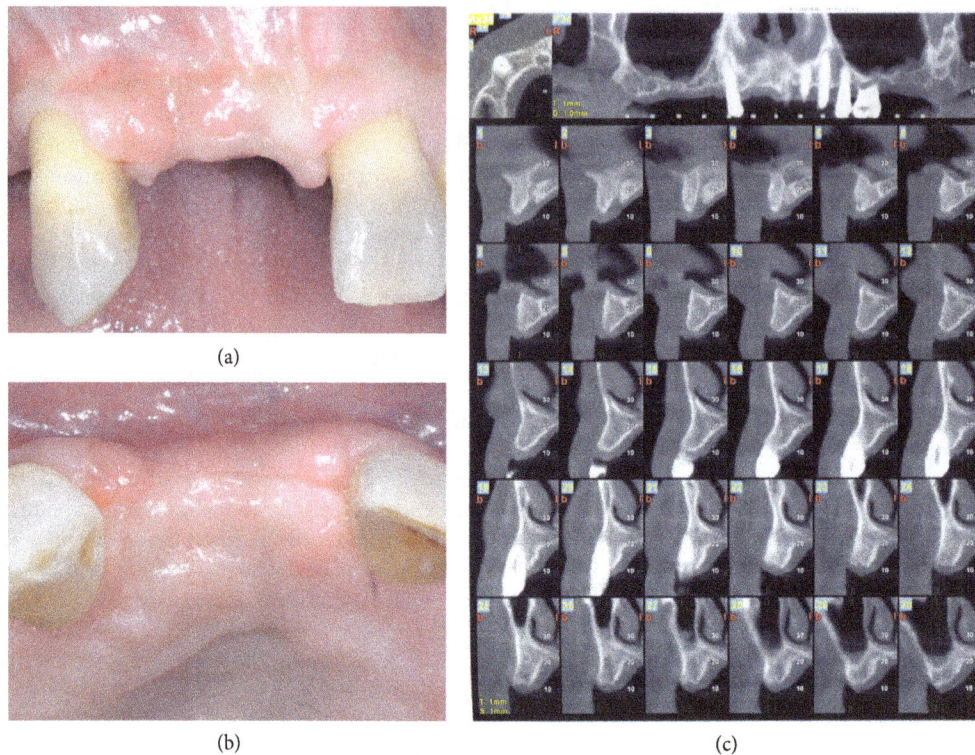

(a)

(b)

(c)

FIGURE 3: One year after the ridge reconstruction procedure ridge regeneration was achieved. Buccal view (a); occlusal view (b); cone-beam computed tomographic scan (c).

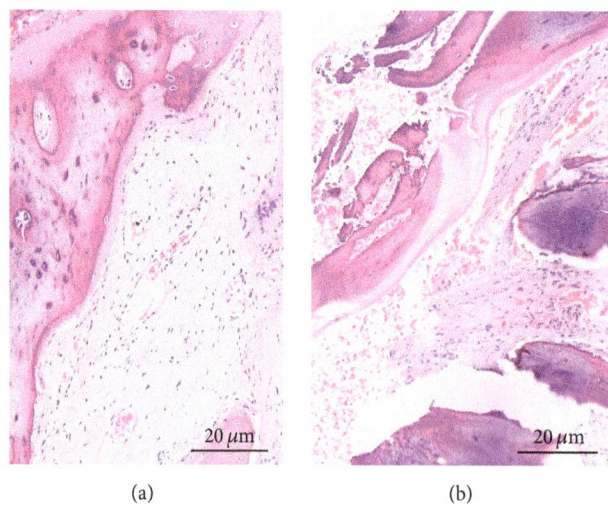

(a)

(b)

FIGURE 4: Bone biopsy illustrating socket healing 4 months after the ridge reconstruction procedure. Hematoxylin and eosin staining. Total magnification: ×100 ((a), central incisor; (b), lateral incisor).

in buccal-bone-deficient alveolar sockets during the first 8 weeks of healing [6].

The present results may be explained by the combined use of d-PTFE membrane and type I collagen materials. The optimal antimicrobial effects and durability of d-PTFE membrane protect the clot from both mechanical and chemical stress. Due to its submicron porosity (<0.3 μm) preventing or minimizing bacterial penetration, the d-PTFE membrane

may provide a reasonably microbe-free environment to the underlying collagen material, thereby facilitating its cell adhesive properties [7]. In the present report an equine type I collagen sponge was used as filling material to promote and stabilize clot formation in the early stages of healing and to avoid any interference in the later bone regeneration stages due to the inflammatory response when the filling material starts to degrade. Type I collagen has shown proangiogenic qualities and acceleration of ingrowth, proliferation, and maturation of endothelial cells that encourage physiological bone regeneration [8].

The rationale of the proposed modification of the conventional socket grafting approach relies on the findings by Serino et al. [9]. They used a polylactide-polyglycolide sponge as space filler in alveolar postextraction sockets without primary closure of the surgical wound. The histologic analysis at 6-month follow-up showed mature and well-structured bone with no residual particles of the grafted material. In this regard, it should be noted that studies in humans using demineralized freeze-dried bone allograft or deproteinized natural bovine bone have shown variable amount of particles of the grafted material in the alveolar sockets 4–9 months following their insertion [10–12]. Histologic examinations demonstrated that such biomaterials retard the extraction socket healing when compared to the naturally healing control [13]. Nevertheless, a recent systematic review reported less mid-buccal height loss in 4-wall intact sites grafted with a xenograft but comparable decrease in mid-lingual bone height and in buccolingual width when compared to alloplastic materials during socket preservation procedures [14].

Another aspect to be considered is the lack of requirement of primary closure over the socket. Because of d-PTFE membrane small porosity and minimal inflammation when exposed to the oral environment soft tissue coverage is not needed [15]. This is a significant advantage over e-PTFE and resorbable membranes in ridge augmentation application. The use of d-PTFE membranes without primary closure allows the clinician to preserve the existing keratinized tissue width and to achieve the regeneration of keratinized tissue over the extraction site [15].

4. Conclusion

Although only a single patient was treated using the present technique, clinical and histologic results are encouraging. They do indicate that this postextraction reconstructive procedure, even with open healing, may promote bone formation, improve ridge shape and dimension in severely resorbed alveolar sockets, and simplify later treatment procedures during implant placement. In addition, it can be easily managed without requiring high surgical skill. Further studies with higher patient number and long-term follow-ups are needed to validate this procedure.

Competing Interests

The authors declare that there is no conflict of interests regarding the publication of this paper. Authors' own institution funded the study.

References

[1] L. Schropp, A. Wenzel, L. Kostopoulos, and T. Karring, "Bone healing and soft tissue contour changes following single-tooth extraction: a clinical and radiographic 12-month prospective study," *International Journal of Periodontics and Restorative Dentistry*, vol. 23, no. 4, pp. 313–323, 2003.

[2] R. Horowitz, D. Holtzclaw, and P. S. Rosen, "A review on alveolar ridge preservation following tooth extraction," *Journal of Evidence-Based Dental Practice*, vol. 12, no. 3, pp. 149–160, 2012.

[3] T. Thalmair, S. Fickl, D. Schneider, M. Hinze, and H. Wachtel, "Dimensional alterations of extraction sites after different alveolar ridge preservation techniques—a volumetric study," *Journal of Clinical Periodontology*, vol. 40, no. 7, pp. 721–727, 2013.

[4] S. M. Toloue, I. Chesnoiu-Matei, and S. B. Blanchard, "A clinical and histomorphometric study of calcium sulfate compared with freeze-dried bone allograft for alveolar ridge preservation," *Journal of Periodontology*, vol. 83, no. 7, pp. 847–855, 2012.

[5] B. S. McAllister and K. Haghighat, "Bone augmentation techniques," *Journal of Periodontology*, vol. 78, no. 3, pp. 377–396, 2007.

[6] J.-S. Lee, J.-S. Jung, G.-I. Im, B.-S. Kim, K.-S. Cho, and C.-S. Kim, "Ridge regeneration of damaged extraction sockets using rhBMP-2: An Experimental Study in Canine," *Journal of Clinical Periodontology*, vol. 42, no. 7, pp. 678–687, 2015.

[7] B. K. Bartee and J. A. Carr, "Evaluation of a high-density polytetrafluoroethylene membrane as a barrier material to facilitate guided bone regeneration in the rat mandible," *Journal of Oral Implantology*, vol. 21, no. 2, pp. 88–95, 1995.

[8] T. Twardowski, A. Fertala, J. P. R. O. Orgel, and J. D. San Antonio, "Type I collagen and collagen mimetics as angiogenesis promoting superpolymers," *Current Pharmaceutical Design*, vol. 13, no. 35, pp. 3608–3621, 2007.

[9] G. Serino, S. Biancu, G. Iezzi, and A. Piattelli, "Ridge preservation following tooth extraction using a polylactide and polyglycolide sponge as space filler: A Clinical and Histological Study in Humans," *Clinical Oral Implants Research*, vol. 14, no. 5, pp. 651–658, 2003.

[10] W. Becker, B. E. Becker, and R. Caffesse, "A comparison of demineralized freeze-dried bone and autologous bone to induce bone formation in human extraction sockets," *Journal of Periodontology*, vol. 65, no. 12, pp. 1128–1133, 1994.

[11] D. Carmagnola, P. Adriaens, and T. Berglundh, "Healing of extraction sockets filled with Bio-Oss," *Clinical Oral Implants Research*, vol. 14, no. 2, pp. 137–143, 2003.

[12] D. Cardaropoli and G. Cardaropoli, "Preservation of the postextraction alveolar ridge: a clinical and histologic study," *International Journal of Periodontics and Restorative Dentistry*, vol. 28, no. 5, pp. 469–477, 2008.

[13] F. A. Santos, M. T. Pochapski, M. C. Martins, E. G. Zenóbio, L. C. Spolidoro, and E. Marcantonio, "Comparison of biomaterial implants in the dental socket: histological analysis in dogs," *Clinical Implant Dentistry and Related Research*, vol. 12, no. 1, pp. 18–25, 2010.

[14] G. Avila-Ortiz, S. Elangovan, K. W. O. Kramer, D. Blanchette, and D. V. Dawson, "Effect of alveolar ridge preservation after tooth extraction: a systematic review and meta-analysis," *Journal of Dental Research*, vol. 93, no. 10, pp. 950–958, 2014.

[15] H. D. Barber, J. Lignelli, B. M. Smith, and B. K. Bartee, "Using a dense PTFE membrane without primary closure to achieve bone and tissue regeneration," *Journal of Oral and Maxillofacial Surgery*, vol. 65, no. 4, pp. 748–752, 2007.

Coverage Root after Removing Peripheral Ossifying Fibroma: 5-Year Follow-Up Case Report

Paulo S. G. Henriques,[1] **Luciana S. Okajima,**[1] **Marcelo P. Nunes,**[1] **and Victor A. M. Montalli**[2]

[1]*Department of Periodontology, São Leopoldo Mandic Institute and Research Center, Campinas, SP, Brazil*
[2]*Department of Oral Pathology, São Leopoldo Mandic Institute and Research Center, Campinas, SP, Brazil*

Correspondence should be addressed to Paulo S. G. Henriques; phenriques@mpc.com.br

Academic Editor: Cleverson Silva

When lesions in soft tissue reach the gingival margin, they can produce aesthetic defects during its permanence and after its removal. Periodontal plastic surgery allows the correction of the gingival contour using different techniques. This paper is a case report of a peripheral ossifying fibroma removal in the interproximal area of teeth 21 and 22 in addition to root coverage of the affected area through two surgical phases: keratinized gingival tissue augmentation surgery with free gingival graft concurrent with removal of the lesion and, in a second stage, root coverage by performing coronally advanced flap technique with a follow-up of five years. The initial results achieved, which were root coverage of 100% after 6 months, promoted an adequate gingival contour and prevented the development of a mucogingival defect or a root exposure with its functional and aesthetic consequences. After five years, the results showed long term success of the techniques, where the margin remained stable with complete root coverage and tissues were stable and harmonic in color.

1. Introduction

Peripheral ossifying fibroma is characterized as a hyperplasic gingival mass with calcified foci, supposedly formed by metaplastic bone [1]. The bone is found in the middle of a nonencapsulated proliferation of bulky benign fibroblasts. The lesion may be derived from the connective tissue of the submucosa or the periodontal ligament. There is a tendency for the presence of inflammatory cells in the outer portion of the lesion. The surface often shows ulcerated areas and rarely causes erosion of adjacent bone [2].

The peripheral ossifying fibroma, also known as ossifying fibroid epulis, ossifying fibroma with calcification, peripheral cement-ossifying fibroma, and calcifying fibroblastic granuloma, is also part of the nonneoplastic proliferative lesions [3].

It is considered a reactive lesion, although its pathogenesis is uncertain. This pathology appears as a tissue response to chronic long term stimulation. This can occur when the gum tissue reacts in response to irritants such as biofilm

and subgingival calculus, misplaced teeth, restorations over contour, ill-fitting dentures, root remnants, poorly preserved teeth, foreign bodies in the gingival sulcus, and orthodontic treatment. There is a mesenchymal cell of the periodontal ligament and/or cementum proliferation that are induced by such local irritants. The displacement and mobility of the teeth are uncommon, unless preexisting periodontal disease is found or in cases where the teeth are erupting [4].

Clinically, it appears as a nodular lesion, exophytic, pedunculated in most cases, of streaky reddish coloration of whitish areas, or similar in color to the adjacent mucosa. It features bright and opaque surface in some spots and irregular texture and contours, with slow growth rate, although it is able to reach large dimensions [5].

This injury is located, preferably, in the attached gingiva or exceptionally in the free marginal gingiva. There is a predilection for the anterior portion of the jaws [4, 5]. Sometimes it extends throughout the teeth, involving both the facial and the lingual gum [4]. There may be bleeding when the lesion is touched or even spontaneously, but mainly when it is constantly traumatized. In most cases the patient is asymptomatic [3, 5].

Women are affected more often than men by this injury, which occurs predominantly in the second decade of life [4, 5] and in Caucasians [3, 5], accounting for 9.6% of gingival lesions [6].

Other injuries that have similar clinical appearance to peripheral ossifying fibroma include pyogenic granuloma, peripheral giant cells granuloma, fibrous hyperplasia, and giant cell fibroma [1, 5]. All these injuries are caused by low intensity chronic irritation.

The treatment of choice is local excision, which should include the periodontal ligament, if it is also involved. Furthermore, one should remove any identifiable causative agent [1, 4, 6]. There may be recurrence [4, 6], but its risk is diminished if the excision is performed under the periosteum [2, 6].

The literature provides several ways of removing the lesion, such as the use of Nd:YAG laser or conventional surgery with scalpel [7].

The excisional biopsy necessary for this case is aggressive and may result in a severe periodontal defect because it can involve the entire keratinized adjacent tissue creating a similar Class I or II Miller defect. When trying to recreate the excised tissue, several approaches can effectively increase the present tissue, such as a graft of the subepithelial connective tissue, free gingival graft, derivatives of the enamel matrix, guided tissue regeneration, and coronal or lateral advanced flaps. The choice of technique will depend on the amount of tissue to be recreated [8].

2. Case Report

A 36-year-old female leucoderma patient sought treatment complaining of a lesion located between teeth 21 and 22, painless and compromising the aesthetics of her smile (Figure 1(a)). Intraoral physical examination showed an injury inserted in the interproximal gum, measuring $1.2 \times 0.9 \times 0.5$ cm on the facial surface and $0.7 \times 0.5 \times 0.3$ cm in the palatal face, exophytic and nodular. The radiographic examination showed no related changes (Figure 1(c)).

Surgical techniques were performed as described below: after local anesthesia with 2% lidocaine with epinephrine at a concentration of $1:100,000$, the excision of the lesion was proceeded with a 15C scalpel blade (Figures 1(b) and 1(e)), removing all the gingival and periodontal tissue involved, followed by scaling and root planing of the same teeth (Figure 1(d)).

After excision of the lesion, the removal of a free gingival graft from the palate was performed, which was placed in the exposed conjunctive tissue area to recreate the band of keratinized tissue lost as a result of the lesion itself and its excision. The graft was taken from the palate and its format was similar to the open area of the receiving tissue (Figure 1(f)). The apical and coronal dimension and thickness were measured so that it could be suitable and uniform. The graft was sutured along its entire length (Figure 1(f)). Digital pressure was performed with saline moistened gauze to

remove any blood clot and maintain the graft in intimate contact with the recipient bed.

The material obtained from excisional biopsy was sent for pathological analysis. Histologically, the lesion showed an intact squamous epithelium and in the lamina propria a highly cellular component of fibroblasts was observed with central area of calcification, setting the diagnosis for peripheral ossifying fibroma (Figure 1(g)).

Three months after the procedure (Figure 2(a)), a second surgical procedure was performed in order to cover the exposed root of tooth 22. The biomechanical preparation of the surface of the root was accomplished with scaling and root planing (Figure 2(b)) and application of EDTA 24% neutral pH (Pref-Gel®, Straumann). The coronally advanced flap technique, described by de Sanctis and Zucchelli (2007) [9], was the selected technique: two horizontal beveled incisions were performed, mesial and distal to the recession, located at one end of the anatomical papillae and equal to the height of the recession plus 1 mm; two oblique incisions, slightly divergent, starting at the end of the two horizontal incisions and extending to the alveolar mucosa (Figure 2(c)). The coronal portion of the flap is partially divided, while the portion apical to the recession is a full thickness flap, exposing 3-4 mm of bone (Figure 2(d)). The relaxing vertical incisions are elevated in partial thickness. Apical bone exposure is held in the partial thickness flap, ending where it is possible to passively move the flap in coronal direction and coronally in the cementum-enamel junction. At this time simple sutures are performed throughout the flap (Figure 2(e)).

After the initial results were achieved, root coverage of 100% was obtained after 6 months (Figure 2(f)), and suitable gingival contour was promoted which prevented the development of a mucogingival defect or root exposure with its functional and aesthetic consequences. After five years (Figure 2(g)) the margin remained at its initial position, with no relapse in the exhibition of the cementum-enamel junction; and tissues were stable and characterized by color harmony, demonstrating the success of the chosen techniques.

3. Discussion

The gingiva when subjected to local chronic irritation or trauma reacts with localized hyperplasia that can be composed of mature collagen, cellular fibroblastic tissue, mineralized tissue, endothelial tissue, and multinucleated giant cells (3). Clinical and histological examinations are essential to achieve a diagnosis and ensure a complete treatment plan, which, in this case, included not only the removal of the lesion, but also reconstruction of the anterior esthetic zone impaired when performing the biopsy.

5-year follow-up of this case showed no recurrence of the lesion. Our findings are in accordance with Silva et al. (2007) [10], who presented a case report of a surgical excision of a peripheral ossifying fibroma coincident with central odontogenic fibroma with an uneventful follow-up of one year.

Excisional biopsies when performed frequently result in mucogingival defects, which may produce esthetic problems and increase the chance of hyperesthesia [11].

(a)

(b)

(c)

(d)

(e)

(f)

(g)

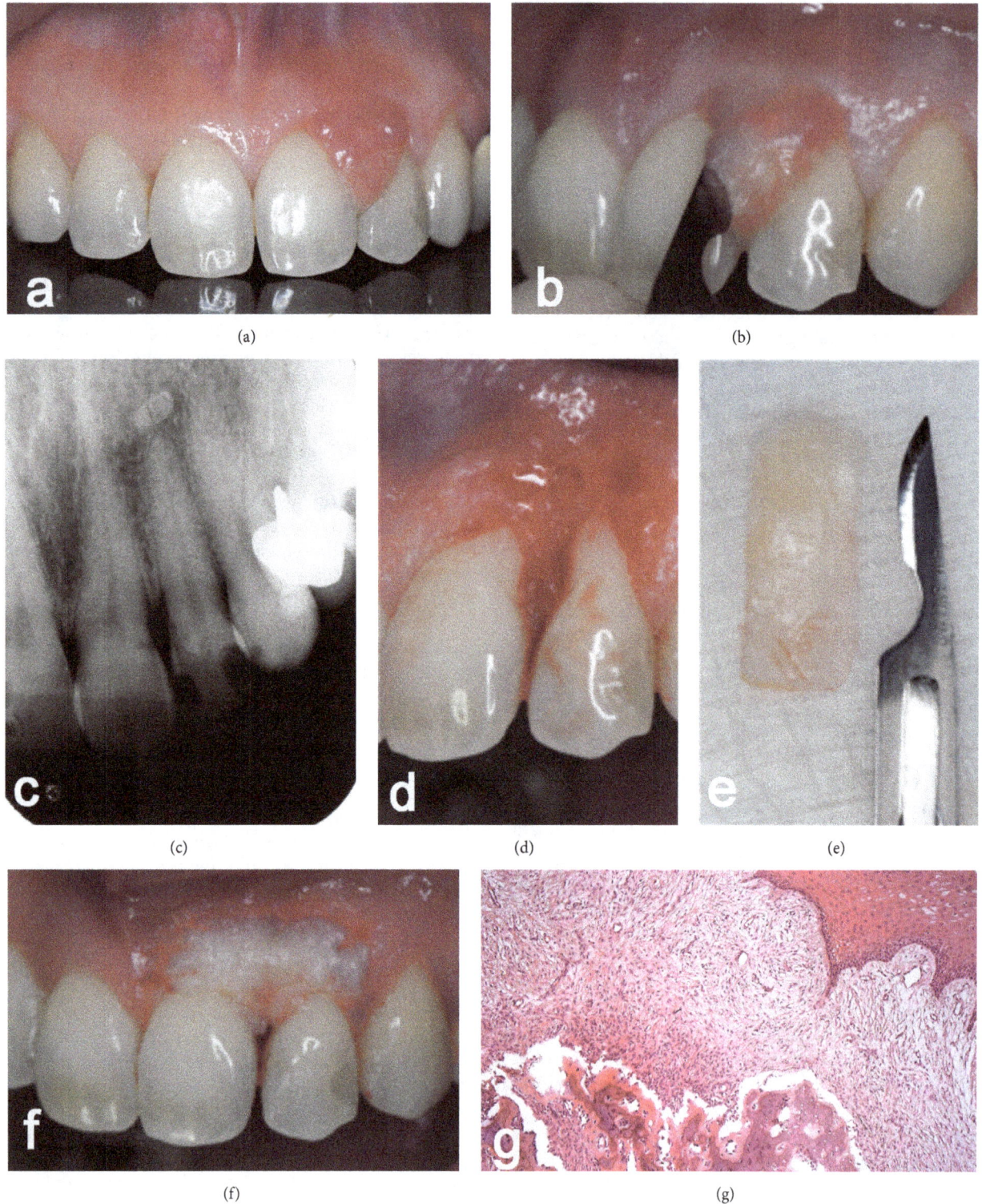

FIGURE 1: (a) Intraoral physical examination showed an injury inserted in the interproximal gum; ((b), (d), and (e)) excision of the lesion; (c) radiographic examination with no changes observed. (g) Histological diagnosis of peripheral ossifying fibroma.

Bernimoulin et al. (1975) [12] first described a root coverage technique with free gingival graft placed to increase the zone of keratinized gingiva and flap coronally repositioned later.

Besides having an important role in maintaining gingival health, the attached gingiva protects the periodontium against external injuries, maintains a stable position of the gingival margin, and dispels the physiological forces made

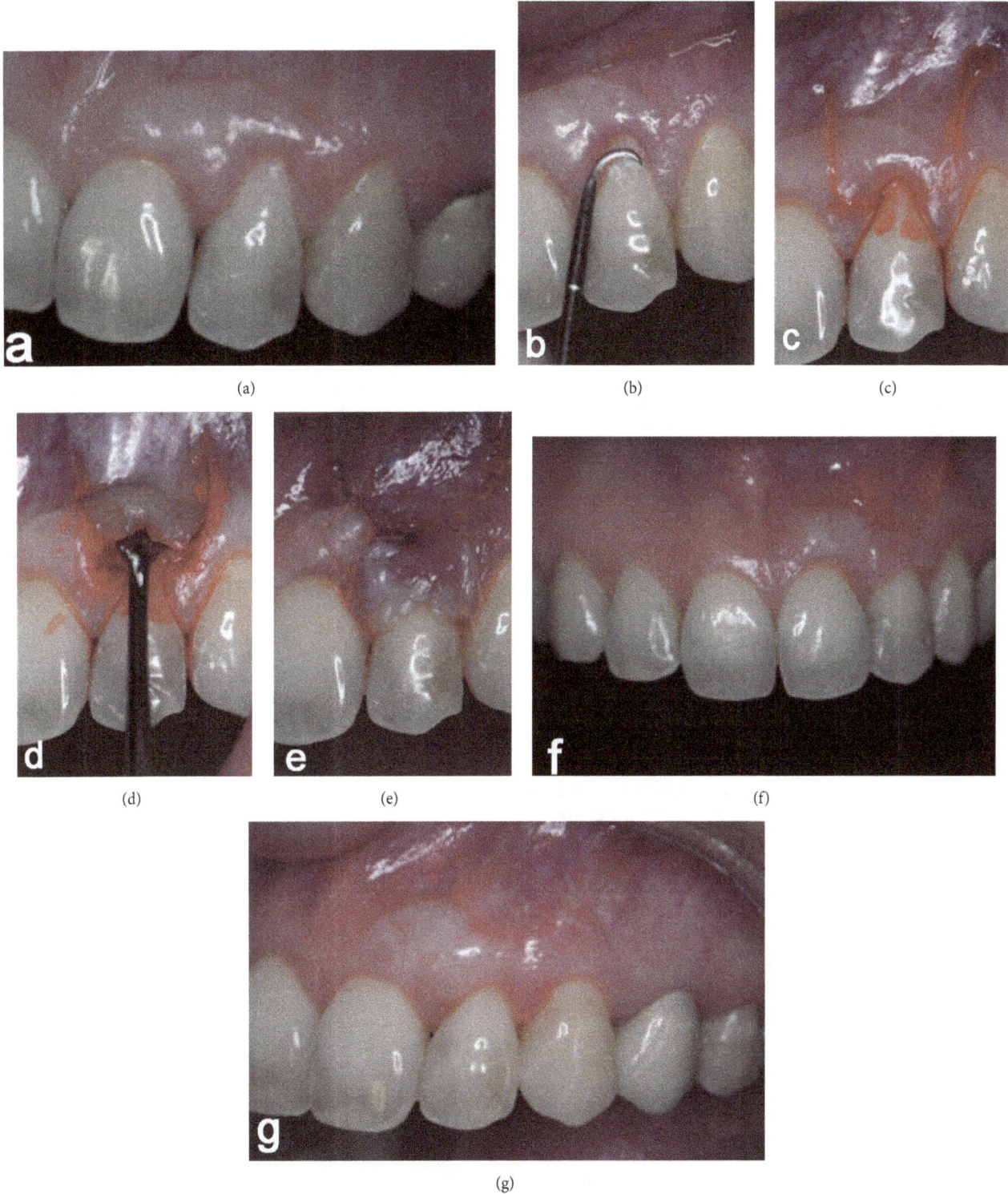

FIGURE 2: (a) After three months of the procedure; ((b), (c), (d), and (e)) a second surgical stage was performed in order to cover the exposed root of tooth 22; (f) root coverage of 100% after 6 months and (g) 5-year follow-up.

by the muscle fibers of the alveolar mucosa against the gum tissues. There is controversy regarding the amount of keratinized tissue to maintain gingival health. Mucogingival techniques are present in the literature to increase the zone of attached gingiva. Among the alternatives, the free gingival graft is a widespread procedure, because of abundant donor site and the possibility of treating multiple teeth. As disadvantages we can cite postoperative discomfort, unpredictable color harmony, and the need for a second donor site [13].

During this treatment, biopsy and the free gingival graft were performed at the same surgical procedure. This decision was made to avoid repetitious postoperative discomfort for the patient and to make oral hygiene procedures more effective in accordance with Anderegg and Metzler (1996) [14] and Keskiner et al. (2016) [15].

The decision of performing first the free gingival graft found evidence in literature which points out that thin adjacent gingiva makes root coverage less predictable [16] and an adequate amount of attached gingiva improves periodontal health [17]. A systematic review [18] stated that the free gingival graft is a successful treatment concept to increase the width of attached gingiva around teeth. In this case report, as described also by other authors [9], clinical increases in the apicocoronal dimensions of keratinized tissue and attached gingiva were observed.

Root exposure, as a side effect of the biopsy, can be corrected after the recreation of keratinized tissue band. The coronally advanced flap technique (CAF) is a great alternative treatment because it presents satisfactory results in long term root coverage, good color harmony of the area treated with the surrounding tissues [19], without an excessive increase in the thickness of the tissue, and complete recovery of the original morphology of the marginal soft tissue. It also presents better postoperative course when compared to coronally advanced flap with connective tissue graft [19]. The only limiting factor to this technique is the need of a band of at least 1 mm keratinized tissue [11]. A systematic review performed in 2008 [20] confirmed that the coronally advanced flap procedure is a safe and reliable approach in periodontal plastic surgery and is associated with consistent recession reduction and frequently with complete root coverage.

Coronally advanced flap can be associated with different materials as membrane barriers [21, 22], grafts, subepithelial connective tissue [19], porcine collagen matrix [23, 24], platelet-rich plasma [25, 26] and platelet-rich fibrin [27, 28].

Consensus Report of the European Workshop on Periodontology in 2014 [29] claimed that periodontal plastic procedures are complex, technique-sensitive interventions that require advanced skills and expertise. The choice of the technique should take in account increased morbidity when having a donor area or increased cost when using allograft materials. When there is enough tissue in the area to provide a well-designed flap for root coverage with stability, there is no need to use a soft tissue graft.

The treatment for gingival recession is considered completely successful when root coverage is associated with a gingival margin and a crevice probing depth that is coronal to the cementoenamel junction [30], as presented in this case report with 5-year follow-up.

4. Conclusion

Peripheral ossifying fibroma is a benign, slowly progressive lesion, with limited growth and histopathologic confirmation is mandatory. Complete surgical excision down to the periosteum is the preferred treatment and close postoperative follow-up is required. Surgical procedures with two stages using free gingival graft and coronally advanced flap present

good results. In the presence of sufficient keratinized tissue, coronally advanced flap shows efficacy in root coverage.

Competing Interests

The authors declare that they have no competing interests.

References

[1] I. Kaplan, Z. Nicolaou, D. Hatuel, and S. Calderon, "Solitary central osteoma of the jaws: a diagnostic dilemma," *Oral Surgery, Oral Medicine, Oral Pathology, Oral Radiology and Endodontology*, vol. 106, no. 3, pp. e22–e29, 2008.

[2] F. R. de Matos, T. G. Benevenuto, C. F. W. Nonaka, L. P. Pinto, and L. B. de Souza, "Retrospective analysis of the histopathologic features of 288 cases of reactional lesions in gingiva and alveolar ridge," *Applied Immunohistochemistry and Molecular Morphology*, vol. 22, no. 7, pp. 505–510, 2014.

[3] A. Buchner, A. Shnaiderman-Shapiro, and M. Vered, "Relative frequency of localized reactive hyperplastic lesions of the gingiva: a retrospective study of 1675 cases from Israel," *Journal of Oral Pathology and Medicine*, vol. 39, no. 8, pp. 631–638, 2010.

[4] S. A. Choudary, A. R. Naik, M. S. Naik, and D. Anvitha, "Multicentric variant of peripheral ossifying fibroma," *Indian Journal of Dental Research*, vol. 25, no. 2, pp. 220–224, 2014.

[5] A. Buchner and L. S. Hansen, "The histomorphologic spectrum of peripheral ossifying fibroma," *Oral Surgery, Oral Medicine, Oral Pathology*, vol. 63, no. 4, pp. 452–461, 1987.

[6] J. D. Walters, J. K. Will, R. D. Hatfield, D. A. Cacchillo, and D. A. Raabe, "Excision and repair of the peripheral ossifying fibroma: a report of 3 cases," *Journal of Periodontology*, vol. 72, no. 7, pp. 939–944, 2001.

[7] G. Mergoni, M. Meleti, S. Magnolo, I. Giovannacci, L. Corcione, and P. Vescovi, "Peripheral ossifying fibroma: a clinicopathologic study of 27 cases and review of the literature with emphasis on histomorphologic features," *Journal of Indian Society of Periodontology*, vol. 19, no. 1, pp. 83–87, 2015.

[8] S. B. Hutton, K. W. Haveman, J. H. Wilson, and K. E. Gonzalez-Torres, "Esthetic management of a recurrent peripheral ossifying fibroma," *Clinical Advances in Periodontics*, vol. 6, no. 2, pp. 64–69, 2016.

[9] M. de Sanctis and G. Zucchelli, "Coronally advanced flap: a modified surgical approach for isolated recession-type defects: three-year results," *Journal of Clinical Periodontology*, vol. 34, no. 3, pp. 262–268, 2007.

[10] C. O. Silva, A. W. Sallum, C. E. do Couto-Filho, A. A. Costa Pereira, J. A. Hanemann, and D. N. Tatakis, "Localized gingival enlargement associated with alveolar process expansion: peripheral ossifying fibroma coincident with central odontogenic fibroma," *Journal of Periodontology*, vol. 78, no. 7, pp. 1354–1359, 2007.

[11] A. F. Bosco, S. Bonfante, D. S. Luize, J. M. D. Bosco, and V. G. Garcia, "Periodontal plastic surgery associated with treatment for the removal of gingival overgrowth," *Journal of Periodontology*, vol. 77, no. 5, pp. 922–928, 2006.

[12] J. P. Bernimoulin, B. L. Lüscher, and H. R. Mühlemann, "Coronally repositioned periodontal flap. Clinical evaluation after one year," *Journal of Clinical Periodontology*, vol. 2, no. 1, pp. 1–13, 1975.

[13] J. Carnio, P. M. Camargo, and P. Q. Pirih, "Surgical techniques to increase the apicocoronal dimension of the attached gingiva:

a 1-year comparison between the free gingival graft and the modified apically repositioned flap," *The International Journal of Periodontics and Restorative Dentistry*, vol. 35, no. 4, pp. 571–578, 2015.

[14] C. R. Anderegg and D. G. Metzler, "Free gingival graft following biopsy: a case report of tissue management," *Journal of Periodontology*, vol. 67, no. 5, pp. 532–535, 1996.

[15] I. Keskiner, B. A. Alkan, and Z. Tasdemir, "Free gingival grafting procedure after excisional biopsy, 12-year follow-up," *European Journal of Dentistry*, vol. 10, no. 3, pp. 432–434, 2016.

[16] J. G. Maynard Jr., "Coronal positioning of a previously placed autogenous gingival graft," *Journal of Periodontology*, vol. 48, no. 3, pp. 151–155, 1977.

[17] N. Lang and H. Löe, "The relationship between the width of keratinized gingiva and gingival," *Journal of Periodontology*, vol. 43, no. 10, pp. 623–627, 1972.

[18] D. S. Thoma, G. I. Benić, M. Zwahlen, C. H. Hämmerle, and R. E. Jung, "A systematic review assessing soft tissue augmentation techniques," *Clinical Oral Implants Research*, vol. 20, supplement 4, pp. 146–165, 2009.

[19] G. Zucchelli, I. Mounssif, C. Mazzotti et al., "Coronally advanced flap with and without connective tissue graft for the treatment of multiple gingival recessions: a comparative short- and long-term controlled randomized clinical trial," *Journal of Clinical Periodontology*, vol. 41, no. 4, pp. 396–403, 2014.

[20] F. Cairo, U. Pagliaro, and M. Nieri, "Treatment of gingival recession with coronally advanced flap procedures: a systematic review," *Journal of Clinical Periodontology*, vol. 35, no. 8, pp. 136–162, 2008.

[21] K. Al Hezaimi, M. Al Askar, D. M. Kim et al., "The feasibility of using coronally advanced flap with an extracellular matrix membrane for treating gingival recession defects: a preclinical study," *International Journal of Periodontics & Restorative Dentistry*, vol. 34, no. 3, pp. 375–380, 2014.

[22] A. Rath, S. Varma, and R. Paul, "Two-stage mucogingival surgery with free gingival autograft and biomend membrane and coronally advanced flap in treatment of class III millers recession," *Case Reports in Dentistry*, vol. 2016, Article ID 9289634, 5 pages, 2016.

[23] A. R. O. Moreira, M. P. Santamaria, K. G. Silvério et al., "Coronally advanced flap with or without porcine collagen matrix for root coverage: a randomized clinical trial," *Clinical Oral Investigations*, 2016.

[24] M. Stefanini, K. Jepsen, M. de Sanctis et al., "Patient-reported outcomes and aesthetic evaluation of root coverage procedures: a 12 months follow-up of a randomized controlled clinical trial," *Journal of Clinical Periodontology*, 2016.

[25] S. M. Biradar, A. Satyanarayan, A. J. Kulkarni, B. Patti, S. K. Mysore, and A. Patil, "Clinical evaluation of the effect of platelet rich plasma on the coronally advanced flap root coverage procedure," *Dental Research Journal*, vol. 12, no. 5, pp. 469–475, 2015.

[26] A. R. Naik, A. V. Ramesh, C. D. Dwarkanath, M. S. Naik, and A. B. Chinnappa, "Use of autologous platelet rich plasma to treat gingival recession in esthetic periodontal surgery," *Journal of Indian Society of Periodontology*, vol. 17, no. 3, pp. 345–353, 2013.

[27] H. G. Keceli, G. Kamak, E. O. Erdemir, M. S. Evginer, and A. Dolgun, "The adjunctive effect of platelet-rich fibrin to connective tissue graft in the treatment of buccal recession defects: results of a randomized, parallel-group controlled trial," *Journal of Periodontology*, vol. 86, no. 11, pp. 1221–1230, 2015.

[28] S. K. Agarwal, R. Jhingran, V. K. Bains, R. Srivastava, R. Madan, and I. Rizvi, "Patient-centered evaluation of microsurgical management of gingival recession using coronally advanced flap with platelet-rich fibrin or amnion membrane: a comparative analysis," *European Journal of Dentistry*, vol. 10, no. 1, pp. 121–133, 2016.

[29] M. S. Tonetti and S. Jepsen, "Clinical efficacy of periodontal plastic surgery procedures: consensus Report of Group 2 of the 10th European Workshop on Periodontology," *Journal of Clinical Periodontology*, vol. 41, supplement 15, pp. S36–S43, 2014.

[30] G. Pini-Prato, C. Magnani, F. Zaheer, R. Rotundo, and J. Buti, "Critical evaluation of complete root coverage as a successful endpoint of treatment for gingival recessions," *The International Journal of Periodontics and Restorative Dentistry*, vol. 35, no. 5, pp. 655–663, 2015.

Oral Health Characteristics and Dental Rehabilitation of Children with Global Developmental Delay

Saurabh Kumar,[1] **Deepika Pai,**[1] **and Runki Saran**[2]

[1]*Department of Pedodontics & Preventive Dentistry, Manipal College of Dental Sciences, Manipal, India*
[2]*Faculty of Dentistry, Melaka Manipal Medical College, Manipal, India*

Correspondence should be addressed to Saurabh Kumar; drsaurabh19@yahoo.co.in

Academic Editor: Giuseppe Colella

Global developmental delay (GDD) is a chronic neurological disturbance which includes defects in one or more developmental domains. The developmental domain can be motor, cognitive, daily activities, speech or language, and social or personal development. The etiology for GDD can be prenatal, perinatal, or postnatal. It can be diagnosed early in childhood as the delay or absence of one or more developmental milestones. Hence the role of pedodontist and pediatricians becomes more crucial in identifying this condition. The diagnosis of GDD requires a detailed history including family history and environmental risk factors followed by physical and neurological examinations. Investigations for GDD include diagnostic laboratory tests, brain imaging, and other evidence-based evaluations. GDD affects multiple developmental domains that not only have direct bearing on maintenance of oral health, but also require additional behavior management techniques to deliver optimal dental care. This paper describes two different spectra of children with GDD. Since the severity of GDD can vary, this paper also discusses the different behavior management techniques that were applied to provide dental treatment in such children.

1. Introduction

According to American Academy of Neurology (AAN) and Child Neurology Society (CNS), global developmental delay (GDD) is a subset of developmental disabilities defined as significant delay in two or more domains of development, including activities of daily living as well as motor, cognitive, speech/language, and personal/social skills [1, 2]. The development delay should be evident in comparison with attainment of skills to their chronological peers. Those deficits are evident in comparison with the skills attainment of chronological peers. Significant delay is defined as performance of two standard deviations or more below the mean on age-appropriate, standardized norm referenced testing [3, 4]. The prevalence of GDD is not precisely estimated [5]. The etiology can be intrapartum asphyxia, cerebral dysgenesis, early severe psychosocial deprivation, antenatal toxin exposure like alcoholism or multidrug exposures, chromosomal disorders including Down syndrome, fragile X syndrome, and Rett's syndrome [6, 7].

Diagnosis of GDD is comprehensive one which must include a detailed history, thorough clinical examination, and appropriate investigations. Most often a diagnosis can be made based on detailed history and clinical evaluation. A thorough prenatal, natal, and postnatal history along with family history is essential and is the first step towards establishing the diagnosis. Clinical examination for GDD includes neuromuscular examination and examination of the spine, reflexes, gait, and vision. In order to diagnose a case of GDD the investigations can be performed selectively or guided by history and clinical features. Most often a clinical diagnosis is sufficient. Hence if required the pediatrician can perform metabolic investigations, neuroimaging, or advanced genetic investigations [8].

Clinical presentation of GDD may not be uniform, as it depends on the domains affected. Clinical features may include one or more of the following dysmorphic features like short stature, macrocephaly, generalized hair growth anomalies, facial asymmetry, flat facial profile, and midface hypoplasia. Epilepsy is a common finding with children having GDD. Oral findings include drug induced gingival hyperplasia if the child is on medication for epilepsy [7]. Due to motor and cognitive developmental delay, children with GDD also display poor oral hygiene and dental caries commensurate to inadequate plaque control. We hereby present two cases of varying intensities of GDD, their oral findings, and behavior management techniques which were applied for dental treatment.

2. Case Reports

2.1. Case 1. A seven-year-old boy reported to our clinic with the chief complaint of multiple decayed teeth. The child was a known case of global developmental delay with seizure disorder. There was no familial history of any neurological problem. Due to the developmental delay in speech, language, and cognition, a thorough oral examination was not possible. The child's behavior was categorized as definitely negative according to Frankl's behavior rating scale. Since the child's ability to cooperate was limited due to presence of GDD additionally the child was a known epileptic, the dental treatment was planned under chairside general anesthesia. After obtaining necessary consents and clearance from the department of pediatrics and anesthesiology the child was scheduled for dental rehabilitation under chairside general anesthesia (Figure 1). Oral examination under general anesthesia revealed mixed dentition with multiple decayed teeth and poor oral hygiene (Figure 2). The dental treatment including oral prophylaxis, pit and fissure sealant (Clinpro Sealant, 3M ESPE) application on all the permanent first molars, the Glass ionomer cement (Fuji IX) restorations of the carious primary second molars, and bifluoride varnish (VOCO) application was done under general anesthesia (Figure 3).

2.2. Case 2. A six-year-old male child was referred by his pediatrician for dental treatment of decayed teeth. He was a known case of global developmental delay since the age of two years as his parents found that his milestones like walking and speech were delayed. Mother gave the history of her son who had difficulty in learning at school. He was attending special school and also was being rehabilitated at center for children with neuromuscular disorders. Upon review with his pediatrician we learnt that he had a mild degree of developmental delay and predominance in the development of speech and communication but was rehabilitated enough to vocalize in English fairly well. Frankl's behavior rating for this child was positive. On examination the carious lesions were present on the primary molars and maxillary incisors (Figures 4 and 5). Oral prophylaxis was accomplished with behavior management and physical restraining. However owing to uncontrolled tongue movement and instable jaw movements the restorations including stainless steel crown placement were done under oral sedation with Pedicloryl (dosage: 0.5–1 mg/kg) (Figures 6 and 7). APF gel was applied as a preventive protocol. The patient was advised to use powered toothbrushes for maintaining oral hygiene. He was reviewed periodically at every 3 months interval.

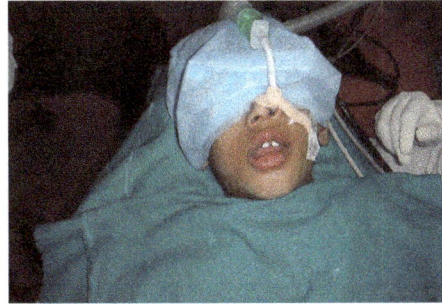

FIGURE 1: Dental treatment under general anesthesia (Case 1).

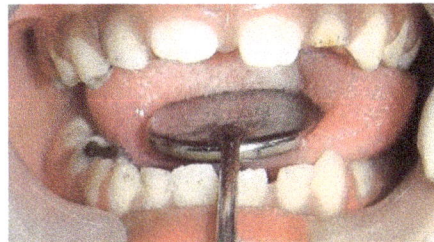

FIGURE 2: Preoperative photograph (Case 1).

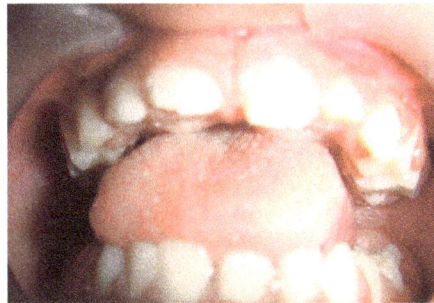

FIGURE 3: Postoperative photograph (Case 1).

3. Discussion

As the clinical presentation of GDD may be heterogeneous the oral findings depend on the developmental domains affected. Hence both the treatment needs and behavior management techniques depend on individual case presentation. Developmental domains such as gross/fine motor skills, speech and language, cognitive development, social/personal development, and activities of daily living are affected by GDD [1].

Functional motor disability can lead to uncontrolled movements of head and neck and also involuntary movements of tongue that can interfere in delivering optimal dental treatment. Excessive drooling of saliva and poor manual dexterity due to motor disability can also influence the effectiveness of tooth brushing. Occupational therapy towards neuromuscular coordination and training can improve the motor disability over time [9]. Delay or deficiencies in development of speech, language, and cognition definitely act as a hindrance to appropriate delivery of oral care. If social/personal development is affected, the child may not

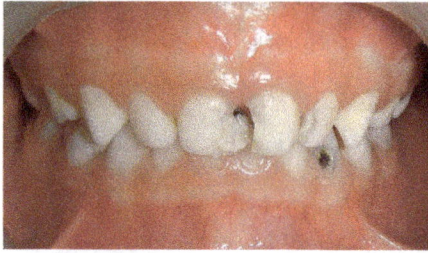

FIGURE 4: Preoperative photograph (Case 2).

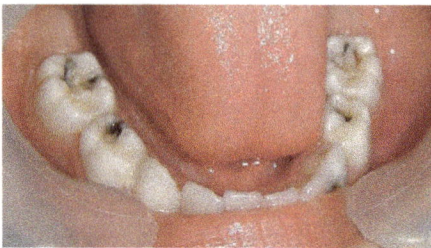

FIGURE 6: Postoperative photograph (Case 2).

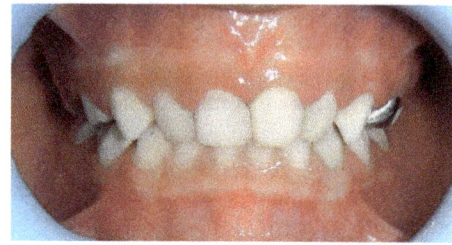

FIGURE 5: Preoperative photograph (Case 2).

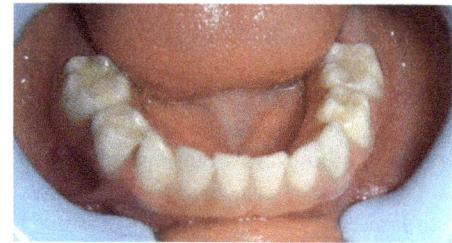

FIGURE 7: Postoperative photograph (Case 2).

be attending school or may not want to visit a dentist too. The pedodontist should build a good rapport with such children so as to be familiar with the child. Tooth brushing is a routine daily activity; hence if the domain of daily activities remains affected in a child with GDD, they are definitely vulnerable for poor oral hygiene and so it increases their risk for development of dental caries. In such situations powered toothbrushes act as an excellent method for achieving satisfactory plaque control [10].

A universal behavior management protocol cannot be adopted for children with GDD. As in our cases, Case 1 was an extreme case of GDD with epilepsy with developmental delay in multiple domains. Hence general anesthesia was considered the best management option for complete dental rehabilitation. Unlike the first case the child in Case 2 was a mild case of GDD, had no other underlying systemic illness detected, and also was adequately rehabilitated at neurology center. This facilitated chair side oral examination and minimally invasive treatments like oral prophylaxis. Since salivary contamination and unstable head and neck movements would compromise the quality of the restoration, the restorations of decayed teeth were done under oral sedation.

The objective of treatment planning in cases with GDD therefore should encompass the assessment of level of cooperating ability for delivering oral care, a thorough review of the underlying medical conditions, and possible drug therapy for the systemic conditions along with oral health status of the individual.

4. Conclusion

Since pediatricians and pedodontist are the first of the health care providers to examine a child for developmental milestones. A careful history and examination can lead to early detection of GDD. Adequate rehabilitation of these children at occupational therapy centers can also enable them to improve the quality of life at large along with their oral health. Hence we emphasize the role of pedodontist in early detection of GDD and helping these children gain better oral and general health.

Disclosure

Deepika Pai is the co-first author and Runki Saran is the coauthor.

Competing Interests

The authors declare that they do not have any conflict of interests regarding the publication of this paper.

Authors' Contributions

Saurabh Kumar and Deepika Pai have equal contribution to this article and hence both are declared as first authors.

References

[1] M. Shevell, S. Ashwal, D. Donley et al., "Practice parameter: evaluation of the child with global developmental delay: report of the quality standards subcommittee of the American Academy of Neurology and The Practice Committee of the Child Neurology Society," *Neurology*, vol. 60, no. 3, pp. 367–380, 2003.

[2] AAN Guideline Summary for clinicians, http://www.childneurologysociety.org/.

[3] A. Majnemer and M. I. Shevell, "Diagnostic yield of the neurologic assessment of the developmentally delayed child," *The Journal of Pediatrics*, vol. 127, no. 2, pp. 193–199, 1995.

[4] M. I. Shevell, A. Majnemer, P. Rosenbaum, and M. Abrahamow-icz, "Etiologic yield of subspecialists' evaluation of young children with global developmental delay," *Journal of Pediatrics*, vol. 136, no. 5, pp. 593–598, 2000.

[5] M. Yeargin-Allsopp, C. C. Murphy, J. F. Cordero, P. Decouflé, and J. G. Hollowell, "Reported biomedical causes and associated medical conditions for mental retardation among 10 year old children, metropolitan Atlanta, 1985 to 1987," *Developmental Medicine and Child Neurology*, vol. 39, no. 3, pp. 142–149, 1997.

[6] M. Shevell, "Global developmental delay and mental retardation or intellectual disability: conceptualization, evaluation, and etiology," *Pediatric Clinics of North America*, vol. 55, no. 5, pp. 1071–1084, 2008.

[7] R. B. Patil, P. Urs, S. Kiran, and S. D. Bargale, "Global devel-opmental delay with sodium valproate-induced gingival hyper-plasia," *BMJ Case Reports*, 2014.

[8] L. McDonald, A. Rennie, J. Tolmie, P. Galloway, and R. McWilliam, "Investigation of global developmental delay," *Archives of Disease in Childhood*, vol. 91, no. 8, pp. 701–705, 2006.

[9] A. B. Sorsdahl, R. Moe-Nilssen, H. K. Kaale, J. Rieber, and L. I. Strand, "Change in basic motor abilities, quality of move-ment and everyday activities following intensive, goal-directed, activity-focused physiotherapy in a group setting for children with cerebral palsy," *BMC Pediatrics*, vol. 10, article 26, 2010.

[10] M. C. Doğan, A. Alaçam, N. Aşici, M. Odabaş, and G. Sey-daoğlu, "Clinical evaluation of the plaque–removing ability of three different toothbrushes in a mentally disabled group," *Acta Odontologica Scandinavica*, vol. 62, no. 6, pp. 350–354, 2009.

31

Cone Beam CT in Diagnosis and Surgical Planning of Dentigerous Cyst

Naira Figueiredo Deana[1] and Nilton Alves[2,3]

[1]Magister Program in Dentistry, Faculty of Dentistry, Universidad de La Frontera, Temuco, Chile
[2]CIMA-Research Center in Applied Morphology, Universidad de La Frontera, Temuco, Chile
[3]Faculty of Dentistry, Universidad de La Frontera, 1145 Francisco Salazar Avenue, P.O. Box 54-D, Temuco, Chile

Correspondence should be addressed to Nilton Alves; niltonnalves@yahoo.com.br

Academic Editor: Daniel Torrés-Lagares

Diagnosis and preoperative planning are critical in the execution of any surgical procedure. Panoramic radiography is a routine method used in dentistry to assist clinical diagnosis; however, with this technique 3D anatomical structures are compressed into 2D images, resulting in overlapping of structures which are of interest in the diagnosis. In this study we report the case of a patient who presented with a dentigerous cyst of expressive dimensions in the body of the mandible region. The surgery was planned and executed after observing the margins of the lesion by Cone Beam Computed Tomography (CBCT). We conclude that CBCT is a precise method to help diagnosis; it provides greater accuracy in surgical treatment planning through 3D image display, allowing more effective results.

1. Introduction

The dentigerous (or follicular) cyst (DC) is the second most common type of dental cyst and the most common in jaw development [1]. Benn and Altini [2] propose the existence of two types of dentigerous cysts: one of a developing nature and the other inflammatory. From a clinical point of view, dentigerous cysts are generally asymptomatic, slow-growing, associated with the crown of an impacted or unerupted permanent tooth, and characterised by retarded eruption of the tooth [1]. However they may grow large enough to cause destruction of the cortical bone, resulting in fluctuation, spontaneous pain, exudation, and rapid development of the pathology, which are signs of acute inflammation round the margins of the cyst [3].

Diagnosis of the lesion should not be based on X-ray evidence alone, but also on clinical evidence, particularly microscopic examination of the sample [2].

Periapical and panoramic X-rays are the most commonly used imaging examinations in dentistry for diagnosis and surgical planning. However the information acquired in these examinations is limited, since the three-dimensional anatomy of the area X-rayed is shown in two dimensions, with superimposed planes. Although these methods produce acceptable images in the mesiodistal direction, observation in the vestibulolingual direction is difficult. There may also be geometrical distortion of the structures X-rayed when we use these imaging methods [4]. A very efficient imaging technique for diagnosing DC is Magnetic Resonance Imaging (MRI), since it allows cysts to be distinguished from tumoral lesions [5], ensuring safe, efficient performance [6]; however MRI is a very high-cost examination with limited availability, making it impractical for routine clinical use.

In the last decade a new technology—Cone Beam Computerised Tomography (CBCT)—has offered dental surgeons three-dimensional reproduction of images of mineralised maxillofacial tissues, with minimum distortion and significantly lower doses of radiation than conventional CT [7].

The object of this study was to report a clinical case of a dentigerous cyst in which the diagnostic hypothesis and the decision on the treatment plan were based on CBCT.

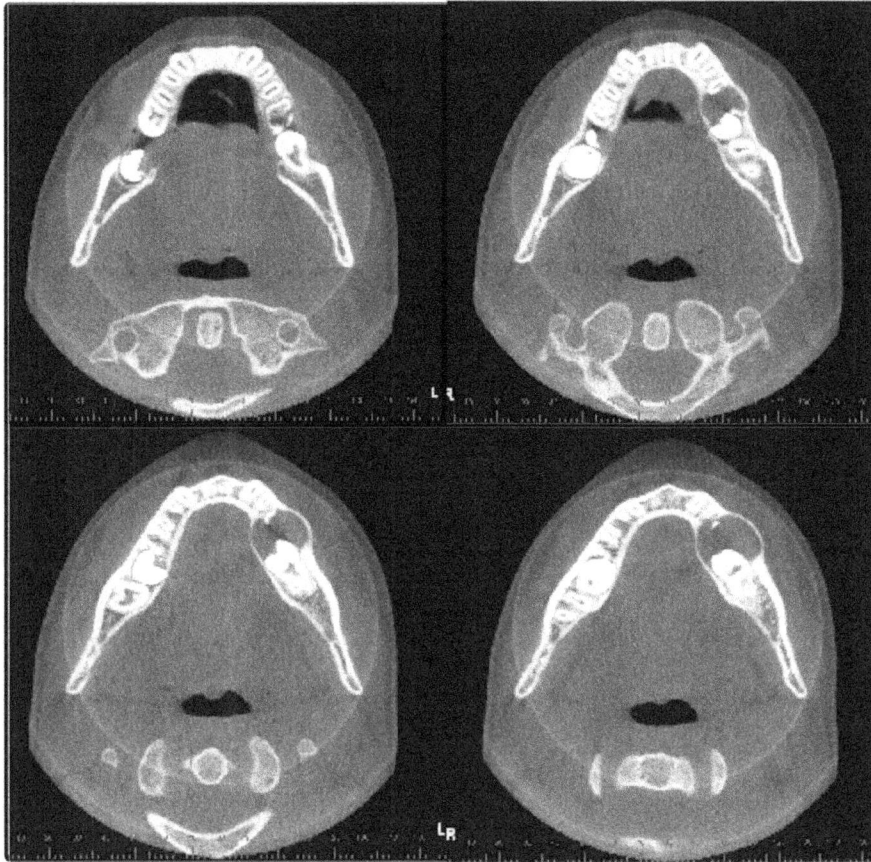

FIGURE 1: CBCT image, axial sections, showing bulging of osseous cortices in the region of the left permanent mandibular second molar.

2. Case Report

Male patient, 28 years, Brazilian, white, attended a private dental practice complaining of increased volume in the vestibular region of the left mandibular second molar and slight discomfort when eating. The patient reported that the increase had evolved slowly over approximately one year, with no apparent cause and no pain. In clinical examination, the absence of the left mandibular second molar was observed, with an increase in volume in the vestibular region.

CBCT was carried out to evaluate the case. The CBCT images were obtained with i-CAT® Next Generation, 120 Kv, 18.5 mA, FOV 16 × 6 cm. The data were converted into 3D images with volume representation by the Vision Standalone software. In the axial sections an extensive, hypodense image was observed in the body of the mandible region, left side, containing the permanent mandibular second molar; bulging of both osseous cortices was also found (Figure 1). In the coronal sections a hypodense image was observed in the body of the mandible region, left side, associated with the left permanent mandibular second molar, with radicular reabsorption of the left permanent mandibular first molar (Figure 2). In orthoradial reconstructions from the left mandibular first premolar to the left permanent mandibular first molar an extensive hypodense area was observed with radicular reabsorption of the left mandibular

second premolar and the left permanent mandibular first molar (Figure 3). A 3D reconstruction was made of the vestibular and lingual views (Figure 4).

The diagnostic hypothesis based on the clinical and imaging examinations was of a dentigerous cyst of the circumferential radiographic type. Because the lesion presented with relatively unaggressive comportment, with large size and limits, and was located very close to important anatomical structures, we decided on conservative surgical treatment, that is, decompression of the cyst and subsequent enucleation.

The procedure practised on the patient started with aspiration puncture, which confirmed the presence of an intralesional liquid content. After confirmation of a cyst-type lesion, an incision was made to give access to the cyst capsule and to promote biopsy. The surgical piece obtained was sent for histopathological examination, resulting in the histological diagnosis of a dentigerous cyst.

3. Discussion

Dentigerous cysts account for 30.7% of all odontogenic cysts in the Brazilian population [8], being commoner in men than in women (2.33 : 1) [9], with no racial predilection, most frequent in the second and third decades of life [2, 10] due to the chronology of dental eruption [11]. They tend

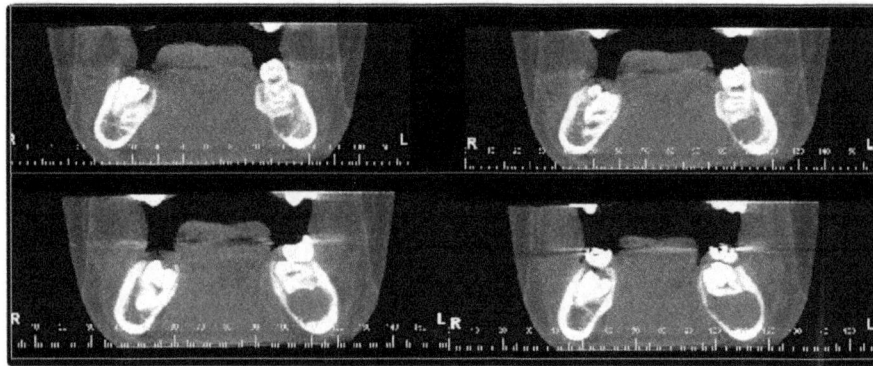

FIGURE 2: CBCT image, coronal sections, showing hypodense image associated with the left permanent mandibular second molar, with radicular reabsorption of the left permanent mandibular first molar.

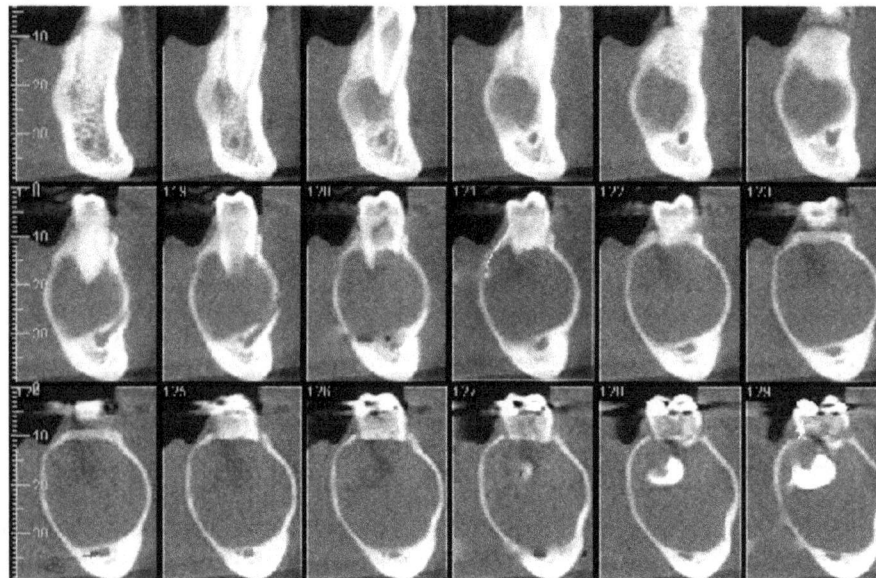

FIGURE 3: CBCT image: orthoradial reconstructions from the left mandibular first premolar to the left permanent mandibular first molar. An extensive hypodense area can be observed with radicular reabsorption of the left mandibular second premolar and the left permanent mandibular first molar.

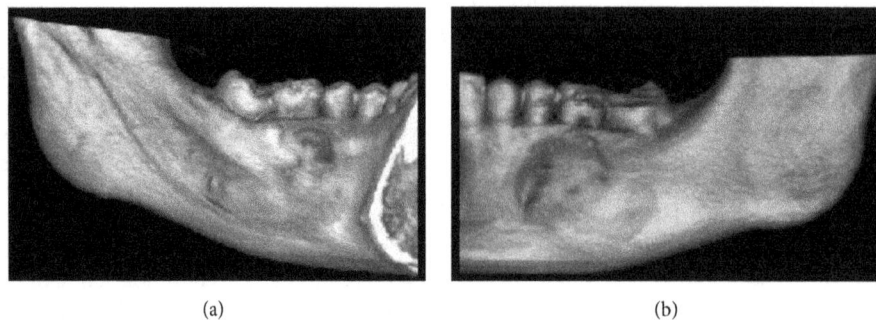

(a) (b)

FIGURE 4: CBCT image, 3D reconstructions. Observe the body of the mandible in the region of the left permanent mandibular first molar. Internal (lingual) view (a) and external (vestibular) view (b).

to be solitary; bilateral dentigerous cysts usually occur in association with syndromes like cleidocranial dysplasia and mucopolysaccharidosis (Type VI) [11].

Dentigerous cysts are usually located in the region of the maxillary canines and the mandibular third molars [2, 12, 13]; in the case reported the cyst was associated with the left mandibular second molar. In general the patients present with impacted teeth or slow-growing, asymptomatic swellings [11]. In the present case the patient reported slow, asymptomatic growth and also presented unerupted left mandibular second molar.

Hyomoto et al. [14] analysed the factors which interfere with the spontaneous eruption of mandibular premolars associated with this type of cyst and concluded that impacted teeth tend to erupt more easily in the presence of inflammatory infiltrate, suggesting that the higher the number of inflammatory cells, the greater the possibility of eruption of the tooth associated with a cyst. For Carvalho and Luna [15], this finding may explain the fact that the depth of the impaction is insufficient to determine the failure of the tooth to erupt spontaneously. Thus the characteristics of the impaction are of fundamental importance in enabling the dentist to select a suitable treatment plan [15].

CBCT has been widely used in dentistry to provide basic information on dental and maxillofacial structures for diagnosis and surgical planning [16]. According to Cha et al. [17] CBCT can be a much-needed improvement in diagnosis and treatment planning. However it must be noted that all tomographic examinations must be carried out under the basic principles of justification (weighing benefits against risks) and optimisation (keeping doses as low as possible) [18], because of the radiation to which the patient is subjected during the examination. There is controversial evidence on the risk of cancer associated with higher radiation levels; however most authorities assume the risk of cancer resulting from X-ray exposure; the risk is higher in younger individuals [19, 20]. The radiation dose to which the patient is subjected in CBCT is 40% lower than in conventional CT and 3 to 7 times higher than in panoramic radiography. The CBCT dose varies substantially depending on the device, FOV, and selected technique factors [21, 22]. Ludlow et al. [22] carried out a study comparing the effective dose of three types of commercially available CBCT equipment, observing that the NewTom 3G emitted the lowest radiation dose, followed by the I-CAT and the CB Mercuray. Pauwels et al. [23] carried out a study to estimate the effective dose absorbed by each organ, using 14 types of CBCT machine (3D Accuitomo 170, Kodak 9000 3D, Galileos Comfort, I-CAT New Generation, Iluma Elite, Kodak 9500, NewTom VG, NewTom VGi, Scanora 3D, Veraviewepocs 3D, Promax 3D, Pax-Uni 3D, Picasso Trio, and SkyView) and different protocols and geometries. These authors conclude that the radiation dose emitted by most machines is in the range of 20 to 100 Sv, confirming that the radiation emitted by CBCT is higher than in the 2D radiographic methods used in dentistry but considerably lower than the doses reported for the common Multislice Computed Tomography protocols. Pauwels et al. [23] observed a big difference in the dose absorbed by the salivary glands, thyroid glands, oral mucous,

and the extrathoracic pathways; it is moreover significantly greater with a large FOV than with a medium or small FOV. In the present study the CBCT examination was carried out using a medium FOV, and the patient was not subjected to the highest radiation dose. The same machine can emit different radiation doses for the same examination, depending on operator choices [18, 23]. The Kv and mAs configuration, combined with a large visual field, can also determine a high radiation dose [24]. However it should be noted that when a better quality image is needed, higher exposure factors will be recommended [25].

Dentigerous cysts are usually discovered during routine X-ray examinations or when X-ray is indicated to determine the reason for a failed tooth eruption [26]. Panoramic radiography is a low-cost imaging method widely used in routine dentistry; however it produces a two-dimensional image which only allows two dimensions of the lesion to be observed and does not show its relation to adjacent anatomical structures [27, 28]. Furthermore, because of the superposition of a large tissue volume, extraoral X-ray images often do not provide reliable information on the internal structure of the lesion. Observation of the third dimension, that is, the buccolingual extension of the lesion, requires additional X-rays taken at 90 degrees to the original view [28]. Correct identification of lesions is often impossible in two-dimensional viewing of the image, which may lead to incorrect selection of treatment plan and finally incorrect performance by the dentist. CBCT offers the advantage of a multiplane image (axial, coronal, and sagittal planes) which gives important information on the presence and extension of bone reabsorption, sclerosis of neighbouring bone, cortical expansion, and internal or external calcifications, as well as showing the proximity to other important anatomical structures [28]. Three-dimensional radiographic techniques are of inestimable assistance, not only in differential X-ray diagnosis but also in determining the displacement space of the mandibular canal [29]. We agree with Huumonen et al. [30] and Cohenca et al. [31] when they say that the CBCT image allows in-depth observation of a determined region, eliminating overlapping and so avoiding one of the main limitations of X-rays, the lack of depth. CBCT also offers advantages over Multislice Computed Tomography, including lower radiation emissions, lower cost, and greater accuracy in detecting thinning and/or perforation of the buccal plate and tooth displacement [32]. However it should be noted that CBCT presents the disadvantage of not being indicated for soft tissue analysis. Magnetic Resonance Imaging (MRI) is a noninvasive imaging technique which offers excellent tissue contrast [33] and is becoming increasingly important in oral and maxillofacial surgery. MRI assists in lesion diagnosis because it can reliably differentiate between odontogenic cysts, keratocystic odontogenic tumors, and ameloblastoma, while panoramic radiography and computerised tomography (conventional and cone beam) cannot differentiate between these types of lesion [34]. MRI provides useful information on the relations between the lesion and adjacent structures, as well as offering better tissue contrast and the ability to acquire images along arbitrary planes [35]. MRI presents the additional advantage of not subjecting the patient to ionising radiation; however it is an expensive examination due to the very high cost of the equipment, which puts it beyond the reach of private clinics.

Imaging is an essential part of preparation for most surgical procedures [18]. Preoperative examination of odontogenic lesions prevents complications in surgery and functional deterioration after surgery and reduces surgical stress [32, 36]. In surgical planning for a dentigerous cyst, it may be necessary to measure the lesion from different angles [28], requiring more advanced radiological imaging. CBCT offers great accuracy in measuring osseous components, with less than 1% error as compared to the gold standard method [37]. The CBCT images obtained in the case reported here allowed the margins and limits of the lesion and adjacent structures to be examined, showing details of the relationship between the lesion and the mandibular canal and also the radicular reabsorption of the left mandibular second premolar and the left mandibular first molar. After examining the margins of the lesion in the CBCT images we observed that the patient presented a cystic lesion of expressive magnitude in the body of the mandible region, left side, very close to important anatomical structures. This finding allowed careful planning of surgery, which helped to reduce the time taken in the procedure and the patient's recovery.

In general, surgery is recommended for dentigerous cysts because they often block tooth eruption, become large, displace teeth, destroy bone, and invade vital structures; in some cases they may cause fractures [12, 26]. In selecting the treatment method for a dentigerous cyst, the size and location of the cyst, the age of the patient, the dentition involved, and the participation of vital structures must all be considered [38]. Small cysts which present no risk of lesion to important anatomical structures can easily be enucleated and sent for pathological examination, preserving the tooth and the affected region [15, 38]; this is the technique most frequently used by dental surgeons [10, 12, 13]. Enucleation of the cyst with tooth extraction is indicated for teeth such as the 3rd molar, but if the cyst is very extensive or involves teeth which are important aesthetically or for occlusion, tooth extraction is not indicated. Extraction of the impacted tooth is indicated when the tooth is useless or space is required for eruption [38]. Marsupialisation and decompression are indicated when there are tooth displacement and bone loss [39, 40]. The advantage of marsupialisation is that an impacted tooth can enter into eruption more rapidly [41]; however its main disadvantage is that the pathological tissue remains in situ [39, 42], with the possibility of a more aggressive lesion in the residual tissue [42]. Both enucleation and decompression will relieve the pressure on the cyst, allowing the retained tooth to erupt normally if root formation is incomplete; otherwise the teeth are assisted by orthodontic treatment [38]. In our study, due to the size and wide limits of the cyst, as well as the fact that it was very close to important anatomical structures, we opted for decompression and subsequent enucleation.

According to Neville et al. [12], the level of recurrence of dentigerous cysts is low (3.7%); however patients are recommended to have periodical clinical and imaging monitoring, so we duly informed our patient of the importance of long-term check-ups.

In conclusion we may say that CBCT is a very useful complementary tool for diagnosis and surgery planning in cases of dentigerous cyst. Three-dimensional viewing of the structures using this imaging method offers greater accuracy in planning surgical treatment, thus allowing more effective results to be achieved.

Competing Interests

The authors declare that they have no conflict of interests.

References

[1] J. A. Regezi, J. J. Sciubba, and R. C. K. Jordan, *Oral Pathology: Clinical Pathologic Correlations*, Saunders, Philadelphia, Pa, USA, 4nd edition, 2003.

[2] A. Benn and M. Altini, "Dentigerous cysts of inflammatory origin: a clinicopathologic study," *Oral Surgery, Oral Medicine, Oral Pathology, Oral Radiology, and Endodontics*, vol. 81, no. 2, pp. 203–209, 1996.

[3] L. M. Lin, D. Ricucci, J. Lin, and P. A. Rosenberg, "Nonsurgical root canal therapy of large cyst-like inflammatory periapical lesions and inflammatory apical cysts," *Journal of Endodontics*, vol. 35, no. 5, pp. 607–615, 2009.

[4] R. K. P. Lima, N. B. Faria-Júnior, J. M. Guerreiro-Tanomaru, and M. Tanomaru-Filho, "Diagnosis and planning in apical surgery: use of cone-beam tomography," *South Brazilian Dentistry Journal*, vol. 7, no. 4, pp. 474–480, 2010.

[5] U. N. Yilmaz, F. Yaman, and S. S. Atilgan, "MR T_1 and T_2 relaxations in cysts and abscesses measured by 1.5 T MRI," *Dentomaxillofacial Radiology*, vol. 41, no. 5, pp. 385–391, 2012.

[6] A. S. Pinto, A. L. Costa, N. d. Galvão, T. L. Ferreira, and S. L. Lopes, "Value of magnetic resonance imaging for diagnosis of dentigerous cyst," *Case Reports in Dentistry*, vol. 2016, Article ID 2806235, 6 pages, 2016.

[7] W. C. Scarfe, M. D. Levin, D. Gane, and A. G. Farman, "Use of cone beam computed tomography in endodontics," *International Journal of Dentistry*, vol. 2009, Article ID 634567, 20 pages, 2009.

[8] R. L. Avelar, A. A. Antunes, R. W. F. Carvalho, P. G. C. F. Bezerra, P. J. Oliveira Neto, and E. S. S. Andrade, "Odontogenic cysts: a clinicopathological study of 507 cases," *Journal of Oral Science*, vol. 51, no. 4, pp. 581–586, 2009.

[9] P. V. Deepthi, V. T. Beena, S. K. Padmakumar, R. Rajeev, and R. Sivakumar, "A study of 1177 odontogenic lesions in a South Kerala population," *Journal of Oral and Maxillofacial Pathology*, vol. 20, no. 2, pp. 202–207, 2016.

[10] E. Ustuner, S. Fitoz, C. Atasoy, I. Erden, and S. Akyar, "Bilateral maxillary dentigerous cysts: a case report," *Oral Surgery, Oral Medicine, Oral Pathology, Oral Radiology, and Endodontics*, vol. 95, no. 5, pp. 632–635, 2003.

[11] D. Q. Freitas, L. M. Tempest, E. Sicoli, and F. C. Lopes-Neto, "Bilateral dentigerous cysts: review of the literature and report of an unusual case," *Dentomaxillofacial Radiology*, vol. 35, no. 6, pp. 464–468, 2006.

[12] W. Neville, D. D. Damm, C. M. Allen, and J. E. Bouquot, *Patologia Oral & Maxilofacial*, Editora Guanabara Koogan S/A, Rio de Janeiro, Brazil, 2nd edition, 2008.

[13] W. G. Shafer, M. K. Hine, and B. M. Levy, *Tratado de Patologia Bucal*, Guanabara Koogan, Rio de Janeiro, Brazil, 4nd edition, 1987.

[14] M. Hyomoto, M. Kawakami, M. Inoue, and T. Kirita, "Clinical conditions for eruption of maxillary canines and mandibular premolars associated with dentigerous cysts," *American Journal of Orthodontics and Dentofacial Orthopedics*, vol. 124, no. 5, pp. 515–520, 2003.

[15] I. K. F. de Carvalho and A. H. B. Luna, "Spontaneous eruption of premolar associated with a dentigerous cyst," *Case Reports in Dentistry*, vol. 2016, Article ID 5323978, 5 pages, 2016.

[16] K. Tsiklakis, K. Syriopoulos, and H. C. Stamatakis, "Radiographic examination of the temporomandibular joint using cone beam computed tomography," *Dentomaxillofacial Radiology*, vol. 33, no. 3, pp. 196–201, 2004.

[17] J.-Y. Cha, J. Mah, and P. Sinclair, "Incidental findings in the maxillofacial area with 3-dimensional cone-beam imaging," *American Journal of Orthodontics and Dentofacial Orthopedics*, vol. 132, no. 1, pp. 7–14, 2007.

[18] K. Horner, "Cone-beam computed tomography for oral surgical applications: where is the evidence?" *Oral Surgery*, vol. 6, no. 3, pp. 112–128, 2013.

[19] B. F. Wall, R. Haylock, J. T. M. Jansen, M. C. Hillier, D. Hart, and P. C. Shrimpton, *HPA-CRCE-028—Radiation Risks from Medical X-Ray Examinations as a Function of the Age and Sex of the Patient*, Chilton, Health Protection Agency, 2011.

[20] S. F. Mobbs, C. R. Muirhead, and J. D. Harrison, *HPA-RPD-066—Risks from Ionising Radiation*, Health Protection Agency, Chilton, Wiss, USA, 2010.

[21] N. L. Frederiksen, B. W. Benson, and T. W. Sokolowski, "Effective dose and risk assessment from film tomography used for dental implant diagnostics," *Dentomaxillofacial Radiology*, vol. 23, no. 3, pp. 123–127, 1994.

[22] J. B. Ludlow, L. E. Davies-Ludlow, S. L. Brooks, and W. B. Howerton, "Dosimetry of 3 CBCT devices for oral and maxillofacial radiology: CB Mercuray, NewTom 3G and i-CAT," *Dentomaxillofacial Radiology*, vol. 35, no. 4, pp. 219–226, 2006.

[23] R. Pauwels, J. Beinsberger, B. Collaert et al., "Effective dose range for dental cone beam computed tomography scanners," *European Journal of Radiology*, vol. 81, no. 2, pp. 267–271, 2012.

[24] M. Loubele, R. Jacobs, F. Maes et al., "Radiation dose vs. image quality for low-dose CT protocols of the head for maxillofacial surgery and oral implant planning," *Radiation Protection Dosimetry*, vol. 117, no. 1–3, pp. 211–216, 2006.

[25] S. Lofthag-Hansen, A. Thilander-Klang, and K. Gröndahl, "Evaluation of subjective image quality in relation to diagnostic task for cone beam computed tomography with different fields of view," *European Journal of Radiology*, vol. 80, no. 2, pp. 483–488, 2011.

[26] J. A. Regezi, J. J. Sciubba, and M. A. Pogrel, *Atlas of Oral and Maxillofacial Pathology*, Saunders, Philadelphia, Pa, USA, 2000.

[27] R. B. Junqueira, F. S. Verner, E. M. Vilela, K. L. Devito, M. G. A. M. Chaves, and A. M. R. Carmo, "Tomografia computadorizada de feixe cônico como instrumento complementar de diagnóstico e planejamento cirúrgico de cisto radicular: relato de um caso clínico," *Revista de Odontologia da UNESP*, vol. 40, no. 6, pp. 338–343, 2011.

[28] M. Ahmad, J. Jenny, and M. Downie, "Application of cone beam computed tomography in oral and maxillofacial surgery," *Australian Dental Journal*, vol. 57, pp. 82–94, 2012.

[29] S. McCrea, "Adjacent dentigerous cysts with the ectopic displacement of a third mandibular molar and supernumerary (forth) molar: a rare occurrence," *Oral Surgery, Oral Medicine, Oral Pathology, Oral Radiology and Endodontology*, vol. 107, no. 6, pp. e15–e20, 2009.

[30] S. Huumonen, T. Kvist, K. Gröndahl, and A. Molander, "Diagnostic value of computed tomography in re-treatment of root fillings in maxillary molars," *International Endodontic Journal*, vol. 39, no. 10, pp. 827–833, 2006.

[31] N. Cohenca, J. H. Simon, R. Roges, Y. Morag, and J. M. Malfaz, "Clinical indications for digital imaging in dento-alveolar trauma. Part 1: traumatic injuries," *Dental Traumatology*, vol. 23, no. 2, pp. 95–104, 2007.

[32] M. Shweel, M. I. Amer, and A. F. El-Shamanhory, "A comparative study of cone-beam CT and multidetector CT in the preoperative assessment of odontogenic cysts and tumors," *Egyptian Journal of Radiology and Nuclear Medicine*, vol. 44, no. 1, pp. 23–32, 2013.

[33] M. Lenz, H. Greess, U. Baum, M. Dobritz, and B. Kersting-Sommerhoff, "Oropharynx, oral cavity, floor of the mouth: CT and MRI," *European Journal of Radiology*, vol. 33, no. 3, pp. 203–215, 2000.

[34] M. Minami, T. Kaneda, K. Ozawa et al., "Cystic lesions of the maxillomandibular region: MR imaging distinction of odontogenic keratocysts and ameloblastomas from other cysts," *American Journal of Roentgenology*, vol. 166, no. 4, pp. 943–949, 1996.

[35] M. Hisatomi, J.-I. Asaumi, H. Konouchi, H. Shigehara, Y. Yanagi, and K. Kishi, "MR imaging of epithelial cysts of the oral and maxillofacial region," *European Journal of Radiology*, vol. 48, no. 2, pp. 178–182, 2003.

[36] Y. Nakagawa, K. Kobayashi, H. Ishii et al., "Preoperative application of limited cone beam computerized tomography as an assessment tool before minor oral surgery," *International Journal of Oral and Maxillofacial Surgery*, vol. 31, no. 3, pp. 322–327, 2002.

[37] J. B. Ludlow, W. S. Laster, M. See, L. J. Bailey, and H. G. Hershey, "Accuracy of measurements of mandibular anatomy in cone beam computed tomography images," *Oral Surgery, Oral Medicine, Oral Pathology, Oral Radiology and Endodontology*, vol. 103, no. 4, pp. 534–542, 2007.

[38] M. H. K. Motamedi and K. T. Talesh, "Management of extensive dentigerous cysts," *British Dental Journal*, vol. 198, no. 4, pp. 203–206, 2005.

[39] S. Takagi and S. Koyama, "Guided eruption of an impacted second premolar associated with a dentigerous cyst in the maxillary sinus of a 6-year-old child," *Journal of Oral and Maxillofacial Surgery*, vol. 56, no. 2, pp. 237–239, 1998.

[40] M. Wong, "Surgical fenestration of large periapical lesions," *Journal of Endodontics*, vol. 17, no. 10, pp. 516–521, 1991.

[41] S. Miyawaki, M. Hyomoto, J. Tsubouchi, T. Kirita, and M. Sugimura, "Eruption speed and rate of angulation change of a cyst-associated mandibular second premolar after marsupialization of a dentigerous cyst," *American Journal of Orthodontics & Dentofacial Orthopedics*, vol. 116, no. 5, pp. 578–584, 1999.

[42] J. R. Hupp Jr., M. R. Tucker, and E. Ellis III, *Contemporary Oral and Maxillofacial Surgery*, Mosby, St. Louis, Mo, USA, 2014.

32

Free Gingival Graft to Increase Keratinized Mucosa after Placing of Mandibular Fixed Implant-Supported Prosthesis

Danny Omar Mendoza Marin,[1] **Andressa Rosa Perin Leite,**[1] **Lélis Gustavo Nícoli,**[2] **Claudio Marcantonio,**[3] **Marco Antonio Compagnoni,**[1] **and Elcio Marcantonio Jr.**[2]

[1]*Araraquara Dental School, Department of Dental Materials and Prosthodontics, Universidade Estadual Paulista (UNESP), Araraquara, SP, Brazil*
[2]*Araraquara Dental School, Department of Diagnosis and Surgery, Universidade Estadual Paulista (UNESP), Araraquara, SP, Brazil*
[3]*Araraquara Dental School, Department of Postgraduate Studies in Implantology, University Center of Araraquara (UNIARA), Araraquara, SP, Brazil*

Correspondence should be addressed to Marco Antonio Compagnoni; compagno@foar.unesp.br

Academic Editor: Jamil A. Shibli

Insufficiently keratinized tissue can be increased surgically by free gingival grafting. The presence or reconstruction of keratinized mucosa around the implant can facilitate restorative procedure and allow the maintenance of an oral hygiene routine without irritation or discomfort to the patient. The aim of this clinical case report is to describe an oral rehabilitation procedure of an edentulous patient with absence of keratinized mucosa in the interforaminal area, using a free gingival graft associated with a mandibular fixed implant-supported prosthesis. The treatment included the manufacturing of a maxillary complete denture and a mandibular fixed implant-supported prosthesis followed by a free gingival graft to increase the width of the mandibular keratinized mucosa. Free gingival graft was obtained from the palate and grafted on the buccal side of interforaminal area. The follow-up of 02 and 12 months after mucogingival surgery showed that the free gingival graft promoted peri-implant health, hygiene, and patient comfort. *Clinical Significance.* The free gingival graft is an effective treatment in increasing the width of mandibular keratinized mucosa on the buccal side of the interforaminal area and provided an improvement in maintaining the health of peri-implant tissues which allows for better oral hygiene.

1. Introduction

Fixed implant-supported prosthesis is an alternative treatment in prosthodontics mandibular rehabilitation [1]. However, the maintenance and health of the peri-implant soft tissue is necessary for the longevity of dental implants [2] and prosthesis. The soft tissue healing following implant surgery may result in the establishment of a border tissue composed of either keratinized or nonkeratinized mucosa [3].

A study showed that an amount ≥2 mm of keratinized mucosa (KM) is needed to maintain the health of periodontal tissues providing a soft tissue seal around natural teeth [4]. However, peri-implant health with presence or absence of a minimal zone of keratinized tissue around dental implants has been studied and the literature showed divergent theories

[5]. A literature review showed no significant association between "inadequate" keratinized tissue with higher plaque scores and mucosal inflammation [3]. Other studies showed that absence of adequate KM around dental implants is associated with increased plaque accumulation, mucosal inflammation, mucosal recession, and attachment loss [6, 7]. Furthermore, patient discomfort when performing oral hygiene was reported to be painful as a result of KM absence surrounding the implant, as well as mechanical irritation due to the mobility of the nonkeratinized tissue under function [3, 8, 9].

The weak sealing ability of the peri-implant nonkeratinized tissue [10], the critical bacterial plaque control in some patients [7], pain, and discomfort are the main reasons for justifying a gingival graft on the implant site [11] with absence

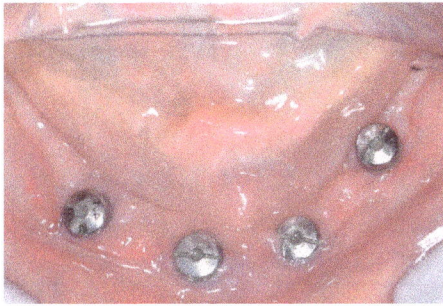

FIGURE 1: Initial appearance of the gingival tissue around the implants.

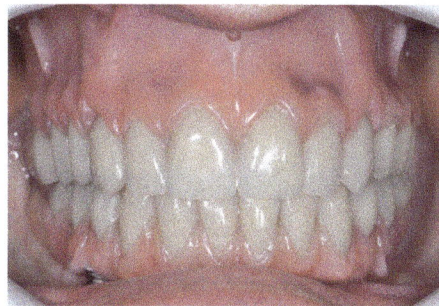

FIGURE 2: Checking the fitting of prostheses in mouth.

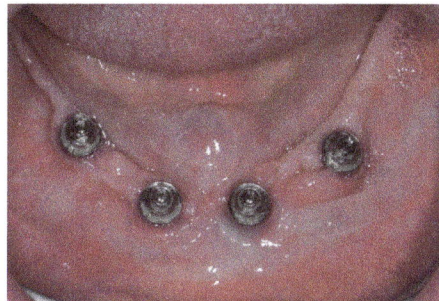

FIGURE 3: Plaque accumulation on the prosthetic components after 30 days of installation of definitive prostheses.

of KM using a mandibular fixed implant. Thus, the aim of this clinical case report is to describe an oral rehabilitation procedure of an edentulous patient with absence of KM in the interforaminal area, using a free gingival graft associated with a mandibular fixed implant-supported prosthesis.

2. Case Description

A 60-year-old, nonsmoking, female patient in good general health came to the Department of Dental Materials and Prosthodontics at Araraquara Dental School complaining that her maxillary complete denture was unstable. Clinical and radiographic examinations revealed an old maxillary complete denture and four osseointegrated dental implants in the interforaminal area with their healing caps. In addition, it was verified on the mandible the absence of KM on the buccal side of interforaminal area, shallow vestibule, presence of bacterial place around the healing caps, and complaint of painful symptoms in the gingival tissue around the implants (Figure 1). In addition, the manufacturing of a mandibular fixed implant-supported prosthesis was also needed.

Considering the patient's age, health, and comfort, as a first step, the proposed treatment was the manufacturing of a new conventional maxillary complete denture and a mandibular fixed implant-supported prosthesis. After 30 days, as a second step, a free gingival graft associated with the mandibular fixed implant-supported prosthesis was indicated for maintenance of peri-implant tissue after 30 days of installation of the new prostheses because the patient had pain and difficulty during hygienization of the mandibular prosthesis and presence of plaque accumulation.

All procedures for manufacturing of a new conventional maxillary complete denture in combination with a mandibular fixed implant-supported prosthesis were used. A record base with an occlusion rim was used to reestablish occlusal planes and the occlusal vertical dimension and record patient's centric relation. Afterwards, the definitive casts were mounted in a semiadjustable articulator and artificial acrylic teeth were set and after evaluated in the patient. A mandibular multifunctional guide was manufactured for definitive impression and occlusal registration. Four miniabutments (Micro Unit Abutment, Conexão Sistemas de Prótese, São Paulo, Brazil) were installed on the implants and the impression was performed using impression coping

(Impression Coping Micro Unit Abutment, Conexão Sistemas de Prótese, São Paulo, Brazil) and occlusal records were performed on the multifunctional guide. Heat-polymerized polymethyl methacrylate resin (Lucitone 550, Dentsply International Inc., New York, USA) was used for manufacturing the maxillary complete denture and mandibular fixed implant-supported prosthesis. Afterwards, both prostheses were installed and the fitting and adaptation were checked. (Figure 2).

After 30 days, the patient returned for maintenance of the prostheses and plaque accumulation was observed in the peri-implant area on the prosthetic components (Figure 3). In addition, pain and difficulty during hygienization of the mandibular prosthesis were verified. Therefore, a free gingival graft surgery was performed to provide a KM in the peri-implant area, thus, minimizing the sensitivity during hygiene. The patient was anesthetized locally with mepivacaine 2% associated with epinephrine 1 : 100,000 (Mepiadre-New DFL Ind. e Com. S.A., Rio de Janeiro, Brazil). An intrasulcular incision was performed and a partial-thickness flap was made on the buccal side of the interforaminal area around the four dental implants (Figure 4). A sterile paper was used to make a template with the same size of the recipient bed, which was transferred to the palate in order to remove two free 1.5 mm thick gingival grafts (Figure 5).

A free gingival graft [12, 13] was obtained from the right and left side portions of the palate, approximately 2 mm below the gingival margin. One portion of the graft was placed covering the left surgical area and fixed by compression sutures using absorbable thread (Vicryl–Ethicon, Johnson &

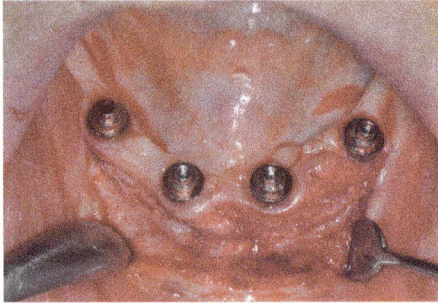

FIGURE 4: Partial-thickness flap on the buccal side of the interforaminal area around the implants.

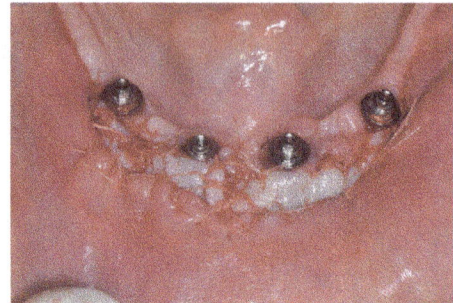

FIGURE 6: Free gingival graft placed around the implants.

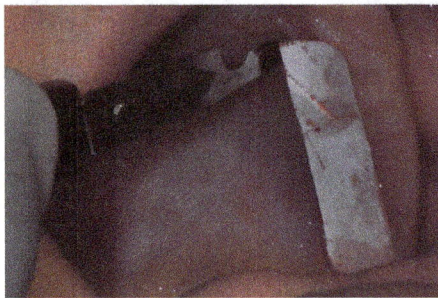

FIGURE 5: A sterile paper to make a map with the size of the recipient bed and transferred to the palate.

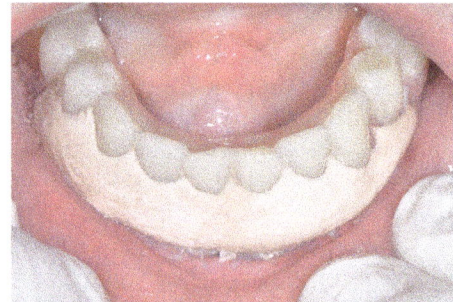

FIGURE 7: Surgical cement in the recipient bed and stabilized on the mandibular prosthesis.

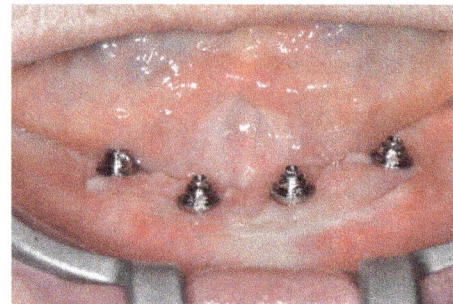

FIGURE 8: Six months of follow-up after surgery showed a good health of peri-implant tissues and absence of plaque accumulation.

Johnson do Brasil, São José dos Campos, Brazil) to remain stable and in close contact with the periosteal bed. The same protocol described above was applied to the second portion of the graft on the right surgical area (Figure 6).

The palatal donor sites were sutured using 4-0 silk threads (Ethichon–Johnson & Johnson Medical Limited, New Brunswick, NJ) to promote hemostasis and clot stabilization. Following, surgical cement (Coe-Pack-GC Europe N.V.) was added onto the palatal donor sites along with the new maxillary complete denture to aid in healing by second intention and provide comfort to the patient during the postoperative period. The mandibular fixed implant-supported prosthesis was installed in the mouth and surgical cement was added in the recipient bed and stabilized on the mandibular prosthesis (Figure 7).

Postoperative care included a 0.12% chlorhexidine rinse twice daily for 2 weeks, 500 mg of amoxicillin 3 times a day for 7 days, 100 mg of nimesulide 2 times a day for 3 days, and 500 mg of paracetamol as needed for pain. Surgical cement was replaced in the conventional maxillary denture after 48 h and 7 days, respectively, to avoid food impact between the prosthesis and mucosa. In mandible, surgical cement was replaced after 7 days after the surgical procedures. The surgical cement was removed completely in both prostheses after 14 days. Sutures of donor and recipient sites were removed after 14 days and healing took place without postoperative discomfort to the patient. Patient was recalled after 1, 3, and 6 months for follow-up, when instructions regarding home oral hygiene techniques were reinforced.

After a 6-month period of follow-up (Figure 8), it was observed an improvement of thickness and a 3 mm increase in the height of keratinized mucosa, promoting a good peri-implant health and facilitating the hygiene procedures. After one year of follow-up, the patient reported being satisfied with the treatment and an improvement in the ease of cleaning the mandibular prosthesis without any complaint of painful symptoms in the peri-implant area.

3. Discussion

The absence of KM, around the peri-implant tissue [14], could lead to an inadequate oral hygiene, plaque accumulation, mucosal inflammation, bleeding on probing, mucosal recession, and alveolar bone loss that could negatively influence the long-term maintenance of dental implants and prosthesis

[9, 15]. Several surgical procedures have been used to increase KM around implant including free gingival grafts, connective tissue grafts, pedicle grafts, and apically positioned flaps [16–18].

Free gingival graft is a successful and predictable technique [19] that could prevent hard and soft tissue problems developed after implant rehabilitation [20]. This procedure can be performed previous to implant placement, during the second stage surgery in implants or after placing of the final prosthesis [19]. Free gingival graft previous to implant placement or during the second stage surgery can result in a greater waiting time for realization of rehabilitation treatment [21]. The patient cannot wear this prosthesis during healing graft period and this could have an impact on their physiological functions, especially in patients who suffer from pain and discomfort through several surgical stages [21].

Furthermore, the pain and difficulty during hygienization of the prosthesis could lead to plaque accumulation around the peri-implant tissues [22, 23] and cause discomfort to the patient and mucosal inflammation. An adequate width of keratinized tissue around implants could provide a prosthetic favorable environment, facilitate precise prosthetic procedures, and allow adequate oral hygiene maintenance by the patient, which would help to prevent gingival recession [5]. In addition, wider zones of KM can offer more resistance to the forces of mastication and frictional contact that occur during oral hygiene procedures [15].

One limitation of this technique is that it involves two surgical sites, causing morbidity in both. However, with adequate medication, stabilization of the surgical cement, obtained in this case by the use of both prostheses, and a good follow-up during the first 15 days of healing, we can minimize this limitation. In addition, some percentage of shrinkage should be expected and periodical controls must be performed [19, 24].

In this clinical case report, the patient experienced discomfort, restriction during oral hygiene performance, and plaque accumulation after 30 days of use of the final prosthesis due to a lack of KM, requiring a free gingival graft. The free gingival graft, which was performed after placing of the final prosthesis, allowed the stability of the surgical cement, protection of recipient bed, and immovability of the graft and reestablished physiological functions once the patient was able to continue wearing the prosthesis. Considering the patient's age and health, the use of a free gingival graft was considered a viable and satisfactory treatment option with good outcomes during a 6- and 12-month period of follow-up.

4. Conclusion

The free gingival graft, after placing of the final prosthesis and diagnosis of pain and difficulty during hygienization of mandibular prosthesis, was effective in increasing the width of mandibular keratinized mucosa on the buccal side of the interforaminal area and provided an improvement in maintaining the health of peri-implant tissues, which allows for better oral hygiene.

Competing Interests

No potential conflict of interests relevant to the present article was reported.

References

[1] C. Huard, M. Bessadet, E. Nicolas, and J.-L. Veyrune, "Geriatric slim implants for complete denture wearers: clinical aspects and perspectives," *Clinical, Cosmetic and Investigational Dentistry*, vol. 5, pp. 63–68, 2013.

[2] B.-S. Kim, Y.-K. Kim, P.-Y. Yun et al., "Evaluation of peri-implant tissue response according to the presence of keratinized mucosa," *Oral Surgery, Oral Medicine, Oral Pathology, Oral Radiology and Endodontology*, vol. 107, no. 3, pp. e24–e28, 2009.

[3] J. L. Wennström and J. Derks, "Is there a need for keratinized mucosa around implants to maintain health and tissue stability?" *Clinical Oral Implants Research*, vol. 23, supplement 6, pp. 136–146, 2012.

[4] N. P. Lang and H. Löe, "The relationship between the width of keratinized gingiva and gingival health," *Journal of Periodontology*, vol. 43, no. 10, pp. 623–627, 1972.

[5] S. J. Narayan, P. K. Singh, S. Mohammed, and R. K. V. Patel, "Enhancing the zone of keratinized tissue around implants," *Journal of Indian Prosthodontist Society*, vol. 15, no. 2, pp. 183–186, 2015.

[6] D. Boynueğri, S. K. Nemli, and Y. A. Kasko, "Significance of keratinized mucosa around dental implants: a prospective comparative study," *Clinical Oral Implants Research*, vol. 24, no. 8, pp. 928–933, 2013.

[7] G.-H. Lin, H.-L. Chan, and H.-L. Wang, "The significance of keratinized mucosa on implant health: a systematic review," *Journal of Periodontology*, vol. 84, no. 12, pp. 1755–1767, 2013.

[8] M. L. A. Kaptein, G. L. De Lange, and P. A. Blijdorp, "Peri-implant tissue health in reconstructed atrophic maxillae—report of 88 patients and 470 implants," *Journal of Oral Rehabilitation*, vol. 26, no. 6, pp. 464–474, 1999.

[9] M. Adibrad, M. Shahabuei, and M. Sahabi, "Significance of the width of keratinized mucosa on the health status of the supporting tissue around implants supporting overdentures," *The Journal of Oral Implantology*, vol. 35, no. 5, pp. 232–237, 2009.

[10] I. Ericsson and J. Lindhe, "Probing depth at implants and teeth. An experimental study in the dog," *Journal of Clinical Periodontology*, vol. 20, no. 9, pp. 623–627, 1993.

[11] M. A. Salonen, K. Oikarinen, K. Virtanen, and H. Pernu, "Failures in the osseointegration of endosseous implants," *The International Journal of Oral & Maxillofacial Implants*, vol. 8, no. 1, pp. 92–97, 1993.

[12] B. Langer and L. Langer, "Overlapped flap: a surgical modification for implant fixture installation," *The International journal of periodontics & restorative dentistry*, vol. 10, no. 3, pp. 208–215, 1990.

[13] B. Langer and D. Y. Sullivan, "Osseointegration: its impact on the interrelationship of periodontics and restorative dentistry: part I," *The International Journal of Periodontics and Restorative Dentistry*, vol. 9, pp. 84–105, 1989.

[14] Q. Wu, Y. Qu, P. Gong, T. Wang, T. Gong, and Y. Man, "Evaluation of the efficacy of keratinized mucosa augmentation techniques around dental implants: a systematic review," *Journal of Prosthetic Dentistry*, vol. 113, no. 5, pp. 383–390, 2015.

[15] A. Bouri Jr., N. Bissada, M. S. Al-Zahrani, F. Faddoul, and I. Nouneh, "Width of keratinized gingiva and the health status of the supporting tissues around dental implants," *International Journal of Oral and Maxillofacial Implants*, vol. 23, no. 2, pp. 323–326, 2008.

[16] G. Wiesner, M. Esposito, H. Worthington, and M. Schlee, "Connective tissue grafts for thickening peri-implant tissues at implant placement. One-year results from an explanatory split-mouth randomised controlled clinical trial," *European Journal of Oral Implantology*, vol. 3, no. 1, pp. 27–35, 2010.

[17] C. E. Nemcovsky and O. Moses, "Rotated palatal flap. a surgical approach to increase keratinized tissue width in maxillary implant uncovering: technique and clinical evaluation," *International Journal of Periodontics and Restorative Dentistry*, vol. 22, no. 6, pp. 607–612, 2002.

[18] J. Carnio and P. M. Camargo, "The modified apically repositioned flap to increase the dimensions of attached gingiva: the single incision technique for multiple adjacent teeth," *International Journal of Periodontics and Restorative Dentistry*, vol. 26, no. 3, pp. 265–269, 2006.

[19] A. Elkhaweldi, C. R. Soler, R. Cayarga, T. Suzuki, and Z. Kaufman, "Various techniques to increase keratinized tissue for implant supported overdentures: retrospective case series," *International Journal of Dentistry*, vol. 2015, Article ID 104903, 7 pages, 2015.

[20] E. Büyükerkmen and E. Oncu, "Gingival graft prior to and after delivery of implant-supported prostheses," *Clinical Oral Implants Research*, vol. 25, p. 627, 2014.

[21] J.-Y. Sohn, J.-C. Park, K.-S. Cho, and C.-S. Kim, "Simultaneous placement of an interpositional free gingival graft with nonsubmerged implant placement," *Journal of Periodontal and Implant Science*, vol. 44, no. 2, pp. 94–99, 2014.

[22] C. Marcantonio, L. G. Nicoli, E. Marcantonio Junior, D. L. Zandim-Barcelos, and S. Patil, "Prevalence and possible risk factors of peri-implantitis: a concept review," *The Journal of Contemporary Dental Practice*, vol. 16, pp. 750–757, 2015.

[23] S. Renvert and I. Polyzois, "Risk indicators for peri-implant mucositis: a systematic literature review," *Journal of Clinical Periodontology*, vol. 42, pp. S172–S186, 2015.

[24] J.-J. Yan, A. Y.-M. Tsai, M.-Y. Wong, and L.-T. Hou, "Comparison of acellular dermal graft and palatal autograft in the reconstruction of keratinized gingiva around dental implants: a case report," *International Journal of Periodontics and Restorative Dentistry*, vol. 26, no. 3, pp. 287–292, 2006.

Necrotizing Sialometaplasia of the Hard Palate in a Patient Treated with Topical Nonsteroidal Anti-Inflammatory Drug

Alessandro Gatti, Emanuele Broccardo, Giuseppe Poglio, and Arnaldo Benech

Unit of Oral and Maxillofacial Surgery, Maggiore della Carità University Hospital, Novara, Italy

Correspondence should be addressed to Emanuele Broccardo; broccardo1@gmail.com

Academic Editor: Kenji Yamagata

Necrotizing sialometaplasia is a rare, benign, self-limiting, necrotizing process involving the minor salivary glands, mainly the mucoserous glands of the hard palate. It is thought to be the result of an ischemic event of the vasculature supplying the salivary gland lobules. Some predisposing factors such as smoking, use of alcohol, denture wearing, recent surgery, traumatic injuries, respiratory infections, systemic diseases bulimia, and anorexia have been described. Herein we present a case of necrotizing sialometaplasia of the hard palate in a patient without known predisposing factors, in our opinion, resulting from the use of topical anti-inflammatory drug. After diagnosis, the patient underwent treatment with chlorhexidine gluconate and a full palatal acrylic guard to protect the exposed bone from food residues during meals. After the sixth week the lesion regressed.

1. Introduction

Necrotizing sialometaplasia (NS) is a rare, benign, self-limiting, necrotizing process involving the minor salivary glands, in most cases the mucoserous glands of the hard palate. This lesion was first described in 1973 by Abrams et al. [1]. However, it may be confused with malignant lesions both histopathologically and clinically, in particular squamous cell carcinoma and mucoepidermoid carcinoma [2].

Etiologically NS is thought to be the result of an ischemic event of the vasculature supplying the salivary gland lobules. However, some predisposing factors related to these lesions have been described, including smoking, use of alcohol, denture wearing, recent surgery, other traumatic injuries, respiratory infections, systemic diseases [3–5], bulimia, and anorexia [6]. In the literature no cases of NS are described in relation to the use of anti-inflammatory drugs.

We describe a case of necrotizing sialometaplasia of the hard palate in a patient treated with topical anti-inflammatory drug, in the absence of other predisposing factors.

2. Clinical Report

A 47-year-old woman presented with a painless swelling in the hard palate, which appeared 2 days before. The patient reported pain during swallowing. There was no history of alcohol intake, smoking, systemic disease, trauma, or recent surgery. The only relevant fact that we found in the patient's history was the excessive use of flurbiprofen oral spray for 5 weeks, which she reported as prevention for sore throat. No diagnosis of pharyngitis was made. The patient reported over 6 daily administration for 5 weeks. Physical examination revealed a deep crateriform ulcer of the palatal mucosa, measuring 20 mm in diameter, located at the left side of the midline of the hard palate. The ulcer appeared with sharp margins without evidence of mucosal erythema (Figure 1), and the underlying bone was exposed without any sign of infection and erosion. A computed tomography scan showed a mucosal lesion without bone involvement (Figure 2) and laterocervical reactive lymphadenopathy. An incisional biopsy of the lesion was performed under local anesthesia. The histopathological examination showed a

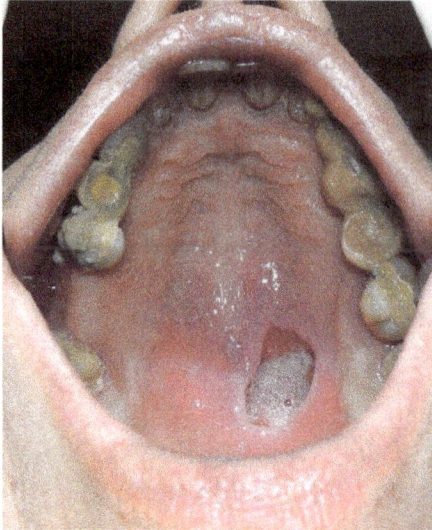

FIGURE 1: Deep crateriform ulcer of the palatal mucosa, located at the left side of the midline of the hard palate.

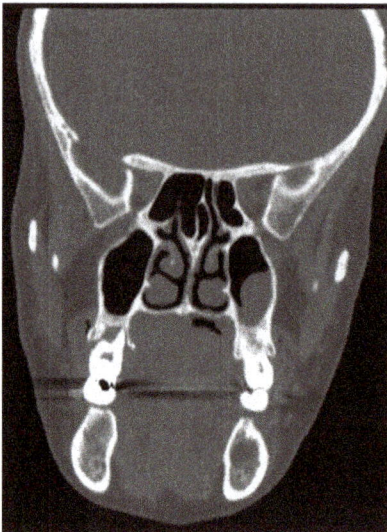

FIGURE 2: Computed tomography scan showing a mucosal lesion without bone involvement (coronal view).

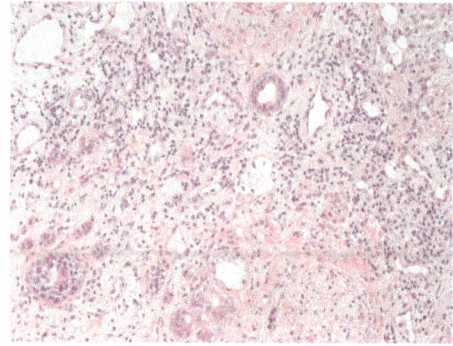

(a)

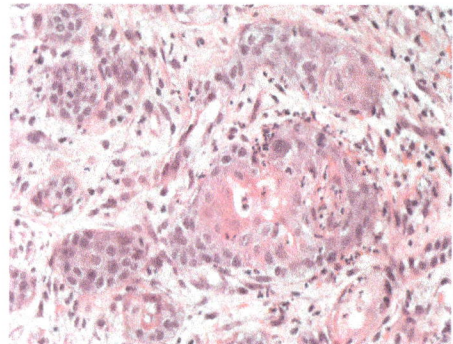

(b)

FIGURE 3: Photomicrographs of the histological specimen, showing a reactive inflammatory process involving the minor salivary glands, associated with focal necrosis of the lobules and areas of squamous metaplasia of the salivary ducts. (a) H&E, 20x magnification and (b) H&E, 40x magnification.

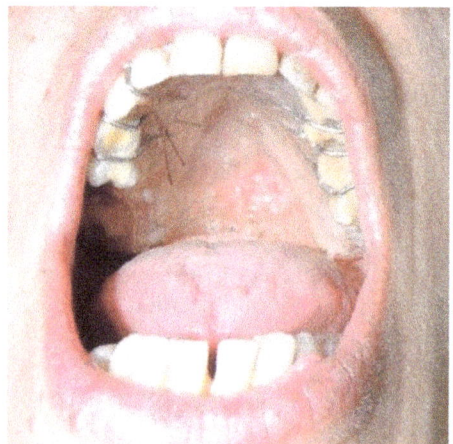

FIGURE 4: Full palatal acrylic guard lined with silicone placed to protect the exposed bone and to reduce the pain on swallowing.

reactive inflammatory process involving the minor salivary glands, associated with focal necrosis of the lobules and areas of squamous metaplasia of the salivary ducts (Figure 3).

The patient underwent treatment with chlorhexidine gluconate gel 3 times a day; a full palatal acrylic guard was fabricated, lined with silicone and placed to protect the exposed bone from food residues during meals and to reduce the pain on swallowing (Figure 4). A weekly follow-up was carried out for 8 weeks. After the first week the pain during swallowing was resolved. After the sixth week the lesion regressed (Figure 5).

3. Discussion

Necrotizing sialometaplasia was first described in 1973, by Abrams et al. [1]. This lesion is a benign inflammatory condition which can be found at any site in the body that contains elements of salivary gland. In the literature cases of NS located at the lung and at the paranasal sinuses are reported, but

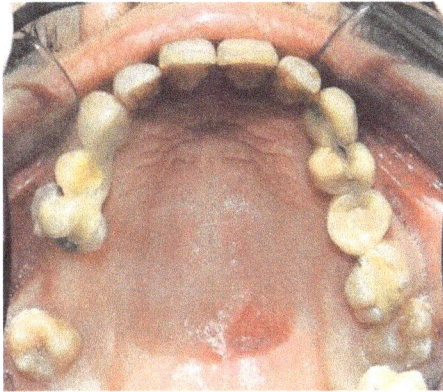

FIGURE 5: Regression of the lesion at sixth week of follow-up.

most of the cases have still been reported in the oral cavity [7]. The etiology of NS has not been fully understood, but an underlying cause appears to be the gland tissue ischemia. The appearance of these lesions is believed to be related to a physicochemical or biological injury on the blood vessels that would produce an ischemic event and consequently necrosis, inflammation, and metaplasia of the ducts [4].

Anneroth and Hansen, in their study [8], have described the pathogenesis of NS, dividing it into five histologic stages: infarction, sequestration, ulceration, the reparative stage, and the healed stage.

Numerous risk factors have been described to explain the onset of local ischemia of the palate. Local trauma is considered the most frequent of them. Before extraction of maxillary teeth, the injection of local anesthetic with adrenaline to the hard palate may contribute to ischemia through pharmacologic vasoconstriction [9]. Surgery may also represent a form of local trauma, either as an accidental traumatic event during intubation or extubation or due to prolonged local pressure. Poor-fitting prostheses are also considered a predisposing factor; in fact the damage may result from a prolonged compression on the palate [7]. Alcohol, tobacco, or cocaine abuse may decrease blood flow to the mucosa, especially if these factors coexist [4]. Other possible predisposing factors cited in the literature are chemical irritation resulting from bulimia and chronic vomiting; there may be a combination of mechanical and chemical factors such as the low pH of the gastric contents and the use of fingers to mechanically induce vomiting [6]. Radiation, respiratory infections or allergies, previous adenoidectomy or surgery for other lesions, and adjacent tumours may produce compression and consequently ischemia [3].

Some systemic diseases are considered as a predisposing factor such as diabetes, HIV [10], due to reduced immunity defense, and drepanocytic anaemia, with an increase in blood viscosity that favours ischemia.

Recently Senapati et al. demonstrated that necrotizing sialometaplasia could be a manifestation of a localized vasculitis [11].

In the literature, to our knowledge, a case of NS associated with the use of topical nonsteroidal anti-inflammatory drugs has never been described.

Nonsteroidal anti-inflammatory drugs normally elicit therapeutic anti-inflammatory, analgesic, and antipyretic effects by inhibition of prostaglandins synthesis. They, for the most part, competitively inhibit cyclooxygenases, the enzymes that catalyze the synthesis of cyclic endoperoxides from arachidonic acid to form prostaglandins [12, 13].

Prostaglandins and their derivatives, such as prostacyclin and thromboxane, are involved in physiological functions such as protection of the stomach mucosa, aggregation of platelets, and regulation of kidney function. In addition, they have a well-documented pathophysiological role in inflammation, fever, and pain [13].

Prostaglandins are in fact potent mediators of inflammation that results in edema, pain, and vasodilation. The inhibition of these compounds is associated with analgesia and a reduction in inflammation [12].

Nevertheless, in 2006, Cannon et al. [14] demonstrated that prolonged use of systemic nonsteroidal anti-inflammatory drugs increases the risk of cardiovascular events. Suppression of prostacyclin and prostaglandin E2, mediated by this class of drugs, is the most thoroughly developed explanation for the cardiovascular hazard; in fact, prostacyclin is a prostanoid that acts as a restraint on mediators of platelet activation, hypertension, and atherogenesis, including thromboxane A2.

In our case the patient had abused topical flurbiprofen, a nonsteroidal anti-inflammatory drug, which also contained alcohol as excipient. The patient reported more than 6 daily doses for more than one month.

We suppose that the synergistic action of nonsteroidal anti-inflammatory drug and alcohol, acting as local microenvironmental factors on the palatal mucosa for a long time, had resulted in an ischemic event of the vasculature supplying a salivary gland.

The treatment of necrotizing sialometaplasia does not require surgery; in fact this kind of lesion is a self-limiting condition. When risk factors are removed, healing is obtained within 4–8 weeks [3]. In this case we have treated the patients with chlorhexidine gel 3 times daily to control the inflammation and, thanks to the use of a full palatal acrylic guard, the storage of food residues inside the ulcer with consequent risk of inflammation and pain has been avoided. The healing has been regularly obtained after 6 weeks.

To the best of our knowledge, this is the first case of NS associated with the use of topical nonsteroidal anti-inflammatory drug. We suppose that the prolonged use of topical anti-inflammatory drugs may be considered as a predisposing factor to NS. More extensive histopathological and clinical studies are necessary to confirm this hypothesis and to clarify the correct pathogenesis of this rare, benign disease.

Competing Interests

The authors declare that there is no conflict of interests regarding the publication of this paper.

References

[1] A. M. Abrams, R. J. Melrose, and F. V. Howell, "Necrotizing sialometaplasia. A disease simulating malignancy," *Cancer*, vol. 32, no. 1, pp. 130–135, 1973.

[2] Y. Kimura, K. Matsuzaka, K. Matsuoka, T. Muramatsu, Y. Yokoyama, and T. Inoue, "A case report of necrotizing sialometaplasia with immunohistological findings and a review of the literature," *Oral Medicine & Pathology*, vol. 15, no. 3, pp. 87–90, 2011.

[3] R. B. Brannon, C. B. Fowler, and K. S. Hartman, "Necrotizing sialometaplasia. A clinicopathologic study of sixty-nine cases and review of the literature," *Oral Surgery, Oral Medicine, Oral Pathology*, vol. 72, no. 3, pp. 317–325, 1991.

[4] T. A. Imbery and P. A. Edwards, "Necrotizing sialometaplasia: literature review and case reports," *Journal of the American Dental Association*, vol. 127, no. 7, pp. 1087–1092, 1996.

[5] I. Kaplan, M. Alterman, S. Kleinman et al., "The clinical, histologic, and treatment spectrum in necrotizing sialometaplasia," *Oral Surgery, Oral Medicine, Oral Pathology and Oral Radiology*, vol. 114, no. 5, pp. 577–585, 2012.

[6] H. Schöning, R. Emshoff, and A. Kreczy, "Necrotizing sialometaplasia in two patients with bulimia and chronic vomiting," *International Journal of Oral and Maxillofacial Surgery*, vol. 27, no. 6, pp. 463–465, 1998.

[7] L. Ylikontiola, M. Siponen, T. Salo, and G. K. B. Sándor, "Sialometaplasia of the soft palate in a 2-year-old girl," *Journal of the Canadian Dental Association*, vol. 73, no. 4, pp. 333–336, 2007.

[8] G. Anneroth and L. S. Hansen, "Necrotizing sialometaplasia. The relationship of its pathogenesis to its clinical characteristics," *International Journal of Oral Surgery*, vol. 11, no. 5, pp. 283–291, 1982.

[9] S. Ghali, K. R. Knox, J. Verbesey, U. Scarpidis, K. Izadi, and P. A. Ganchi, "Effects of lidocaine and epinephrine on cutaneous blood flow," *Journal of Plastic, Reconstructive and Aesthetic Surgery*, vol. 61, no. 10, pp. 1226–1231, 2008.

[10] A. D. Silva, C. A. B. Silva, C. Furuse, R. C. Nunes e Souza, M. H. M. da Costa, and V. C. de Araújo, "Necrotizing sialometaplasia in a patient who is HIV positive: a case report," *Special Care in Dentistry*, vol. 30, no. 4, pp. 160–162, 2010.

[11] S. Senapati, S. C. Samal, R. Kumar, and S. Patra, "Necrotizing sialometaplasia: manifestation of a localized unclassified vasculitis," *Indian Journal of Pathology and Microbiology*, vol. 59, no. 2, pp. 232–234, 2016.

[12] G. A. Green, "Understanding NSAIDs: from aspirin to COX-2," *Clinical Cornerstone*, vol. 3, no. 5, pp. 50–58, 2001.

[13] R. M. Botting, "Inhibitors of cyclooxygenases: mechanisms, selectivity and uses," *Journal of Physiology and Pharmacology*, vol. 57, supplement 5, pp. 113–124, 2006.

[14] C. P. Cannon, S. P. Curtis, G. A. FitzGerald et al., "Cardiovascular outcomes with etoricoxib and diclofenac in patients with osteoarthritis and rheumatoid arthritis in the Multinational Etoricoxib and Diclofenac Arthritis Long-term (MEDAL) programme: a randomised comparison," *The Lancet*, vol. 368, no. 9549, pp. 1771–1781, 2006.

34

Differential Diagnosis of Parotid Lipoma in a Breast Ca Patient

Melda Misirlioglu, Yagmur Yilmaz Akyil, Mehmet Zahit Adisen, and Alime Okkesim

Department of Oral and Maxillofacial Radiology, Faculty of Dentistry, Kırıkkale University, Kırıkkale, Turkey

Correspondence should be addressed to Yagmur Yilmaz Akyil; dtyagmuryilmaz@gmail.com

Academic Editor: Gavriel Chaushu

Lipomas are common benign tumors usually detected on the torso, neck, upper thighs, and upper arms. However, they are rarely found in the parotid gland region. Because of their rarity at this site, they are not often considered in the differential diagnosis of parotid tumors. This report describes a rare case of a lipoma in the superficial lobe of parotid gland. A 71-year-old female patient admitted to our department complaining about swelling and pain in the posterior area of the left mandibular region since one month. Her medical history included mastectomy after breast CA fifteen years ago. Clinical examination revealed a smooth-surfaced, soft, and painful mass, with well-defined margins in the left mandibular region. Differential diagnosis of metastasis, inflammatory neck swellings, and benign salivary gland tumors were considered for the patient. Advanced imaging methods such as ultrasonography and contrast tomography revealed that the lesion was a lipoma of parotid gland. A surgical intervention under general anesthesia was planned for the removal of the mass; however patient refused the surgical treatment. Patient was placed on six-month periodic recall. This article reviews the radiographic appearance and differential diagnoses of lipoma in this rare location.

1. Introduction

The ordinary lipomas are the most common neoplasms of mesenchymal origin [1, 2]. They result due to proliferation of normal adipose tissue. Only 15% of lipomas are found in the head and neck region and they usually occur subcutaneously in the posterior neck [1]. Less commonly they can be found in the anterior neck, infratemporal fossa, submandibular space, pharynx, larynx, and parotid gland and in or around the oral cavity [2, 3]. The incidence of lipoma among parotid tumors ranges from 0.6% to 4.4%, with most series reporting an incidence of 1% [4]. The most common origin of these tumors, in the parotid gland, can be single or multiple and is rarely observed in the deep lobe less than superficial lobe. Lipomas are asymptomatic tumors. However if they grow to a large size, they can interfere with mastication and speaking [5]. Lipomas of parotid generally occur in the sixth decade. Advanced imaging methods such as ultrasonography (US), magnetic resonance imaging (MRI), and computed tomography (CT) are used for diagnosis of lipomas [1, 6]. This report describes differential diagnosis of a parotid lipoma in a breast CA patient detected with advanced imaging methods such as US and contrast tomography.

2. Case Report

A 71-year-old woman patient presented to the Department of Oral and Maxillofacial Radiology with a primary complaint of swelling and pain in the posterior area of the left mandibular region since one month. Patient history revealed that the swelling had been slowly increasing in size. The patient had pain at left side of her face but she cannot distinguish the exact localization. Her medical history included mastectomy after breast CA fifteen years ago. She also has diabetes and is using insulin. Clinical examination revealed a smooth-surfaced, soft, and painful mass, with well-defined margins in the left mandibular region (Figure 1). The swelling was not fixed to the skin and the underlying bone. In her panoramic radiographic examination, root remnant was detected in the left maxillary molar area, possibly related to pain in her face (Figure 2). After taking informed consent of the patient, she was referred to US for differential diagnosis of soft tissue pathologies including metastasis, inflammatory neck swellings, and benign salivary gland tumors. US of the neck region showed bilateral submandibular and parotid glands were normal in size with homogen ecogenity. Thyroid gland was normal with normal ecogenity. However, there

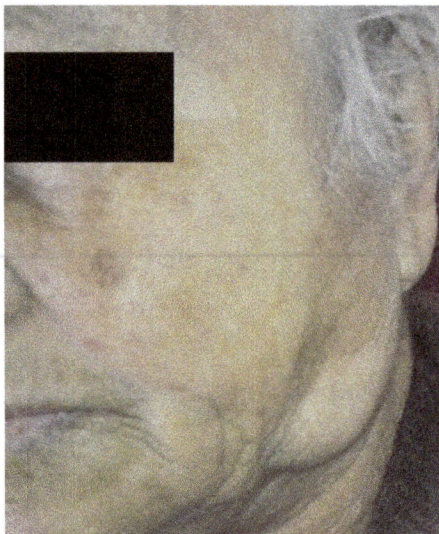

FIGURE 1: Patient extra-oral photograph showed a smooth-surfaced, soft, and painful mass, with well-defined margins in the right mandibular region.

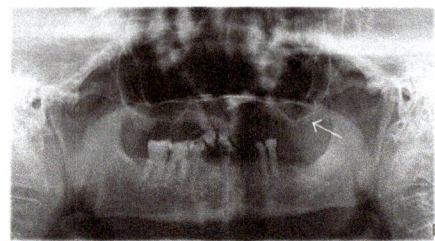

FIGURE 2: Panoramic radiograph of this patient; root remnant (white arrow) was detected in the left maxillary molar area.

was a 40 × 18 mm size, well-defined, hypoechoic solid lesion in her superficial lobe of the parotid gland. The lesion had echogenic septas and acoustic empowerment over the posterior region (Figure 3). Hence a pleomorphic adenoma was suspected and contrast CT was requested. In contrast to CT images, lesion was diagnosed as lipoma due to well-demarcated, hypodense density (Figure 4). A surgical intervention under general anesthesia was planned for the removal of the mass; however patient refused the surgical treatment. Hence, only root remnant was extracted under local anesthesia. Follow-up examination was uneventful and pain was regressed. Patient was placed on a periodic recall.

3. Discussion

Lipoma of salivary glands is quite rare with the highest frequency reported in parotid gland that presents normally adipose tissue. Heredity, obesity, diabetes, trauma, radiation, endocrine disorder, insulin injection, and corticosteroid therapy are occasionally implicated as a possible etiologic factors of lipoma [3, 6].

Diagnostic imaging techniques such as US, MRI, and CT help to differentiate lipomas from other soft tissue lesions while identifying the nature and exact location of lesion. For the masses in the salivary glands area, sialography, US, and radionuclide scanning are all of value [7]. US can give a clear and fast diagnosis of lipoma [8]. It can be used as the initial study and shows a homogenous lesion that can be ovoid or lobulated [1]. Lipomas are hypoechoic relative to the adjacent muscle and contain linear echoic lines with no distal enhancement or attenuation. In most cases, they have a clearly identified capsule [8]. In order to determine whether the mass has a glandular origin, the radionuclide scan or the sialogram are usually performed. These imaging techniques can localize the mass inside or outside the salivary gland [7, 9]. Moreover, the radionuclide scan can identify the functional activity of the mass [7]. CT of the neck, which is a helpful imaging method, may differentiate solid masses from cystic masses. It can also be performed for identification of free nodal lesions, localization of the masses within salivary glands, and differentiation of congenital vascular lesions from the lymph nodal chain [1, 7]. Contrast-enhanced high resolution CT is another useful radiological technique in differential diagnosis [10]. While a positive density is observed in normal parotid tissue, a well-demarcated hypodense density (−50 to −150 Hounsfield units) can be identified in lipomatous tissue in contrast-enhanced images [1, 10]. In MRI examinations, lipomas show a similar signal intensity with subcutaneous fat, characterized by a high T1 and low T2 signal intensity [10]. Lipomatous lesions can be clearly distinguished from other types of tumors with the fat suppression sequence of MRI, which provides superior soft tissue definition. It can also reveal the accurate relationship of tumor with facial nerve [10].

The principle consideration in the differential diagnosis of a mass in the parotid region is whether the salivary gland neoplasia is benign or malign. The primary differential diagnosis of neck masses as benign lesions in the subcutaneous location is a sebaceous cyst or an abscess. Sebaceous cysts are also rounded and subcutaneous. Abscesses typically have overlying induration and erythema [11]. Other benign connective tissue lesions in differential diagnosis include granular cell tumor, traumatic fibroma, neurofibroma, and salivary gland lesions (mucocele and mixed tumor) [5]. Lymphadenopathy is also a common finding in neck area, caused by bacterial or viral infections of the upper respiratory tract. Moreover, cervical tularemia, tuberculosis, brucellosis, or cat scratch disease has to be considered in differential diagnosis of neck masses. Granulomatous inflammatory disease usually occurs in specific age groups and locations. So, the physician should keep this in mind when evaluating a neck mass in clinical examination [7, 12, 13]. Sialolipoma is a new variant of salivary gland lipoma, consisting of both adipose and glandular tissues. Lipoma and sialolipoma can be differentiated from one another microscopically by the lack of entrapment of normal salivary gland acini and ducts [13, 14].

Unless proven otherwise, any unknown neck mass, particularly symptom-free, located unilaterally and related with a known lymph node groups, must be evaluated as a metastatic lesion [7]. Liposarcoma, malignant counterpart of lipoma, is especially important to consider in differential diagnosis [15]. Nevertheless, it is rarely found in this region. MRI can

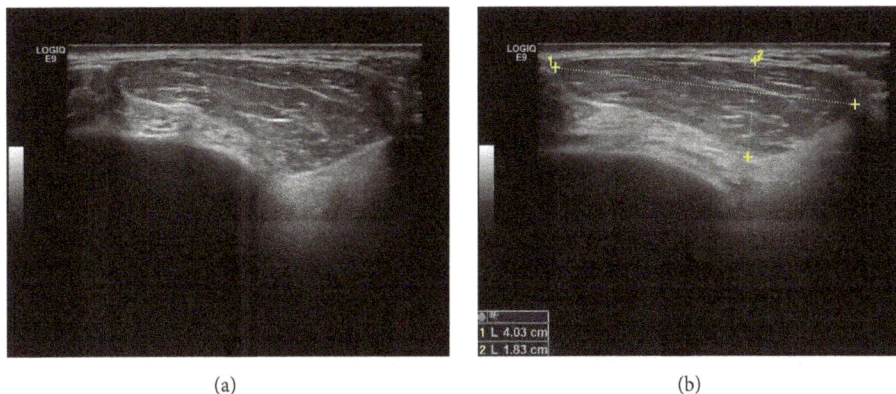

FIGURE 3: (a) Ultrasound image of the patient showing a well-defined, hypoechoic solid lesion in her superficial lobe of the parotid gland. The lesion had echogenic septas and acoustic empowerment over the posterior region. (b) The lesion was measured approximately 40 × 18 mm in size.

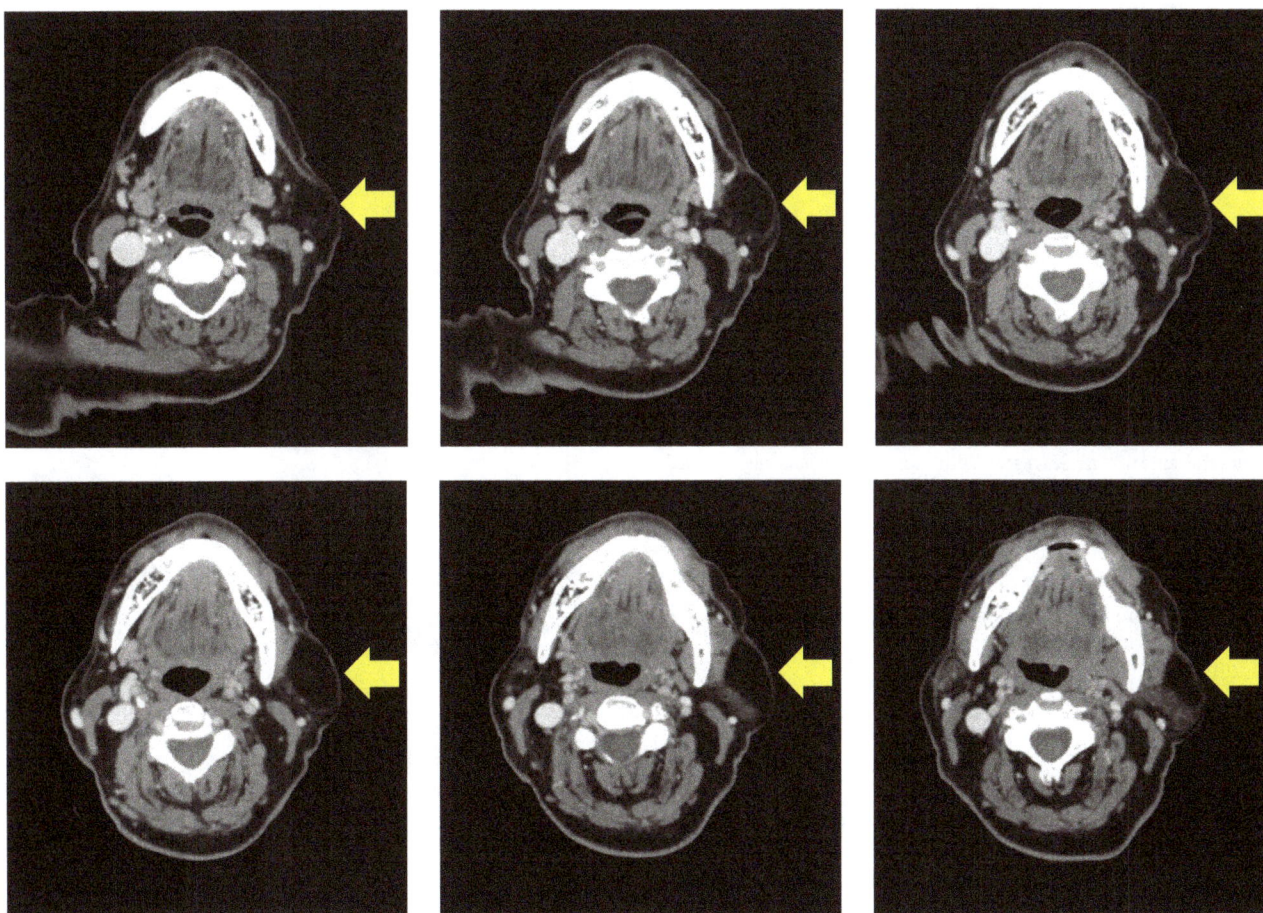

FIGURE 4: CT scans showed a low density homogeneous capsulated mass with sharp margins in the superficial lobe of the left parotid gland.

accurately distinguish between lipomas and liposarcomas [9]. While lipoma shows a homogeneous appearance in MRI images, liposarcoma appears more heterogeneous and is enhanced following injection of contrast medium [1]. Hence MRI with contrast enhancement can be performed to rule out the possibility of liposarcoma, when the patient is decided to be followed up.

Lipomas usually are not treated, because most of them are asymptomatic. Only for esthetic reasons or complaints like paresthesia, lipoma has to be removed surgically [16]. In this case, patient claimed to have pain in lesion area; however the pain was relieved after extraction of inflamed root fragments. Also diabetes may be effective as a cause of pain in this case. Differential diagnosis of neck swellings become very important in suspicious cases. The spread of head and neck carcinoma is similar to inflammatory disease, generally following an orderly lymphatic spread. Metastasis lymph node is also seen similar to this neck swelling [7]. In this case our patient's medical history included breast CA and neck swelling was suspicious about the metastasis. However advanced imaging methods revealed the presence of lipoma in parotid gland. This case emphasizes the need for the oral health care professionals to be familiar with the clinical manifestations and radiological findings of neck swellings and differential diagnosis of lipomas with other benign and malignant lesions.

Competing Interests

The authors declared that they have no conflict of interests.

Acknowledgments

The authors would like to acknowledge the patient and her relatives for their kind cooperation.

References

[1] M. Mesolella, F. Ricciardiello, F. Oliva, T. Abate, A. M. Lullo, and A. Marino, "Parotid lipoma: a case report," *Case Reports in Clinical Medicine*, vol. 3, no. 7, pp. 437–442, 2014.

[2] P. M. Som, M. P. Scherl, V. M. Rao, and H. F. Biller, "Rare presentations of ordinary lipomas of the head and neck: a review," *American Journal of Neuroradiology*, vol. 7, no. 4, pp. 657–664, 1986.

[3] F. Grecchi, I. Zollino, V. Candotto et al., "A case of lipoma of lateral anterior neck treated with surgical enucleation," *Dental Research Journal*, vol. 9, supplement 2, pp. S225–S228, 2012.

[4] Y. Kimura, N. Ishikawa, K. Goutsu, K. Kitamura, and S. Kishimoto, "Lipoma in the deep lobe of the parotid gland: a case report," *Auris Nasus Larynx*, vol. 29, no. 4, pp. 391–393, 2002.

[5] S. Nayak and P. Nayak, "Lipoma of the oral mucosa: a case report," *Archives of Orofacial Sciences*, vol. 6, no. 1, pp. 37–39, 2011.

[6] J.-W. Ryu, M.-C. Lee, N.-H. Myong et al., "Lipoma of the parotid gland," *Journal of Korean Medical Science*, vol. 11, no. 6, pp. 522–525, 1996.

[7] W. F. McGuirt, "Differential diagnosis of neck masses," in *Otolaryngology: Head Neck Surgery*, pp. 1686–1700, Mosby, St. Louis, Mo, USA, 1998.

[8] B. Hohlweg-Majert, M. C. Metzger, J. Dueker, W. Schupp, and D. Schulze, "Salivary gland lipomas: ultrasonographic and magnetic resonance imaging," *Journal of Craniofacial Surgery*, vol. 18, no. 6, pp. 1464–1466, 2007.

[9] D. M. Yousem, M. A. Kraut, and A. A. Chalian, "Major salivary gland imaging," *Radiology*, vol. 216, no. 1, pp. 19–29, 2000.

[10] İ. B. Arslan, S. Uluyol, S. Genç, T. Eruyar, S. Bulgurcu, and İ. Çukurova, "Diagnostic dilemma of parotid lipomas: imaging versus fine needle aspiration cytology," *Bosnian Journal of Basic Medical Sciences*, vol. 14, no. 4, pp. 250–253, 2014.

[11] M. K. Mittal, A. Malik, B. Sureka, and B. B. Thukral, "Cystic masses of neck: a pictorial review," *The Indian Journal of Radiology and Imaging*, vol. 22, no. 4, pp. 334–343, 2012.

[12] M. A. Furlong, J. C. Fanburg-Smith, and E. L. B. Childers, "Lipoma of the oral and maxillofacial region: site and sub-classification of 125 cases," *Oral Surgery, Oral Medicine, Oral Pathology, Oral Radiology and Endodontology*, vol. 98, no. 4, pp. 441–450, 2004.

[13] R. Köse and İ. İynen, "Lipoma of the superficial lobe of parotid gland: a case report and review of the literature," *European Journal of Plastic Surgery*, vol. 33, no. 4, pp. 215–218, 2010.

[14] T. Nagao, I. Sugano, Y. Ishida et al., "Sialolipoma: a report of seven cases of a new variant of salivary gland lipoma," *Histopathology*, vol. 38, no. 1, pp. 30–36, 2001.

[15] G. Keskin, E. Ustundag, and C. Ercin, "Multiple infiltrating lipomas of the tongue," *Journal of Laryngology and Otology*, vol. 116, no. 5, pp. 395–397, 2002.

[16] N. Fakhry, J. Michel, A. Varoquaux et al., "Is surgical excision of lipomas arising from the parotid gland systematically required?" *European Archives of Oto-Rhino-Laryngology*, vol. 269, no. 7, pp. 1839–1844, 2012.

35

A Giant-Cell Lesion with Cellular Cannibalism in the Mandible: Case Report and Review of Brown Tumors in Hyperparathyroidism

Lorenzo Azzi,[1] **Laura Cimetti,**[2] **Matteo Annoni,**[3] **Diego Anselmi,**[4]
Lucia Tettamanti,[1] **and Angelo Tagliabue**[1]

[1]*Department of Surgical and Morphological Sciences, University of Insubria, ASST dei Sette Laghi, Unit of Oral Pathology, Dental Clinic, Varese, Italy*
[2]*Department of Surgical and Morphological Sciences, University of Insubria, ASST dei Sette Laghi, Unit of Pathologic Anatomy, Varese, Italy*
[3]*Department of Surgical and Morphological Sciences, University of Insubria, ASST dei Sette Laghi, Unit of General Surgery 1, Varese, Italy*
[4]*Meditel, Medical Centre, Unit of Radiology, Saronno, Italy*

Correspondence should be addressed to Lorenzo Azzi; lorenzoazzi86@hotmail.com

Academic Editor: Junichi Asaumi

A small radiolucent area in the mandible was discovered in a 58-year-old woman with no oral complaints. The patient's history included only hypertension. The lesion was considered as an inflammatory cyst and was enucleated. Three months later, a CT revealed the presence of a cyst-like lesion in the mandible with thin expanded buccal cortical plate, localized erosion, and a polylobate appearance on the lingual aspect of the cortical plate. The histological diagnosis of the lesion was central giant-cell granuloma (CGCG). The lesion was thoroughly enucleated. Nevertheless, another X-ray carried out six months later revealed multiple bilateral osteolytic areas throughout the jaw. In addition, widespread cortical plate erosion was observed, as well as signs of root resorption and periodontal enlargement. There was no sign of neurological involvement, although the nerves appeared to be dislocated. After full blood chemistry analysis and detailed collection of radiographs, the final diagnosis was brown tumors in primary hyperparathyroidism. This case report demonstrates how dental clinicians may be the first-line specialists who identify a complex systemic disease before other clinicians. Finally, it highlights the role of cellular cannibalism in predicting the clinical aggressiveness of brown tumors as well as in other giant-cell lesions.

1. Introduction

General dentists commonly believe that small, homogeneous, radiolucent areas, which are sometimes observed during X-ray examinations, are almost certainly odontogenic cysts.

Indeed, cleavage and enucleation are only occasionally followed up with histopathological analysis. Although odontogenic cysts are very common lesions in routine practice, with radicular cysts accounting for more than 50% of cases, it should be remembered that many other diseases can affect the jaws, some more frequently than others [1].

Some of these lesions might be more aggressive, with a multilocular shape, root resorption, cortical expansion, and thinning, as well as multiple radiolucencies at times.

By way of an example, keratocystic odontogenic tumor (KCOT) [2, 3], aneurysmal bone cysts [4], intrabony haemangiomas [5], florid cemento-osseous dysplasia [6], Paget's disease [7], Langerhans cells histiocytosis [8, 9], and multiple myeloma may be detected in the jaws.

In addition, local metastasis from a primary carcinoma arising in a cyst, a primary carcinoma of the bone [10], or distant metastasis from unknown primary sites [11] can also occur within the jaws.

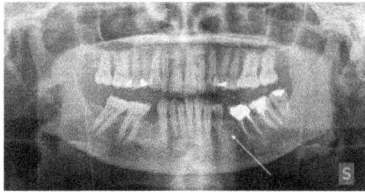

FIGURE 1: Initial clinical manifestation. A small radiolucent area (arrow) is revealed near mobile dental element 34. Chronic periodontitis is present.

Even though most of the pathological entities mentioned above are very rare individually, it should be remembered that it is not uncommon to detect one of them in clinical practice.

Besides, detailed clinical and histopathological evaluation is imperative and must be performed when a radiolucency is detected by chance during an X-ray examination, even if it strongly resembles an odontogenic cyst.

Moreover, multidisciplinary diagnostic work may be required to further investigate whether there are any systemic implications or misdiagnosed malignancies underlying an osteolytic lesion of dubious origin.

This paper aims at reporting a case of an apparently innocuous cyst-like lesion of the mandible in a middle-aged woman and the subsequent diagnostic and therapeutic management which required the involvement of a multidisciplinary team.

2. Case Presentation

A 58-year-old woman with no oral complaints visited our dental surgery for a routine check-up.

Chronic periodontitis was detected, associated with mobility of the left permanent mandibular first premolar. The orthopantomogram only showed a small radiolucent area adjacent to the dental element (Figure 1). The patient's history only included hypertension with the use of an ACE inhibitor and a diuretic drug. The tooth was extracted and the patient was seen again three months later to evaluate the bone healing process, with a view to fitting a dental implant after a full dental-hygiene program. The CT scan revealed the presence of a radiolucent cyst-like lesion in the mandible with thin expanded buccal cortical plate and localized erosion and a polylobate appearance on the lingual aspect of the cortical plate (Figures 2(a)–2(c)). The left permanent mandibular second incisor and canine gave a negative result during pulp testing. The teeth were extracted and the bony lesion underwent thorough curettage.

The histological description of the sample reported the presence of an aggressive lesion with widely distributed giant cells (Figures 3(a)–3(d)). Moreover, several giant cells displayed scattered cannibalistic processes, in the absence of bizarre figures like those reported in complex cannibalism of OSCC (Figures 3(e) and 3(f)).

The pathologist provided the diagnosis of central giant-cell granuloma (CGCG).

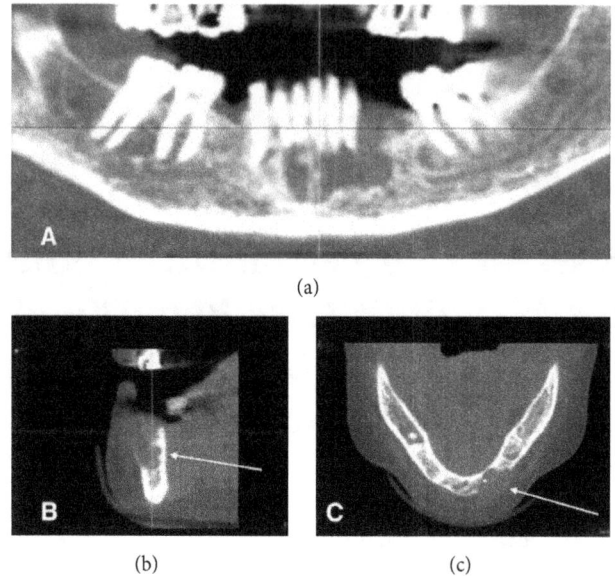

FIGURE 2: Relapse of the lesion. (a) The next examination, three months later, revealed the presence of a radiolucent cyst-like lesion in the mandible with mildly defined and irregular borders. (b) The CT radial view showed lingual cortical plate with a polylobate appearance and erosion of the buccal cortical plate (arrow). (c) The CT axial view highlighted the buccal erosion of the cortical plate (arrow).

Nevertheless, another X-ray carried out six months later revealed multiple bilateral radiolucencies throughout the jaw, in both the molar and the premolar regions. In addition, widespread cortical plate erosion was observed and the left permanent mandibular first molar showed signs of root resorption, while the right permanent mandibular second molar showed periodontal ligament enlargement. There was no sign of neurological involvement, although the nerves appeared to be dislocated (Figures 4(a)–4(d)).

2.1. Differential Diagnosis. Given the latest clinical and radiographic presentation of the lesion, several pathological entities were considered for differential diagnosis.

2.1.1. Keratocystic Odontogenic Tumor (KCOT). KCOT is associated with frequent multiple relapses of the lesion after unsuccessful complete curettage, but the histological predominance of giant cells within the pathologic tissue excluded this hypothesis [2].

2.1.2. Aggressive or Malignant Ameloblastoma. The same consideration was made as regards an aggressive variant of ameloblastoma, since its histological appearance is completely different, even if its radiographic behavior can be similar [12].

2.1.3. Aneurysmal Bone Cyst. Aneurysmal bone cysts may contain many giant cells but show far more cellular pleomorphism, hyperchromatism, and a variety of other cells often of indeterminate appearance [4].

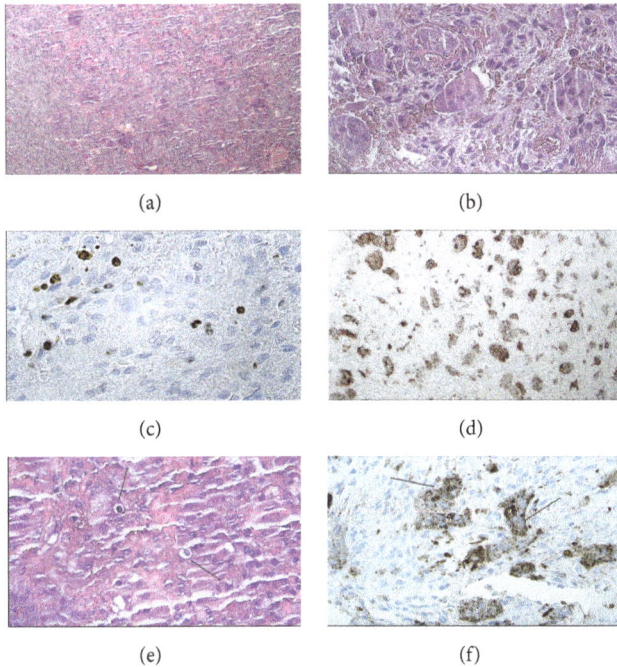

FIGURE 3: Central giant-cell granuloma (CGCG). (a) A lobulated mass of proliferating connective tissue containing many giant cells. (b) A larger view of the giant cell containing more than ten nuclei each. (c) Ki-67 indicates a low mitotic index. The lesion is defined as locally aggressive but cannot be considered as a true neoplasm. (d) CD68 antibody indicates the giant cells deriving from the monocytic-macrophagic line. (e) The so-called "cannibal cells" (arrows) indicate an aggressive CGCG and could suggest likely recurrence. (f) A larger view of the monocytic-derived cannibal giant cells highlighted with CD68.

2.1.4. Fibroosseous Lesions.

Fibrous dysplasia may present some giant-cell foci, but its radiographic appearance, histological features, and behavior are distinctive [13].

Giant-cell lesions can be present in Paget's disease, but in this case there was no sign of pagetoid bone [7].

2.1.5. Osteosarcoma.

Osteosarcoma contains numerous giant cells but displays far more cellular pleomorphism, hyperchromatism, and a variety of other cells often of indeterminate appearance [14].

2.1.6. Metastasis from a Distant Malignancy.

Metastasis from a misdiagnosed primary malignancy could arise in the jaw, but this is rare and should produce neurological complications in the early stages, with more aggressive destructive behavior in the jaws and alveolar ridges. Histological analysis could be used to determine the primary tissue from which the malignancy originated [11].

2.2. Clinical Management.

The multiple lesions described in Figures 4(a)–4(d) required maxillofacial evaluation for surgery, but a decision was made to verify whether the pathology was limited to the mandible or whether other body areas were involved. As the patient had had X-rays of other

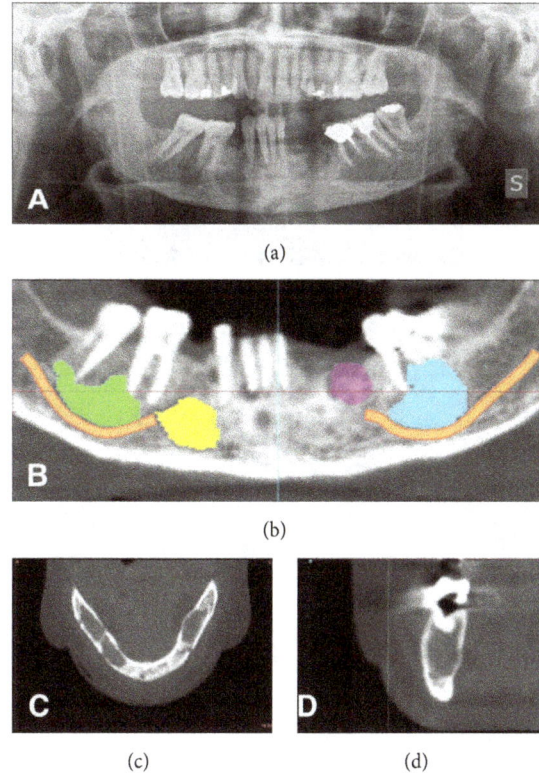

FIGURE 4: Radiographic appearance after six months. (a) Multiple osteolytic areas involving the mandible bilaterally revealed by another orthopantomogram (b–d) and CT scan six months after.

areas of the body during the same period, they were collected together and compared.

MRI and CT scans of the patient's left knee revealed the presence of a cyst-like, polylobate lesion in the kneecap, with regular borders, cortical thinning, and localized erosion (Figures 5(a) and 5(b)). The radiologist affirmed that the lesion was very similar to those discovered in the mandible. Furthermore, chondrocalcinosis was noted in the right shoulder. The patient reported asthaenia, muscular tension, and mild depression. It was advisable to complete the head examination by prescribing an X-ray of the cranial vault, which showed multiple osteolytic areas with a salt-and-pepper appearance (Figure 5(c)).

A full blood chemistry analysis, including a full range of bone metabolism parameters, was prescribed. The alkaline phosphatase levels were found to be raised (374 U/L) and mild anaemia was present (RBC 3.51 $10^6/\mu$L; Hb 10.1 g/dL; HCT 31.6%). However, the most important alterations involved the parathormone (PTH 1014 pg/mL) and calcium (13.1 mg/dL) levels (Table 1).

With this data, the final diagnosis was brown tumors, with suspected primary hyperparathyroidism. Due to hypercalcemia, the patient was admitted immediately and underwent perfusion with saline water to prevent the risk of complications to the neurological and cardiovascular districts. Once hypercalcemia was treated, a neck ultrasound revealed the presence of a nonhomogeneous tumefaction involving the

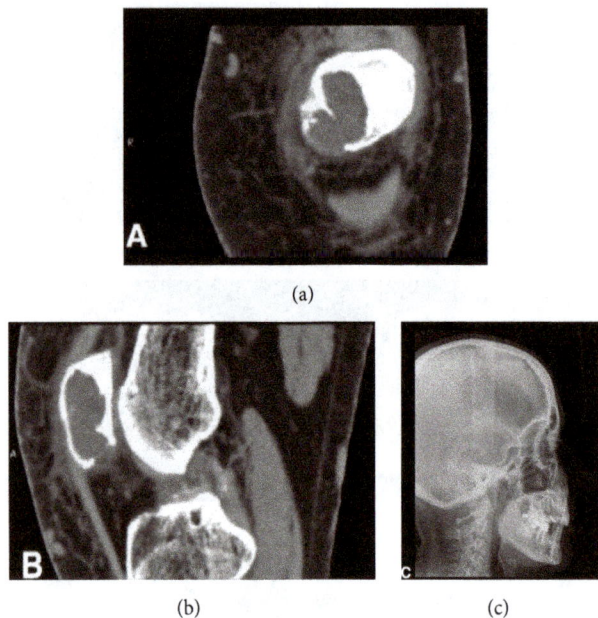

(a)

(b)   (c)

FIGURE 5: Systemic correlation. (a and b) A CT scan of the left knee highlighted the presence of an osteolytic, cyst-like, polylobate lesion which resembles those encountered in the mandible. (c) "Salt-and-pepper" appearance of the cranial vault.

TABLE 1: Blood chemistry analysis. Bone metabolism was altered, parathormone was critically raised, and the calcium levels posed a high risk of heart failure.

Investigation	Results	Normal values
ESR	26 mm	<15
Alkaline phosphatase	374 U/L	40–150
Parathormone	*1014* pg/mL	15–68
Calcium	13,1 mg/dL	8,4–10,2

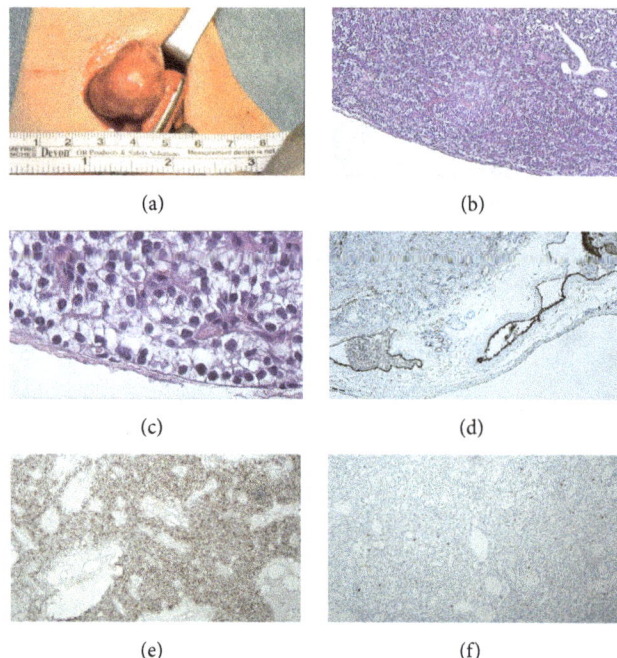

(a)   (b)

(c)   (d)

(e)   (f)

FIGURE 6: Parathyroid adenoma. (a) The patient underwent minimally invasive video-assisted parathyroidectomy (MIVAP) with intraoperative PTH determinations (baseline and 20 minutes after tumor removal) and continuous intraoperative nerve monitoring. A left inferior parathyroid adenoma was successfully removed. The baseline PTH measurement was 678 pg, and 20 minutes after excision the PTH serum level was 47 pg. Postoperative progress was uneventful. The patient was discharged the day after the operation with the appropriate prescriptions. (b and c) Parathyroid adenoma with clear cells at a low and high grade of amplification; a thin fibrous capsule is present. (d) CD34 endothelial staining showed no evidence of angioinvasion. (e) PTH staining confirmed the functional activity of the tumor. (f) Ki-67 expression was low, confirming the benign nature of the tumor.

left inferior parathyroid gland, while the other glands were normal in size and trophism. This finding ruled out the presence of primary parathyroid hyperplasia. Primary hyperparathyroidism is often associated with adenoma, but also a functional carcinoma could not be ruled out until histopathological evaluation.

General surgeons proceeded to remove the parathyroid lesion, which received a histopathological diagnosis of atypical parathyroid adenoma (Figures 6(a)–6(f)).

Another two orthopantomograms carried out 4 months and 2 years later, respectively, showed advanced and complete healing of the bony lesions in the mandible (Figure 7). The patient was able to avoid maxillofacial surgery with resection, which would not have resolved the problem, since the origin of the condition was primary hyperparathyroidism.

3. Discussion

Hyperparathyroidism is defined as excessive parathyroid hormone (PTH) production. PTH is normally produced by the parathyroid glands in response to a decrease in serum

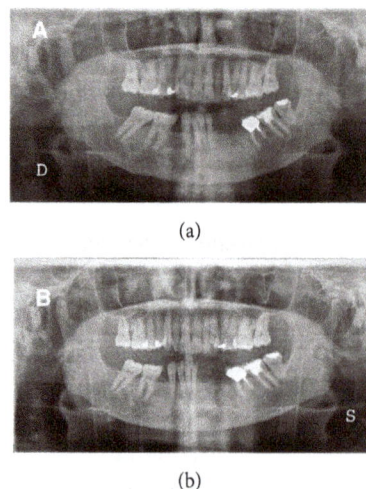

(a)

(b)

FIGURE 7: Radiographic appearance after four months and two years. (a) Signs of bone healing after four months after surgical excision of the parathyroid adenoma. (b) Complete recovery of the bony tissue two years after the operation.

calcium levels. Hyperparathyroidism can be classified as primary, secondary, and, according to several authors, tertiary.

Primary hyperparathyroidism is uncontrolled PTH production not associated with feedback regulation of the serum ionized calcium level. Most patients with primary hyperparathyroidism are over 60 years old [15]. Women are two to four times more likely to have this condition than men. The condition is typically identified during routine serological testing, and the majority of patients are relatively asymptomatic.

3.1. Aetiology. Primary hyperparathyroidism is usually the result of parathyroid adenoma (80–90% of cases), parathyroid hyperplasia (10–15% of cases), or, very rarely, functional parathyroid carcinoma (1% of cases).

Parathyroid adenoma is usually limited to a single gland, with a fibrous capsule generally separating it from the surrounding normal gland tissue, which could appear atrophic in some instances.

Microscopically, the adenoma can be composed of chief cells, oxyphilic cells, or clear cells.

Parathyroid hyperplasia can be divided into chief-cell hyperplasia and clear-cell hyperplasia.

Chief-cell hyperplasia is usually linked to type 1 or 2a multiple endocrine neoplasia (MEN) and is characterized by an increase in volume of all four parathyroid glands. On the contrary, the less frequent clear-cell hyperplasia is not hereditary and it is not linked to MEN. It is characterized by an enormous increase in volume of the glands, due to the combination of hyperplasia and hypertrophy involving the clear cells.

Parathyroid carcinoma is rare and can be differentiated from an adenoma since it shows a trabecular structure and spindle-shaped neoplastic cells, as well as a high mitotic index. It is aggressive and leads to cervical lymph node enlargement and vocal cord paralysis. It can sometimes be a functional carcinoma, producing PTH [16].

Independently of the three abovementioned conditions, the result is an uncontrolled increase in PTH serum levels, which is defined as primary hyperparathyroidism.

3.2. Clinical Features. Primary hyperparathyroidism is a complex condition which involves several body districts and requires a multidisciplinary approach both for diagnosis and for treatment.

The increased serum PTH level leads to excessive osteoclastic activity, with the release of calcium, phosphorus, and hydroxyproline due to the generalized demineralization of the bone district.

The clinical signs and symptoms of primary hyperparathyroidism are the expression of the main feature of the pathology, hypercalcemia. The increased calcium level may cause salt to be deposited in the soft tissues, with the consequent involvement of sclera (band keratitis), tendons (calcific tendonitis), joint cartilage (chondrocalcinosis and arthralgia), kidney parenchyma (nephrocalcinosis), and the pancreas.

PTH stimulates calcium tubular resorption, but serum levels exceeding 12 mg/dL lead to the onset of hypercalciuria.

On the other hand, PTH promotes phosphorus renal elimination, and so hypophosphaturia and hypophosphataemia are observed. Kidney stones are the most common sign of kidney involvement in primary hyperparathyroidism. Furthermore, PTH increases calcium absorption in the bowel due to the augmented conversion of 25(OH) D into 1,25(OH)2 D.

As a result, hypercalcemia is maintained, as mentioned above, by increased bone resorption, increased calcium absorption in the bowel, and inadequate kidney elimination of calcium.

Hypercalcemia leads to functional alterations in the central nervous system, with ideation disorders, recent memory loss, emotional lability, and sleepiness.

In severe cases, a state of confusion, drowsiness, and coma may occur.

Other clinical signs and symptoms of hypercalcemia are intense asthaenia and fatigue, especially along the proximal musculature of the limbs, vomiting, epigastric pain, duodenal ulcer, hypertension, and, in the case of hypercalcemic crisis, bradycardia and heart failure.

A variety of osseous changes may occur in conjunction with hyperparathyroidism. One of the first clinical signs of the disease can be seen during radiographic examination, in the subperiosteal resorption of the phalanges of the index and middle fingers. Generalized loss of the lamina dura surrounding the roots of teeth is also seen as an early manifestation of the condition. Alterations in trabecular pattern characteristically develop next. A decrease in trabecular density and blurring of the normal trabecular density occur, often resulting in a "ground glass" appearance.

3.3. Brown Tumors, Giant-Cell Lesions, and Cellular Cannibalism. With persistent disease, other osseous lesions develop, such as the so-called brown tumors of hyperparathyroidism [17]. These lesions derive their name from the colour of the tissue specimen, which is usually dark red-brown because of the abundant haemorrhaging and haemosiderin deposits within the tumor. These lesions appear radiographically as well-demarcated unilocular or multilocular radiolucent patches. They commonly affect the mandible, clavicle, ribs, and pelvis. They may be solitary but are often multiple, and long-standing lesions may produce significant cortical expansion. The most severe skeletal manifestation of chronic hyperparathyroidism is known as osteitis fibrosa cystica (Von Recklinghausen's disease of bone [18]), a condition that develops from the central degeneration and fibrosis of long-standing brown tumors. Brown tumors cannot be reliably distinguished from nonendocrine central giant-cell granulomas (CGCGs).

CGCGs of the jaw are uncommon. They account for 0.17% of oral biopsies reported by Waldron and Shafer [19]. They are more common in women, with a 3 : 1 F : M ratio. It should be considered that they are most frequent in patients under 30s, and this feature is useful to distinguish them from brown tumors. The jaw is the most common site. They were first described by Jaffe as giant-cell reparative granulomas [20], as they were thought to represent a reparative process.

However, it has now been ascertained that there is no granuloma formation in the histological sense, and they are not linked to a reparative process after trauma or cyst removal. On the contrary, they may grow rapidly and be mildly destructive instead of reparative. In 40% of cases, CGCGs show an aggressive behavior such as perforation of the cortical bone and root resorption. One distinctive histological feature is the cannibalistic component among the giant cells in the lesion [21]. This variant is known as aggressive CGCG and may have been a suitable diagnosis in this case.

Cellular cannibalism is defined as a large cell enclosing a slightly smaller one within its cytoplasm and is a characteristic morphological feature exclusively seen in aggressive malignancies, such as breast carcinoma, giant-cell carcinoma of the lung, gall bladder carcinoma, endometrial stromal carcinoma, malignant thymoma, and malignant melanoma [22]. It is well correlated with the aggressiveness, degree of anaplasia, invasiveness, and metastatic potential of the malignancy.

Sarode et al. were the first to describe cellular cannibalism in oral squamous cell carcinoma. Besides, they reported bizarre morphological appearances of cannibalism, wherein one malignant cell was engulfing the other and this complex was further engulfed by another cell or one cell was engulfing two cells at a time. This kind of feature was named complex cannibalism [23].

Cannibalism in malignant tumor is caused due to a shift in the metabolic pathway that encourages selection of certain cell phenotypes that are able to survive in the caustic environment. These selected malignant cells are highly virulent and cannibalize other malignant cells to survive and progress in adverse conditions within the microenvironment such as hypoxia, low nutrient supply, and acidity.

However, cellular cannibalism has been reported in a benign tumor called the giant-cell tumor of the tendon sheath [24].

A recent study by S. C. Sarode and G. S. Sarode demonstrated that mean cannibalistic giant-cell frequency was greater in aggressive CGCG compared to nonaggressive CGCG. Thus, the presence of cannibalistic giant cells can be used to predict the biological behavior of giant-cell lesions [21].

The biological behavior of CGCG of the jaw ranges from a quiescent lesion with the absence of symptoms, no root resorption or cortical perforation, slow growth, and low recurrence rate (nonaggressive CGCG) to an aggressive pathological process, characterized by pain, rapid growth, root resorption, cortical perforation, and high tendency to recur (aggressive CGCG).

The mean cannibalistic giant-cells frequency was greater in aggressive CGCG than in nonaggressive CGCG. Thus, it can be used for predicting the biological behavior of CGCG.

In giant-cell lesions, the cannibalistic cells are derived from a monocyte-macrophage lineage and resemble osteoclasts (CD68+). Thus, these cells possess the inherent property of engulfment, which is responsible for the cannibalism of stromal tumor cells and represents high metabolic activity in giant-cell lesions [22].

In this case report, we presented a case of cellular cannibalism within brown tumors of the mandible.

The cannibalistic activity looked classic and the lesions showed the same features of an aggressive CGCG: root resorption, cortical expansion, periodontal enlargement, and multiple relapses. The presence of a cannibalistic activity within the histologic sample confirmed the presence of clinical aggressiveness of the lesion and the relapse which followed surgical excision.

3.4. Diagnosis. Primary hyperparathyroidism is diagnosed by means of blood chemistry testing: raised PTH, hypercalcemia, hypophosphataemia, hyperuricaemia, anaemia, raised ESR, hypomagnesaemia, hypokalaemia, and hyperchloremic acidosis.

An X-ray of the urinary tract can reveal the presence of kidney stones or minor calcifications involving the renal parenchyma.

During the later stages, cranial X-rays show alterations within the bones of the cranial vault, which reveal focal areas of demineralization as opposed to sclerotic sites. This is the so-called salt-and-pepper skull.

Ultimately, it is necessary to identify the primary parathyroid disorder: ultrasound, CT, and ^{201}Tl and ^{99}Tc double-track scintigraphy are used for this purpose [25].

If a parathyroid adenoma is not found, suspected PTH-like peptide (PTHrP) production in a paraneoplastic syndrome must be taken into consideration [26].

3.5. Management and Treatment. Treatment involves surgical excision of the affected parathyroid.

However, hypercalcemia must be treated with saline solution infusion, diuretics, and other symptomatic treatments to restore normal electrolyte levels.

Differential diagnoses of hypercalcemia also include vitamin D intoxication, multiple myeloma, sarcoidosis, vitamin A intoxication, Burnett syndrome (milk-alkali syndrome), thyrotoxicosis, prolonged immobilization, adrenocortical insufficiency, and Paget's disease. In all these cases, PTH levels are below normal, while hypercalcemia may be absent in several cases [27].

When an osteolytic lesion is diagnosed as a CGCG, the dental clinician should consider the differential diagnosis of brown tumor in hyperparathyroidism. Differential diagnosis is only possible by means of blood chemistry analysis, as mentioned above.

The decision to surgically excise brown tumors once hyperparathyroidism has been diagnosed should be made after enucleation of the parathyroid adenoma to prevent unsuccessful surgical procedures, which could lead to deterioration in the condition with more aggressive relapses.

However, dental clinicians are commonly thought to proceed with surgical excision following the initial histological diagnosis of CGCG.

4. Conclusion

This case report and review shows, on the one hand, the importance of multidisciplinary management of giant-cell lesions affecting the jaws, while, on the other hand, it demonstrates how dental clinicians may be the first-line specialists who identify a complex systemic disease before other clinicians. It is therefore essential for dental clinicians to communicate properly and promptly with other specialists in the event of a suspected systemic disease primarily expressed in the oral cavity.

Finally, the presence of cannibalistic activity in the monocyte-macrophage derived giant cells in brown tumors can be considered as a prognostic feature to predict the clinical aggressiveness of the lesion and the recurrence rate.

Disclosure

The clinical case was shown during an oral presentation at the 5th International Conference and Exhibition on Pathology, 9–11 May 2016, Chicago.

Competing Interests

The authors declare that there are no competing interests regarding the publication of this paper.

Acknowledgments

Professor Angelo Tagliabue is Dean of the Department of Surgical and Morphological Sciences, Università degli Studi dell'Insubria. Professor Marina Tettamanti supervised the revision process in the English language.

References

[1] E. Peker, F. Öğütlü, I. Karaca, E. Gültekin, and M. Çakir, "A 5 year retrospective study of biopsied jaw lesions with the assessment of concordance between clinical and histopathological diagnoses," *Journal of Oral and Maxillofacial Pathology*, vol. 20, no. 1, pp. 78–85, 2016.

[2] N. R. Johnson, M. D. Batstone, and N. W. Savage, "Management and recurrence of keratocystic odontogenic tumor: a systematic review," *Oral Surgery, Oral Medicine, Oral Pathology and Oral Radiology*, vol. 116, no. 4, pp. e271–e276, 2013.

[3] T. I. Berge, S. B. Helland, A. Sælen et al., "Pattern of recurrence of nonsyndromic keratocystic odontogenic tumors," *Oral Surgery, Oral Medicine, Oral Pathology and Oral Radiology*, vol. 122, no. 1, pp. 10–16, 2016.

[4] A. B. Urs, J. Augustine, and H. Chawla, "Aneurysmal bone cyst of the jaws: clinicopathological study," *Journal of Maxillofacial and Oral Surgery*, vol. 13, no. 4, pp. 458–463, 2014.

[5] R. Syal, I. Tyagi, A. Goyal, S. Barai, and A. Parihar, "Multiple intraosseous hemangiomas—investigation and role of N-butylcyanoacrylate in management," *Head and Neck*, vol. 29, no. 5, pp. 512–517, 2007.

[6] Y. Higuchi, N. Nakamura, and H. Tashiro, "Clinicopathologic study of cemento-osseous dysplasia producing cysts of the mandible: report of four cases," *Oral Surgery, Oral Medicine, Oral Pathology*, vol. 65, no. 3, pp. 339–342, 1988.

[7] K. Karunakaran, P. Murugesan, G. Rajeshwar, and S. Babu, "Paget's disease of the mandible," *Journal of Oral and Maxillofacial Pathology*, vol. 16, no. 1, pp. 107–109, 2012.

[8] V. Panis, N. Nikitakis, A. Daskalopoulos, T. Maragkou, K. Tsiklakis, and A. Sklavounou, "Langerhans cell histiocytosis mimicking aggressive periodontitis: challenges in diagnosis and

management," *Quintessence International*, vol. 47, pp. 731–738, 2016.

[9] B.-D. Lee, W. Lee, J. Lee, and H.-J. Son, "Eosinophilic granuloma in the anterior mandible mimicking radicular cyst," *Imaging Science in Dentistry*, vol. 43, no. 2, pp. 117–122, 2013.

[10] J.-W. Huang, H.-Y. Luo, Q. Li, and T.-J. Li, "Primary intraosseous squamous cell carcinoma of the jaws. Clinicopathologic presentation and prognostic factors," *Archives of Pathology and Laboratory Medicine*, vol. 133, no. 11, pp. 1834–1840, 2009.

[11] A. A. Owosho, B. Xu, A. Kadempour et al., "Metastatic solid tumors to the jaw and oral soft tissue: a retrospective clinical analysis of 44 patients from a single institution," *Journal of Cranio-Maxillofacial Surgery*, vol. 44, no. 8, pp. 1047–1053, 2016.

[12] R. A. Almeida, E. S. Andrade, J. C. Barbalho, A. Vajgel, and B. C. Vasconcelos, "Recurrence rate following for primary multicystic ameloblastoma: systematic review and meta-analysis," *International Journal of Oral and Maxillofacial Surgery*, vol. 45, pp. 359–367, 2016.

[13] J. Li, H. Li, X. Liu, and Z. Han, "Surgical treatment of polyostotic craniomaxillofacial fibrous dysplasia in adult: a case report and review of the literature," *International Journal of Clinical and Experimental Medicine*, vol. 8, no. 9, pp. 16756–16764, 2015.

[14] L. M. Sun, Q. F. Zhang, N. Tang, X. Y. Mi, and X. S. Qiu, "Giant cell rich osteosarcoma of the mandible with abundant spindle cells and osteoclast-like giant cells mimicking malignancy in giant cell tumor," *International Journal of Clinical and Experimental Pathology*, vol. 8, pp. 9718–9722, 2015.

[15] R. W. Gasser, "Clinical aspects of primary hyperparathyroidism: clinical manifestations, diagnosis and therapy," *Wiener Medizinische Wochenschrift*, vol. 163, pp. 397–402, 2013.

[16] J. Goswamy, M. Lei, and R. Simo, "Parathyroid carcinoma," *Current Opinion in Otolaryngology & Head & Neck Surgery*, vol. 24, no. 2, pp. 155–162, 2016.

[17] K. Triantafillidou, L. Zouloumis, G. Karakinaris, E. Kalimeras, and F. Iordanidis, "Brown tumors of the jaws associated with primary or secondary hyperparathyroidism. A clinical study and review of the literature," *American Journal of Otolaryngology—Head and Neck Medicine and Surgery*, vol. 27, no. 4, pp. 281–286, 2006.

[18] A. Caniggia, C. Gennari, R. Guideri, and L. Cesari, "Comparison between the results of radiocalcium studies and histological findings in a case of primary hyperparathyroidism (osteitis fibrosa cystica generalisata of von Recklinghausen) before and after removal of parathyroid adenoma," *Journal of Clinical Endocrinology and Metabolism*, vol. 26, no. 8, pp. 867–874, 1966.

[19] C. A. Waldron and W. G. Shafer, "The central giant cell reparative granuloma of the jaws. An analysis of 38 cases," *American Journal of Clinical Pathology*, vol. 45, no. 4, pp. 437–447, 1966.

[20] H. L. Jaffe, "Giant-cell reparative granuloma, traumatic bone cyst, and fibrous (fibro-osseous) dysplasia of the jawbones," *Oral Surgery, Oral Medicine, Oral Pathology*, vol. 6, no. 1, pp. 159–175, 1953.

[21] S. C. Sarode and G. S. Sarode, "Cellular cannibalism in central and peripheral giant cell granuloma of the oral cavity can predict biological behavior of the lesion," *Journal of Oral Pathology and Medicine*, vol. 43, no. 6, pp. 459–463, 2014.

[22] G. S. Sarode, S. C. Sarode, S. Gawande et al., "Cellular cannibalism in giant cells of central giant cell granuloma of jaw bones and giant cell tumors of long bones," *Journal of Investigative and Clinical Dentistry*, 2016.

[23] G. S. Sarode, S. C. Sarode, and S. Karmarkar, "Complex canni-balism: an unusual finding in oral squamous cell carcinoma," *Oral Oncology*, vol. 48, no. 2, pp. e4–e6, 2012.

[24] A. Fernandez-Flores, "Cannibalism in a benign soft tissue tumor (giant-cell tumor of the tendon sheath, localized type): a study of 66 cases," *Romanian Journal of Morphology and Embryology*, vol. 53, no. 1, pp. 15–22, 2012.

[25] I. Simón, R. Simó, J. Mesa, S. Aguadé, L. Boada, and D. G. Sureda, "Subtraction scintigraphy with thallium 201 chloride and technetium-99m pertechnetate versus high resolution ultrasonography in the localization of the parathyroid glands in primary hyperparathyroidism," *Medicina Clinica*, vol. 99, no. 20, pp. 774–777, 1992.

[26] H. M. Docherty and D. A. Heath, "Multiple forms of parathy-roid hormone-like proteins in a human tumour," *Journal of Molecular Endocrinology*, vol. 2, no. 1, pp. 11–20, 1989.

[27] P. Machenahalli and K. Shotliff, "Problem based review: the patient with hypercalcaemia," *Acute Medicine*, vol. 14, no. 3, pp. 138–141, 2015.

Laser Photobiomodulation for a Complex Patient with Severe Hydroxyurea-Induced Oral Ulcerations

Marco Cabras,[1] **Adriana Cafaro,**[1] **Alessio Gambino,**[1] **Roberto Broccoletti,**[1]
Ercole Romagnoli,[2] **Davide Marina,**[3] **and Paolo G. Arduino**[1]

[1]*Department of Surgical Sciences, CIR-Dental School, University of Turin, Turin, Italy*
[2]*Department of Surgical and Diagnostic Sciences (DISC), University of Genoa, Genoa, Italy*
[3]*Private Practice, Milan, Italy*

Correspondence should be addressed to Paolo G. Arduino; paologiacomo.arduino@unito.it

Academic Editor: Pia L. Jornet

Patients affected by polycythemia vera (PV), a myeloproliferative neoplasm characterized by an elevated red blood cell mass, are at high risk of vascular and thrombotic complications. Conventional therapeutic options aim at reducing vascular and thrombotic risk; low-dose aspirin and phlebotomy are first-line recommendations, for patients at low risk of thrombotic events, whereas cytoreductive therapy, usually hydroxyurea (HU) or interferon alpha, is recommended for high-risk patients. In the present study, we report the case of a patient with persistent oral ulcerations, possibly related to long-lasting HU treatment, firstly treated with topic and systemic corticosteroids and then more effectively with the addition of low-level laser therapy. Laser photobiomodulation has achieved pain control and has contributed to the healing of oral ulcers without any adverse effect; this has permitted a reduction in the dose of systemic corticosteroids and the suspension of the use of the topic ones, due to the long-term stability of oral health, even after the interruption of low-level laser therapy sessions.

1. Introduction

Patients affected by polycythemia vera (PV), a myeloproliferative neoplasm characterized by an elevated red blood cell mass, are at high risk of vascular and thrombotic complications; they also have reduced quality of life due to a substantial symptom burden that includes pruritus, fatigue, constitutional symptoms, microvascular disturbances, and bleeding. Conventional therapeutic options aim at reducing vascular and thrombotic risk; low-dose aspirin and phlebotomy are first-line recommendations, for patients at low risk of thrombotic events, whereas cytoreductive therapy, usually hydroxyurea (HU) or interferon alpha, is recommended for high-risk patients [1].

Mucocutaneous ulcers are possible complicating adverse effects caused by HU; these lesions can appear right after the beginning of HU therapy or can be a later effect, with similar clinical presentation in both situations. The oral alterations are uncommon, but they could have a greater clinical impact because of severe pain and feeding or speaking impairment [2, 3].

Data from literature suggest that oral ulceration is the first occurring oral side effect of hydroxyurea, usually developing after a variable period of time since administration, ranging between 5 months and up to 3 years. Mucocutaneous lesions have been diagnosed in 167 of 3411 patients on hydroxyurea with Philadelphia-chromosome-negative chronic myeloproliferative neoplasms in a large Italian cohort [4]; of this subgroup, 27 patients presented oral ulcerations. Almost half of these patients needed to discontinue hydroxyurea with resolution of lesions in about one month. The remaining patients received local therapy, consisting of mouthwash with folic acid and vitamin A, and they obtained some symptomatic improvement. However, complete healing was achieved only after HU dose reduction or suspension in an average time frame of three months.

Other studies [5, 6] have reported 12.5% to 13% prevalence of mucocutaneous involvement in smaller cohorts of 40 and

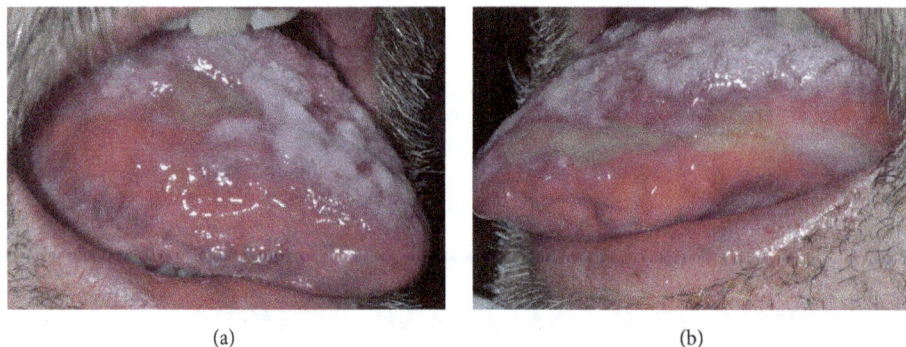

(a)   (b)

FIGURE 1: Erosive lesions presented in (a) and (b) lateral border of the tongue.

158 patients, respectively, including mucosal symptoms, such as pain and burning sensation, atrophy, and ulcers.

Actually, dose reduction or suspension of HU, if possible, can be considered as the most effective available measure [2, 4–6].

In the present study, we report the case of a patient with persistent oral ulcerations, possibly related to long-lasting HU treatment, firstly treated with topic and systemic corticosteroids and then more effectively with the addition of low-level laser therapy.

2. Case Presentation

A 72-year-old male (diagnosed with PV in 1994 and treated with HU since 1995) was referred to the Oral Medicine Section of the Turin University in March 2014 because of severe tongue and lips pain and difficulty in feeding and speaking. At the time being, HU dosage consisted of three 500 mg tablets daily. At physical examination, extensive ulcerations on the tongue and lips were observed (Figure 1). Based on the clinical appearance and the topography of the lesions, a differential diagnosis between HU related ulcers and erosive lichen was posed. However, advice against the execution of the oral biopsy came directly from the oncologist, due to the very high level of platelets (more than $1.000.000/\mu L$) detected in the patient's blood.

Due to the impossibility of solving the diagnostic dilemma through histopathological examination, we opted for an *ex juvantibus* approach and proceeded to administer an appropriate therapy with the intention of improving at first the patient's quality of life.

In agreement with the oncologist, a combined treatment with systemic (oral administration of 75 mg of prednisone daily) and topic corticosteroids (clobetasol 0.05% ointment twice daily) was established. During the following two months, a reduction of symptoms and oral lesions allowed a therapy reduction to 12.5 mg daily of prednisone, with the topic treatment being unchanged.

After a short period of relative wellness, in July 2014 the oral situation worsened again, with diffuse extensive oral ulcerations, high levels of pain, and very poor quality of life, although HU dosage had been unaltered since our first encounter with the patient, four months before. Therapy was modified again: 75 mg of prednisone daily was administered for two weeks and then, in accordance with the oncologist, dosage was reduced to 50 mg daily, but with no reduction of symptoms and pain; tacrolimus ointment (Protopic® 0.1% ointment) was used instead of topical clobetasol, but this was to no avail.

In September 2014, the decision was taken to add photobiomodulation (low-level laser therapy, LLLT) to the pharmacological therapy, with a twice-weekly frequency. A diode laser (GaAlAs) 810 nm (Ora-Laser_D-Light ORALIA Medical GmbH, Germany) was used, with spot size 1.3 cm^2, power setting 100 mW, mean power 50 mW, duty cycle 50%, frequency 10.000 Hz, fluence 6 J/cm^2 (calculated as follows: Fluence = power × time/surface), treatment time 160 seconds, point by point technique, not in contact (distance to the mucosa about 2 mm) perpendicular to the treatment area.

Noncontact mode was specifically chosen in order to prevent the onset of additional pain which could be obtained had we preferred the direct contact between the laser probe and the oral ulcers undergoing the LLLT treatment.

After 2 weeks, a marked improvement was immediately observed with disappearance of pain and the beginning of reepithelialization of the mucosa; at that time, HU dosage consisted of three 500 mg tablets daily interchanged with four 500 mg tablets every other day.

However, due to hospital admission for pulmonary complications, LLLT had to be suspended for 2 months, together with a gradual reduction of prednisone dosage until complete suspension: inevitably, the interruption of these treatments caused a worsening of the oral clinical situation.

After another 4 weeks of photobiomodulation treatment sessions, the lesions had not disappeared completely, but a significant reduction of pain was observed. Due to the improvement of the oral condition, the decision was taken to stop topic corticosteroid treatment continuing with systemic treatment and laser therapy, and the remission of the lingual lesions was obtained.

After another 3 weeks, symptoms and mucosal lesions disappearance, together with functional recovery, were observed (Figure 2).

Since then, photobiomodulation treatment was concluded, together with the gradual reduction of systemic corticosteroid treatment in the following months. In the meantime,

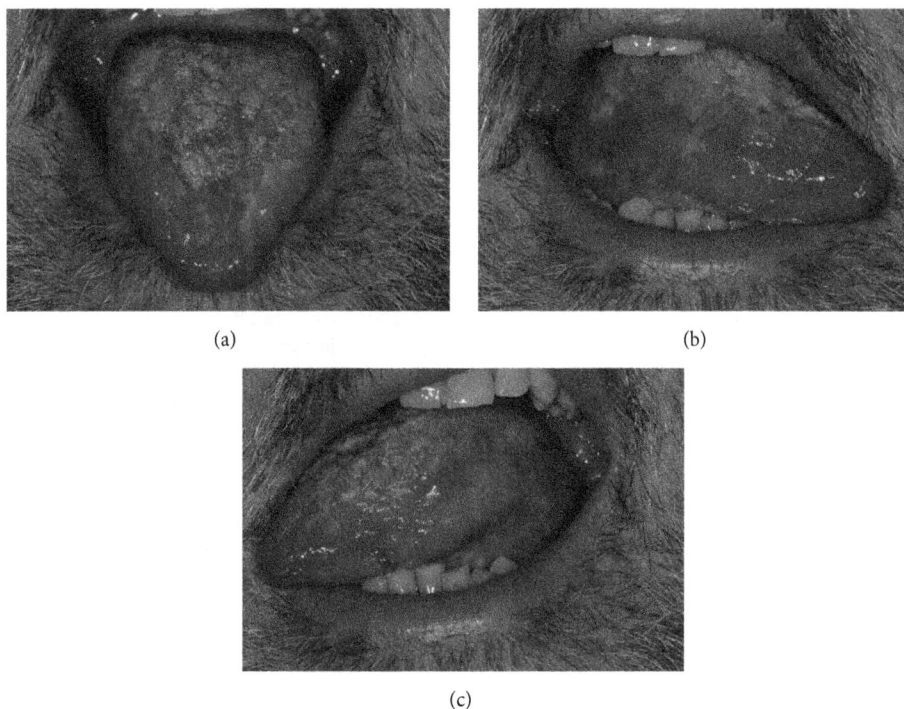

(a)

(b)

(c)

FIGURE 2: (a–c) Complete disappearance of the erosive tongue lesion at the end of the treatment provided.

HU dosage had been maintained, at the aforementioned dosage of three to four 500 mg tablets every other day.

In September 2015, HU was finally substituted with JACAVI; since then, the patient continued to be ulcers-free; *ad libitum* application of topical corticosteroid was prescribed to the patient but has never been used. Our last follow-up visit, conducted in July 2016, showed no signs or symptoms at the oral cavity; meanwhile, prednisone was furthermore reduced to a minimum of 5 mg every other day.

3. Discussion

PV is a classic Philadelphia-chromosome-negative myeloproliferative neoplasm (MPN), characterized primarily by an increase in red blood cell mass together with an excessive proliferation of myeloid and megakaryocytic components in the bone marrow, resulting in high red blood cells and platelet and white blood cells counts.

In the past 10 years, the pathophysiology of this condition has been defined as JAK/STAT pathway activation, almost always due to mutations in JAK2 exon 12 or 14 (JAK2 V617F) [4]. These findings have become indicative not only for diagnosis, so much that the presence of the JAK2 V617F mutation has been introduced as a major criterion in the diagnosis of PV since 2008, but also for treatment, most recently culminating in the approval of JAK inhibitors as an alternative for patients who are resistant or intolerant to HU [1].

Dresler and Stein described the synthesis of HU in 1869; the antitumor activity of this drug was reported in the 1960s, when it was tested against mouse leukemia and other malignancies. In the 1990s, HU was described as an inhibitor of ribonucleotide reductase, an enzyme involved in the synthesis of deoxyribonucleotides: by depleting the pool of deoxyribonucleotides, HU inhibits DNA synthesis, arresting the cell cycle at the G1/S phase [7].

On the other hand, skin and mucosal side effects are not completely understood and usually occur following long-term therapy; cutaneous abnormalities include xerosis, ichthyosiform lesions, dark brown pigmentation of skin folds and nails, and malleolar ulcers as well as malignant tumors [8–10].

Oral lesions are rare complications that can rapidly develop right after the start of the therapy [2] or as the side effect of a long-term exposure [3]; they often appear as painful ulcers, sometimes associated with skin lesions. Glossitis and stomatitis with intense erythema may also be observed [6, 11].

According to literature, there is no specific protocol for management of HU oral ulcers, apart from the dose reduction or suspension of HU itself. In the largest cohort of patients undergoing HU, a mouthwash containing folic acid and vitamin A was prescribed, obtaining symptomatic improvement; however, no details regarding the methods (dosage, timing, etc.) are reported; moreover, the authors declared that healing was achieved only after HU dose reduction or suspension in an average time frame of three months [4].

To our knowledge, only two cases of oral cancer following long-term treatment with HU have been reported [12, 13].

Therapeutic use of laser light was introduced in 1966, when Endre Mester published the first scientific article concerning stimulating and nonthermal effects of ruby laser on mice skin [14].

The energy of certain wavelengths (635–1100 nm) is absorbed by photoacceptor chromophores in the respiratory chain (cytochrome c oxidase) in mitochondria: this results in a change in the redox status of the cell, together with an increase in ATP production and cell proliferation rate [15–17], thanks to the activation of the nucleic acids, proteins, and enzymes regulation paths. It also participates in the regulation of the level of cytokines and growth factors and inflammation and tissue oxygenation mediators.

These biochemical cell changes lead to advantages as an increase in the speed of wound healing and a marked analgesic effect [15–18].

The rationale of using photobiomodulation is related to the possibility of accelerating the healing process of ongoing oral ulcers, as shown and reported by several studies [19–22].

In this case report laser photobiomodulation has achieved pain control and has contributed to the healing of oral ulcers without any adverse effect; this has permitted a reduction in the dose of systemic corticosteroids and the suspension of the use of the topic ones, due to the long-term stability of oral health, even after the interruption of LLLT sessions.

Disclosure

The authors alone are responsible for the content and writing of the paper.

Competing Interests

The authors report no declarations of interest.

References

[1] M. H. Griesshammer, H. Gisslinger, and R. Mesa, "Current and future treatment options for polycythemia vera," *Annals of Hematology*, vol. 94, no. 6, pp. 901–910, 2015.

[2] M. Badawi, S. Almazrooa, F. Azher, and F. Alsayes, "Hydroxyurea-induced oral ulceration," *Oral Surgery, Oral Medicine, Oral Pathology and Oral Radiology*, vol. 120, no. 6, pp. e232–e234, 2015.

[3] R. Mendonça, L. A. Gueiros, K. Capellaro, V. R. P. Pinheiro, and M. A. Lopes, "Oral lesions associated with hydroxyurea treatment," *Indian Journal of Dental Research*, vol. 22, no. 6, pp. 869–870, 2011.

[4] E. Antonioli, P. Guglielmelli, L. Pieri et al., "Hydroxyurea-related toxicity in 3,411 patients with Ph'-negative MPN," *American Journal of Hematology*, vol. 87, no. 5, pp. 552–554, 2012.

[5] A. Martínez-Trillos, A. Gaya, M. Maffioli et al., "Efficacy and tolerability of hydroxyurea in the treatment of the hyperproliferative manifestations of myelofibrosis: results in 40 patients," *Annals of Hematology*, vol. 89, no. 12, pp. 1233–1237, 2010.

[6] C. Vassallo, F. Passamonti, S. Merante et al., "Muco-cutaneous changes during long-term therapy with hydroxyurea in chronic myeloid leukaemia," *Clinical and Experimental Dermatology*, vol. 26, no. 2, pp. 141–148, 2001.

[7] D. Dingli and A. Tefferi, "Hydroxyurea: the drug of choice for polycythemia vera and essential thrombocythemia," *Current Hematologic Malignancy Reports*, vol. 1, no. 2, pp. 69–74, 2006.

[8] N.-P. Hoff, S. Akanay-Diesel, U. Pippirs, K.-W. Schulte, and S. Hanneken, "Cutaneous side effects of hydroxyurea treatment for polycythemia vera," *Hautarzt*, vol. 60, no. 10, pp. 783–787, 2009.

[9] S. Boneberger, R. A. Rupec, and T. Ruzicka, "Ulcers following therapy with hydroxyurea. Three case reports and review of the literature," *Hautarzt*, vol. 61, no. 7, pp. 598–602, 2010.

[10] E. R. de França, M. A. G. Teixeira, K. D. F. Matias, D. E. C. M. Antunes, R. D. A. Braz, and C. E. F. Silva, "Cutaneous effects after prolongaded use of hydroxyurea in polycythemia Vera," *Anais Brasileiros de Dermatologia*, vol. 86, no. 4, pp. 751–754, 2011.

[11] H. Brincker and B. E. Christensen, "Acute mucocutaneous toxicity following high-dose hydroxyurea," *Cancer Chemotherapy and Pharmacology*, vol. 32, no. 6, pp. 496–497, 1993.

[12] E. Estève, C. Georgescu, P. Heitzmann, and L. Martin, "Multiple skin and mouth squamous cell carcinomas related to long-term treatment with hydroxyurea," *Annales de Dermatologie et de Venereologie*, vol. 128, no. 8-9, pp. 919–921, 2001.

[13] M. De Benedittis, M. Petruzzi, C. Giardina, L. Lo Muzio, G. Favia, and R. Serpico, "Oral squamous cell carcinoma during long-term treatment with hydroxyurea," *Clinical and Experimental Dermatology*, vol. 29, no. 6, pp. 605–607, 2004.

[14] E. Mester, "The use of the laser beam in therapy," *Orvosi Hetilap*, vol. 107, no. 22, pp. 1012–1016, 1966.

[15] M. R. Hamblin and T. N. Demidova, "Mechanisms of low level light therapy," in *Proceedings of the Mechanisms for Low-Light Therapy*, vol. 6140 of *Proceedings of SPIE*, San Jose, Calif, USA, January 2006.

[16] A. Amaroli, S. Ravera, S. Parker, I. Panfoli, A. Benedicenti, and S. Benedicenti, "The protozoan, Paramecium primaurelia, as a non-sentient model to test laser light irradiation: the effects of an 808nm infrared laser diode on cellular respiration," *Alternatives to Laboratory Animals*, vol. 43, no. 3, pp. 155–162, 2015.

[17] S. Benedicenti, I. M. Pepe, F. Angiero, and A. Benedicenti, "Intracellular ATP level increases in lymphocytes irradiated with infrared laser light of wavelength 904 nm," *Photomedicine and Laser Surgery*, vol. 26, no. 5, pp. 451–453, 2008.

[18] T. Karu, "Mitochondrial mechanisms of photobiomodulation in context of new data about multiple roles of ATP," *Photomedicine and Laser Surgery*, vol. 28, no. 2, pp. 159–160, 2010.

[19] D. H. Hawkins and H. Abrahamse, "The role of laser fluence in cell viability, proliferation, and membrane integrity of wounded human skin fibroblasts following Helium-Neon laser irradiation," *Lasers in Surgery and Medicine*, vol. 38, no. 1, pp. 74–83, 2006.

[20] J. A. D. A. C. Piva, E. M. D. C. Abreu, V. D. S. Silva, and R. A. Nicolau, "Effect of low-level laser therapy on the initial stages of tissue repair: basic principles," *Anais Brasileiros de Dermatologia*, vol. 86, no. 5, pp. 947–954, 2011.

[21] F. C. F. da Silva Calisto, S. L. da Silva Calisto, A. P. de Souza, C. M. França, A. P. de Lima Ferreira, and M. B. Moreira, "Use of low-power laser to assist the healing of traumatic wounds in rats," *Acta Cirurgica Brasileira*, vol. 30, no. 3, pp. 204–208, 2015.

[22] D. P. Kuffler, "Photobiomodulation in promoting wound healing: a review," *Regenerative Medicine*, vol. 11, no. 1, pp. 107–122, 2016.

Permissions

List of Contributors

Paula Mathias and Thaiane Rodrigues Aguiar
Department of Clinical Dentistry, School of Dentistry, Federal University of Bahia, Salvador, BA, Brazil

Emily Vivianne Freitas da Silva
Department of Dental Materials and Prosthodontics, Aracatuba Dental School, Universidade Estadual Paulista, UNESP, Aracatuba, SP, Brazil

Aline Silva Andrade
Department of Restorative Dentistry, Araraquara Dental School, Universidade Estadual Paulista, UNESP, Araraquara, SP, Brazil

Juliana Azevedo
Department of Clinical Dentistry, School of Dentistry, Bahiana School of Medicine and Public Health, Salvador, BA, Brazil

Alexandra Rubin Cocco and Rudimar Antônio Baldissera
Department of Operative Dentistry, School of Dentistry, Federal University of Pelotas, Pelotas, RS, Brazil

Ângelo Niemczewski Bobrowski
Department of Oral and Maxillofacial Surgery, School of Dentistry, Federal University of Pelotas, Pelotas, RS, Brazil

Luiz Fernando Machado Silveira and Josué Martos
Department of Semiology and Clinics, Faculty of Dentistry, University Federal of Pelotas, Pelotas, RS, Brazil

Zahra Alizadeh Tabari and Tahere Pourseyediyan
Department of Periodontics, Dental School, Qazvin University of Medical Sciences, Qazvin 34157-59811, Iran

Hamed Homayouni
Department of Endodontics, Dental School, Qazvin University of Medical Sciences, Qazvin 34157-59811, Iran

Armita Arvin
Department of Endodontics, Dental School, Yazd University of Medical Sciences, Yazd 8914881167, Iran

Derrick Eiland
Dental Emergency Department, Howard University College of Dentistry, Washington, DC 20001, USA

Nima Moradi Majd
Dental Research Laboratory, Howard University College of Dentistry, Washington, DC 20001, USA

Danielle Lima Corrêa de Carvalho, Fernanda de Paula Eduardo, Letícia Mello Bezinelli and Paulo Henrique Braz-Silva
Department of Stomatology, Division of General Pathology, School of Dentistry, University of São Paulo, São Paulo, SP, Brazil

Alan Motta do Canto
Department of Stomatology, Division of General Pathology, School of Dentistry, University of São Paulo, São Paulo, SP, Brazil
Unit of Oral and Maxillofacial Surgery, Santa Casa de São Paulo, School of Medical Sciences, São Paulo, SP, Brazil

André Luiz Ferreira Costa
Department of Orthodontics and Radiology, University of São Paulo, São Paulo, SP, Brazil

Fatemeh Rezaei
Department of Oral Medicine, School of Dentistry, Kermanshah University of Medical Sciences, Kermanshah, Iran

Hesamedin Nazari
Department of Oral and Maxillofacial Surgery, School of Medicine, Kermanshah University of Medical Sciences, Kermanshah, Iran

Babak Izadi
Department of Pathology, School of Medicine, Kermanshah University of Medical Sciences, Kermanshah, Iran

Antonione Santos Bezerra Pinto
Department of Morphology, Faculty of Medicine, Federal University of Ceará, Fortaleza, CE, Brazil

Moara e Silva Conceição Pinto and Daniel Fernando Pereira Vasconcelos
Department of Histology and Embryology, Faculty of Biomedicine, Federal University of Piauí, Parnaíba, PI, Brazil

CinthyaMelo do Val
Department of Genetic and Applied Toxicology, Lutheran University of Brazil, Canoas, RS, Brazil

Leonam Costa Oliveira
Department of Medical Skills, Faculty of Medicine, Federal University of Piauí, Parnaíba, PI, Brazil

Cristhyane Costa de Aquino
Laboratory of the Biology of Tissue Healing, Ontogeny and Nutrition, Department of Morphology and Institute of Biomedicine, School of Medicine, Federal University of Ceará, Fortaleza, CE, Brazil

Masahiro Yoneda and Takao Hirofuji
Section of General Dentistry, Department of General Dentistry, Fukuoka Dental College, Fukuoka 814-0193, Japan

Hiromitsu Morita
Section of General Dentistry, Department of General Dentistry, Fukuoka Dental College, Fukuoka 814-0193, Japan
Special Patient Oral Care Unit, Kyushu University Hospital, Fukuoka 812-8582, Japan

Akie Hashimoto, Ryosuke Inoue and Shohei Yoshimoto
Special Patient Oral Care Unit, Kyushu University Hospital, Fukuoka 812-8582, Japan

Tatiana Kelly da Silva Fidalgo
Universidade do Estado do Rio de Janeiro, Boulevard Vinte e Oito de Setembro, 175 Vila Isabel, 21941-913 Rio de Janeiro RJ, Brazil
Universidade Salgado de Oliveira, Pólo Niterói, Rua Marechal Deodoro, 263 Centro, 24030-060 Niterói, RJ, Brazil

Carla Nogueira, Andrea Graciene Lopez Ramos Valente and Patricia Nivoloni Tannure
Universidade Veiga de Almeida, Rua Ibituruna 108, Tijuca, 20271-020 Rio de Janeiro, RJ, Brazil

Marcia Rejane Thomas Canabarro Andrade
Department of Specific Formation, School of Dentistry, Universidade Federal Fluminense, Rua Dr. Silvio Henrique Braune 22, 28625-650 Nova Friburgo, RJ, Brazil

José Alcides Arruda, Pamella Álvares, Luciano Silva, Antônio Caubi, Marcia Silveira, Sandra Sayão, Ana Paula Sobral and Alexandrino Pereira dos Santos Neto
Faculdade de Odontologia de Pernambuco, Universidade de Pernambuco, Avenida General Newton Cavalcante, 1650 Aldeia dos Camarás, 54.753-020 Camaragibe, PE, Brazil

Cleomar Donizeth Rodrigues
Faculdades Integradas da União Educacional do Planalto Central, SIGA Área Especial para Indústria, n°2, Setor Leste, 72.445-020, Gama, DG, Brazil

Sapna Rani
Department of Prosthodontics, ITS Dental College, Ghaziabad, India

Jyoti Devi, Chandan Jain, Parul Mutneja and Mahesh Verma
Department of Prosthodontics, MAIDS, Delhi, India

R. K. Morita
Graduate Pontifical Catholic University of Parana, Curitiba, PR, Brazil

M. F. Hayashida
Department of Dentistry, School of Dentistry, University Tuiuti of Parana, Curitiba, PR, Brazil

Y. M. Pupo G. Berger and E. A. G. Betiol
Department of Restorative Dentistry, Federal University of Parana, Curitiba, PR, Brazil

R. D. Reggiani
Graduate Federal University of Parana, Curitiba, PR, Brazil

Resmije Ademi Abdyli, Feriall Perjuci, Ali Gashi, Zana Agani and Jehona Ahmedi
Department of Oral Surgery, Medical Faculty, University of Prishtina, Dental Branch, 10000 Prishtina, Kosovo

Yll Abdyli
Medical Faculty, University of Prishtina, Dental Branch, 10000 Prishtina, Kosovo

Gopinath Thilak Parepady Sundar, Shree Satya and Sourabh M. Gohil
Department of Oral and Maxillofacial Surgery, A.B. Shetty Memorial Institute of Dental Sciences, Mangalore, India

Vishwanath Sherigar
K.S.Hegde Charitable Hospital,Mangalore, India

Sameep S. Shetty
Department of Oral and Maxillofacial Surgery, Manipal College of Dental Sciences, Manipal University, Manipal, India

Lavanya Kalapala, Surapaneni Keerthi sai, Suresh Babburi, Aparna Venigalla, Soujanya Pinisetti and Ajay Benarji Kotti
Department of Oral & Maxillofacial Pathology, Drs. Sudha & Nageswara Rao Siddhartha Institute of Dental Sciences, Chinoutpalli, Gannavaram, India

Kiranmai Ganipineni
Government Dental College, Vijayawada, India

Nayara Romano, Luis Eduardo Souza-Flamini, Isabela Lima Mendonça, Ricardo Gariba Silva and Antonio Miranda Cruz-Filho
Department of Restorative Dentistry, School of Dentistry of Ribeirão Preto, University of São Paulo, Ribeirão Preto, SP, Brazil

Marília Pacífico Lucisano, Paulo Nelson-Filho, Lea Assed Bezerra Silva, Raquel Assed Bezerra Silva, Fabricio Kitazono de Carvalho and AlexandraMussolino de Queiroz
Department of Pediatric Dentistry, School of Dentistry of Ribeirão Preto, University of São Paulo, Ribeirão Preto, SP, Brazil

A. M. Al-Mullahi
Oral Health Department, Sultan Qaboos University Hospital, Sultan Qaboos University, Muscat, Oman

K. J. Toumba
Paediatric Dentistry, Leeds Dental Institute, University of Leeds, Leeds, UK

Rocco Borrello, Elia Bettio, Christian Bacci, Stefano Sivolella, Sergio Mazzoleni and Mario Berengo
1Section of Dentistry, Department of Neurosciences, University of Padova, Padova, Italy

Marialuisa Valente
Department of CardiacThoracic and Vascular Sciences, University of Padova, Padova, Italy

S. Kale, N. Srivastava, V. Bagga and A. Shetty
Department of Oral and Maxillofacial Surgery, Sri Rajiv Gandhi College of Dental Sciences and Hospital, Bangalore, India

S. Lumetti, G. Ghiacci, G. M. Macaluso, C. Galli and E.Manfredi
Centro Universitario di Odontoiatria, SBiBiT, Universit`a degli Studi di Parma, Parma, Italy

M. Amore
Sezione di Psichiatria, Dipartimento di Neuroscienze, Riabilitazione, Oftalmologia, Genetica e Scienze Materno-Infantili, Universit`a degli Studi di Genova, Genova, Italy

E. Calciolari
Centre for Oral Clinical Research, Queen Mary University of London, London, UK

Kenji Yamagata, Kazuhiro Terada, Fumihiko Uchida, Naomi Kanno, Shogo Hasegawa, Toru Yanagawa and Hiroki Bukawa
Department of Oral and Maxillofacial Surgery, Institute of Clinical Medicine, Faculty of Medicine, University of Tsukuba, Tsukuba, Japan

Sachiko Hayashi-Sakai, Takafumi Hayashi, Hideyoshi Nishiyama, Kouji Katsura, Makiko Ike, Yutaka Nikkuni, Miwa Nakayama, Marie Soga and Taichi Kobayashi1
Division of Oral and Maxillofacial Radiology, Niigata University Graduate School of Medical and Dental Sciences, 2-5274 Gakkocho-dori, Chuo-ku, Niigata 951-8514, Japan

Makoto Sakamoto
Department of Health Sciences, Faculty of Medicine, Niigata University, 2-746 Asahimachi-dori, Chuo-ku, Niigata 951-8514, Japan

Jun Sakai
Department of System and Automotive Engineering, Niigata College of Technology, 5-13-7 Kamishinei-cho, Nishi-ku, Niigata 950-2076, Japan

Junko Shimomura-Kuroki
Department of Pediatric Dentistry,The Nippon Dental University, School of Life Dentistry at Niigata, 1-8 Hamaura-cho, Chuo-ku, Niigata 951-8580, Japan

I. Y. Bozo
Department ofMaxillofacial and Plastic Surgery, A.I. EvdokimovMoscow State University ofMedicine and Dentistry,Moscow, Russia

Human Stem Cells Institute, Moscow, Russia
Department of Maxillofacial Surgery, A.I. Burnazyan Federal Medical Biophysical Center, Moscow, Russia

R. V. Deev
Human Stem Cells Institute, Moscow, Russia
I.P. Pavlov Ryazan State Medical University, Ryazan, Russia

A. Y. Drobyshev
Department ofMaxillofacial and Plastic Surgery, A.I. EvdokimovMoscow State University ofMedicine and Dentistry,Moscow, Russia

A. A. Isaev
Human Stem Cells Institute, Moscow, Russia

I. I. Eremin
Central Clinical Hospital with Outpatient Health Center of the Business Administration for the President of the Russian Federation, Moscow, Russia

Cennet Neslihan Eroglu and Serap Keskin Tunc
Oral and Maxillofacial SurgeryDepartment, Faculty of Dentistry, Yuzuncu Yil University, Van, Turkey

Omer Gunhan
Department of Pathology, Gulhane Military Medical Academy, Ankara, Turkey

Antonello Francesco Pavone, ManueleMancini, Roberta Condò, Loredana Cerroni, Claudio Arcuri and Guido Pasquantonio
Department of Clinical and Translational Medicine, University of Rome "Tor Vergata", Rome, Italy

Marjan Ghassemian
University of Sydney, Sydney, NSW, Australia
Catholic University of the Sacred Heart, Rome, Italy
Unit of Oral Surgery and Implant-Prosthetic Rehabilitation, Rome, Italy

Mala Kamboj, Anju Devi and Shruti Gupta
Department of Oral Pathology and Microbiology, Postgraduate Institute of Dental Sciences, Pt. BD Sharma University of Medical Sciences, Rohtak,Haryana, India

Fernando Pedrin Carvalho Ferreira
Cora-Vilhena, Vilhena, RO, Brazil

Maiara da Silva Goulart
Sagrado Coração University, Bauru, SP, Brazil

Renata Rodrigues de Almeida-Pedrin, Ana Claudia de Castro Ferreira Conti and Maurício de Almeida Cardoso
Department of Orthodontics, Sagrado Corac,ão University, Bauru, SP, Brazil

Mario Aimetti, Valeria Manavella, Luca Cricenti and Federica Romano
Department of Surgical Sciences, Periodontology Section, CIR Dental School, University of Turin, Via Nizza 230, 10126 Turin, Italy

Paulo S. G. Henriques, Luciana S. Okajima and Marcelo P. Nunes
Department of Periodontology, São Leopoldo Mandic Institute and Research Center, Campinas, SP, Brazil

Victor A. M. Montalli
Department of Oral Pathology, São Leopoldo Mandic Institute and Research Center, Campinas, SP, Brazil

Saurabh Kumar and Deepika Pai
Department of Pedodontics & Preventive Dentistry, Manipal College of Dental Sciences, Manipal, India

Runki Saran
Faculty of Dentistry, Melaka ManipalMedical College, Manipal, India

Naira Figueiredo Deana
Magister Program in Dentistry, Faculty of Dentistry, Universidad de La Frontera, Temuco, Chile

Nilton Alves
CIMA-Research Center in Applied Morphology, Universidad de La Frontera, Temuco, Chile
Faculty of Dentistry, Universidad de La Frontera, 1145 Francisco Salazar Avenue, P.O. Box 54-D, Temuco, Chile

Danny Omar Mendoza Marin, Andressa Rosa Perin Leite and Marco Antonio Compagnoni
Araraquara Dental School, Department of Dental Materials and Prosthodontics, Universidade Estadual Paulista (UNESP), Araraquara, SP, Brazil

Lélis Gustavo Nícoli and Elcio Marcantonio Jr
Araraquara Dental School, Department of Diagnosis and Surgery, Universidade Estadual Paulista (UNESP), Araraquara, SP, Brazil

Claudio Marcantonio
Araraquara Dental School, Department of Postgraduate Studies in Implantology, University Center of Araraquara (UNIARA), Araraquara, SP, Brazil

Alessandro Gatti, Emanuele Broccardo, Giuseppe Poglio and Arnaldo Benech
Unit of Oral and Maxillofacial Surgery, Maggiore della Carit`a University Hospital, Novara, Italy

Melda Misirlioglu, Yagmur Yilmaz Akyil, Mehmet Zahit Adisen and Alime Okkesim
Department of Oral and Maxillofacial Radiology, Faculty of Dentistry, Kırıkkale University, Kırıkkale, Turkey

Lorenzo Azzi Lucia Tettamanti and Angelo Tagliabue
Department of Surgical and Morphological Sciences, University of Insubria, ASST dei Sette Laghi,Unit ofOral Pathology, Dental Clinic, Varese, Italy

Laura Cimetti
Department of Surgical and Morphological Sciences, University of Insubria, ASST dei Sette Laghi,Unit of Pathologic Anatomy, Varese, Italy

Matteo Annoni
Department of Surgical and Morphological Sciences, University of Insubria, ASST dei Sette Laghi,Unit of General Surgery 1, Varese, Italy

Diego Anselmi
Meditel, Medical Centre, Unit of Radiology, Saronno, Italy

Marco Cabras, Adriana Cafaro, Alessio Gambino, Roberto Broccoletti and Paolo G. Arduino
Department of Surgical Sciences, CIR-Dental School, University of Turin, Turin, Italy

Ercole Romagnoli
Department of Surgical and Diagnostic Sciences (DISC), University of Genoa, Genoa, Italy

Davide Marina
Private Practice, Milan, Italy

Index

A

Alveolar Bone, 1, 27, 29, 83, 85, 117, 127, 133, 155, 176

Alveolar Mucosa, 7, 159, 161

Anesthesia, 7, 12, 20-21, 32, 42, 65, 79, 84, 112-113, 159, 165-166, 179, 183-184

Anterior Teeth, 4, 6, 29, 46-47, 49, 52, 78, 88-89, 117-118, 132-133, 135, 137, 147, 151

Artificial Saliva, 36-39

Artificial Teeth, 31-35

B

Bone Grafting, 12, 14, 122-123, 125-126, 153

Bone Resorption, 75, 93-94, 117, 153-154, 191

Bone Tissue, 42, 93, 122-123, 125-127, 155

Buccal Inclination, 2

Buccal Mucosa, 64, 69, 71, 96, 98-99, 128

C

Calcium Hydroxide, 6-9, 79, 83-86

Collagen Membrane, 99

Complete Maxillary Denture, 31-35

Computed Tomography, 12-13, 26-27, 78-79, 81, 93, 140, 168, 171-173, 179-180

D

Dental Caries, 36, 38-39, 88, 90, 92, 117, 165-166

Dental Implants, 2, 29-30, 105, 108-109, 153, 155, 174-178

Dental Lamina, 16-17, 88, 93

Dental Treatment, 1-3, 8, 25-26, 31-32, 36, 51, 164-165

E

Ectodermal Dysplasia, 25, 27, 29-30

Enamel Removal, 1, 3-4

Endodontic Treatment, 6-7, 9, 12, 37, 42, 78-79, 81, 84-87

Exfoliated Teeth, 116-121

F

Facial Esthetics, 1, 144-145, 147

G

Giant Cell Lesion, 43, 73-74

Gingival Esthetics, 1-2

Gingival Tissue, 8, 54, 79, 158, 175

Gingival Tissues, 52, 79, 137

H

Healing Process, 1, 198

Hyperparathyroidism, 73-75, 77, 187, 189-194

Hyperplasia, 16-17, 159, 165, 167, 190-191

Hypocalcemia, 73

Hypophosphatasia, 91, 116, 120-121

I

Intraoral Swelling, 21, 74

Intravenous Sedation, 31, 35

J

Jawbones, 93, 193

K

Keratocystic Odontogenic Tumor, 21, 187-188, 193

L

Lymph Node, 71, 110-111, 113-114, 184, 186, 191

M

Magnetic Resonance Imaging, 21, 37, 130, 172, 183, 186

Mandibular Bone, 21

Mandibular Teeth, 21, 32

Maxillary Canines, 1-3, 171, 173

Maxillary Incisors, 15, 82, 86, 155, 165

Maxillary Right Central Incisor, 6-8, 83

Mineral Trioxide Aggregate, 6, 9, 83-84, 87

Mpnst, 41-45

N

Neuroendocrine, 110-111, 113-115

O

Odontogenic Myxoma, 21-22, 24

Odontogenic Tumours, 16-17

Oral Care, 31-32, 165-166

Oral Cavity, 23-24, 36-37, 41, 44, 66, 71-73, 77, 93, 104, 110, 113, 115, 129-131, 139, 141, 143, 173, 181, 183, 193, 197

Oral Dyskinesia, 31-35, 107

Oral Hygiene, 16, 20, 26, 29, 38-39, 84, 117, 162, 165-166, 174, 176-177

Oral Manifestations, 22, 76

Oral Parafunction, 103, 105, 107, 109

Oral Rehabilitation, 25, 29-30, 37, 39, 51, 107-109, 174-175

Oral Submucous Fibrosis, 69, 72, 98-99, 101-102

Orthodontic Treatment, 1-2, 4, 36, 60, 145, 147, 152, 154, 172

P

Palatal Mucosa, 93, 180

Parathyroid Gland, 73, 76, 190

Pediatric Dentistry, 36-37, 82-84, 86, 91-92, 116

Periodontal Disease, 15, 26, 36, 39, 153, 155, 158

Periodontal Ligament, 9, 14, 21, 83-86, 154, 158-159, 188

Periodontal Treatment, 11-12, 15, 153

Peripheral Ameloblastoma, 93, 95-97

Peripheral Ceot, 16-18

Permanent Teeth, 5-7, 9, 79-81, 84, 86-88, 90, 92, 119, 138, 145

Plaque Accumulation, 11, 90, 174-177

Plasma Cells, 20, 22-23

Plasmacytoma, 20-24

Pulp Necrosis, 6, 14

R

Radicular Groove, 11-15, 78, 81

Regional Odontodysplasia, 88-92

Restorative Dentistry, 1, 3, 51, 62-63, 78-79, 81, 108, 137-138, 157, 163, 177-178

Root Canal, 6-9, 11-12, 42, 49, 78-79, 81, 83-87, 128, 134, 136, 138, 172

Root Development, 6, 84, 137

S

Salivary Gland, 17, 23, 36, 39, 114, 129, 179-181, 183-184, 186

T

Tardive Dyskinesia, 103, 105, 107, 109

Temporomandibular Joint, 20, 173

Tissue Regeneration, 8, 11-15, 157, 159

Tooth Destruction, 37

Tooth Development, 78

Tooth Extraction, 33, 35, 153-155, 157, 172

Tooth Extractions, 31-33

Tooth Germ, 78, 80

Tooth Pain, 36, 128-129

Tooth Replantation, 83-85, 87

Tooth Structure, 3-4, 9, 49, 51, 56, 59-60, 132-133, 137

Traumatic Injury, 79, 133

Tumour Cells, 69-71, 93-94

Tumour Metastasis, 17